Equine Neonatal Medicine

4th edition

John E. Madigan, D.V.M, M.S., Editor
Diplomate, American College of Veterinary Internal Medicine
Diplomate, American College of Animal Welfare
Professor, Department of Medicine and Epidemiology
School of Veterinary Medicine
University of California-Davis

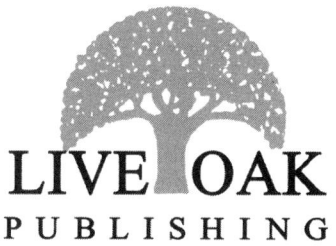

www.equineneonatalmanual.com
P.O. Box 8868, Woodland, Ca 95776

To Drs Bill and Janet Linfoot,
whose guidance and love made being a
veterinarian seem a possiblity

DISCLAIMER NOTICE – Please read the following before utilizing the Manual.

While every effort has been made to assure the accurate dosages of a medication, it is essential that the user read current label recommendations prior to using on a patient. Certain drug dosages and procedures are based on reports, personal experience and unpublished data that may be different than those recommended by the manufacturer. Readers are urged to view the recommendations with this in mind. If the reader is unfamiliar with a drug or a procedure, further and more detailed information should be sought prior to implementation. Please check government regulations for USDA approved drugs. The veterinarian treating a foal is responsible for reviewing each medication dosage or indication and making their own decision for a specific treatment approach to an individual foal.

This is not intended to be a text. It should not be considered the final word nor be the limit of reading needed to be competent in the care of newborn foals. **All material is presented as information and is not meant as specific recommendations. The EC's are not to be considered specific advice or recommendations but are merely for the reader's consideration.** Current textbooks and review articles should be consulted to provide background for those unfamiliar with procedures and drugs. The material in the manual is not the original ideas, thoughts or experiences solely of the authors and editors. It has been obtained by the many researchers, practitioners throughout the world who have presented clinical material on neonatal foals verbally at meetings or in written form. I have chosen to avoid exhaustive reference sections and have often quoted summary presentations of papers or texts which can and should be reviewed for further information. The reader is advised that suggestions and procedures will change rapidly as new information is developed in equine neonatology. The purchaser and/or user of this manual assumes total responsibility for all risks and outcomes related to the use of information, procedures, diagnostic approaches and medical treatments contained in the Manual. The editor and contributors assume no liability for any injury, and/or damage to persons or property arising out of or related to use of material within this Manual.

Copyright, 2013 by Live Oak Publishing, P. O. Box 8868, Woodland, Ca 95776. All rights reserved. No portion of this book may be reproduced, stored in a retrieval system, or transmitted in any form or by any means electronic, without prior written permission from the publisher. Made in the United States of America.

First Edition, 1987
Second Edition, 1991
Second Edition Revised, 1994
Third Edition, 1997
Fourth Edition, 2013

PREFACE – FOURTH EDITION

If you do any foal work, you will likely need this book. It is difficult for all of us to read all published relevant papers and recall specific information at a critical time when we need it when tending to a sick foal. This edition and the 3 previous are written with this need in mind. New methods for disease prevention, new ideas for old conditions, new diseases, drug dosages for neonatal foals, normal values for hematology and clinical pathology are here for practical application. I believe you will find the Manual indispensible to you during the foaling season.

For academic veterinarians, practitioners, veterinary students, technicians and some foal owners the Manual has served as a source of information and education. I have appreciated the many comments from my practitioner colleagues regarding the foals that have been saved by finding information in the Manual that made a difference. The outline form of the popular previous editions is continued along with the use of the EC or editor comments. These are one or two line comments that alert the reader to a pitfall, precaution or experience the editor is aware of relative to the approach to a problem.

The fourth edition has several new sections including information to get you started on a foal with conformation issues or limb deformities. Dr. Hans Castelijns has written these chapters using his tremendous practical experience as a veterinarian and farrier.

I would like to express my sincere thanks and appreciation for all those who have directly contributed to the content of this manual. Notes from courses given by Dr. Gary Magdesian have been a significant source of information to share in portions of the Manual. Dr. Balzs Toth spent considerable time writing and editing portions of many chapters. Dr. Mary Beth Whitcomb has provided highly useful practical ultrasound imaging information. Dr. Hans Castelijns has written chapters on management of limb disorders in foals. The Manual would not have been completed without the diligent proofing and significant contributions by Dr. Kirstie Pickles.

Lastly, this new expanded 4th edition of the Manual is long overdue. It is completed because of the need expressed by those who had access to earlier editions and found it essential to them in their practice of foal medicine. I hope this little book will be a friend in the night, as an aid when presented with a challenging and perplexing foal, or the place you can go to find that piece of information you need to treat a foal. We are doing much better with neonatal foal care today and much of what we have learned is at your fingertips in the Manual.

Best of luck to you with the foals.

John Madigan

CONTRIBUTORS

Monica Aleman, MVZ, PhD, Dipl. ACVIM
Equine Internist- Veterinary Medical Teaching Hospital
School of Veterinary Medicine
University of California
Davis, Ca 95616

Colic in the foal

Gary Carlson, DVM, PhD
Professor Emeritius
School of Veterinary Medicine
University of California-Davis

Fluid therapy

Hans Castelijns, DVM
In 1985 he started his farrier training at the Equine Clinic of Bosh en Duin, Utrecht, the Netherlands, obtaining a farriery diploma released by the region of Tuscany - Italy in 1989.
Doctor of Veterinary Medicine -Perugia - Italy, graduating in 1998 "cum laude" presenting a thesis on "Modern Farrier Techniques in the Prevention and Therapy of lameness in Horses".

Limb Deformities, Flexural Deformities, Angular and Rotational Deviations

John Madigan, DVM, MS Diplomate ACVIM, ACAW
Professor
Department of Medicine and Epidemiology
School of Veterinary Medicine
University of California-Davis

All other chapters

Gary Magdesian DVM, Large Animal Internal Medicine (ACVIM)
Emergency and Critical Care (ACVECC), Clinical Pharmacology (ACVCP)
The Roberta A. and Carla Henry Endowed Chair in Emergency Medicine and Critical Care
Associate Professor Department of Medicine and Epidemiology
School of Veterinary Medicine
University of California-Davis

Source of materials throughout the Manual, for all critical care, fluid therapy, acid-base, resuscitation, CPCR, pharmacology, and much more.

Michael Spensley, DVM
505 Brooke Street
Charles Town, West Virginia 25414

Colostrum Assessment, Blood Administrtion

Balzs Toth, DVM, MS
DVM University of Szent Istvan,
Faculty of Veterinary Science, Budapest, 2005
Masters of Science - Comparative Pathology
University of California-Davis 2010
Resident in Large Animal Internal Medicine 2010-current
Purdue University
College of Veterinary Medicine
West Lafayette, Indiana

Shock, Fluid Therapy, Resuscitation, Parenteral Nutrition, Formulary,

Mary Beth Whitcomb DVM
Associate Professor of Clinical Large Animal Ultrasound
Department of Surgical and Radiological Sciences
School of Veterinary Medicine
University of California-Davis

Fetal ultrasound, Neonatal Ultrasound

W. David Wilson, BVMS, MS, MRCVS
Professor- Dept of Medicine and Epidemiology
School of Veterinary Medicine
University of California –Davis
Director Veterinary Medical Teaching Hospital

Guidelines for Drug Use in Equine Neonates, Drug Formulary, Hematology Reference Values, Blood Chemistry Values, Serum Immunoglobulins versus age.

PRE-FOALING – FOALING, AND POST BIRTH CONSIDERATIONS

1	Management Approaches to the Newborn Foal	1
2	Assessment of Fetal Well Being	8
3	Detection of Impending Parturition	10
4	induction of Parturition	13
5	Normal Equine Labor, Delivery and Newborn Foal Vital Signs	17
6	Dystocia Management Factors for Neonatal Viability	20
7	Post Foaling Procedures-routine (Low Risk Foals)	25
8	Colostrum-Assessment of and Sources for Foals	28
9	Assessment of Passive Immunity	32
10	Plasma Therapy	37

MEDICAL CARE

11	Physical Exam of the Equine Neonate	43
12	Assessment of Maturity – Prematurity	50
13	Assessment of Oxygen Needs	55
14	Transport of the Critically Ill Equine Neonate	63
15	Temperature Regulation of Neonates	66
16	Resuscitation-Pt. 1	69
17	Resuscitation-Pt. 2 Evaluation of Cardiovascular Status	74
18	Shock (SIRS)	80
19	Initial Evaluation and Minimum Data Base	88
20	Daily Plan and Monitoring of the Critical Care Patient	91
21	Daily Nursing Care	95
22	Fluid and Electrolyte Balance	98
23	Parenteral Nutrition	111
24	Enteral Nutrition	117
25	Clinical Signs Observed in the Sick Equine Neonate Considered Normal at Birth	124

MEDICAL DISORDERS OF THE FIRST TWO WEEKS OF LIFE

26	Meconium Retention	126
27	Neonatal Maladjustment syndrome	131
28	Infections	135
29	Rhodococcus Equi Diagnosis, Prevention, and Treatment	146
30	Neonatal Salmonellosis	151
31	Neonatal Seizures	155
32	Immunodeficiencies	162
33	Diarrhea	166
34	Gastroduodenal Ulcers	176
35	Neonatal Isoerythrolysis	182
36	Renal Disorders of Equine Neonates	188
37	Ruptured Bladder & Uroperitoneum	192
38	Septic Arthritis and Osteomeylitis	197
39	Umbilical Problems	204
40	Eye Problems	208
41	Congenital Cardiac Anomalies	211

42	Congenital Anomalies and Genetic Disorders	216
43	White Muscle Disease	229
44	Hypoglycemia	232
45	Hemostatic Disorders	235
46	Endocrine Problems	239
47	Respiratory Distress	243
48	Hernia	248
49	Fractured Ribs	251
50	Colic in the Neonatal Foal	253

PROCEDURES

51	Sedation and Anesthesia	261
52	Ultrasonography of the Fetus and the Neonate	268
53	Thoracic and Abdominal Radiography	313
54	Nasotracheal Intubation	318
55	Transtracheal Aspiration or Wash	320
56	Echocardiography	322
57	Electrocardiography	328
58	Nasogastric Intubation	332
59	Blood culture	335
60	Cerebrospinal Fluid Collection	337
61	Placement and Management of Intravascular Cather	341
62	Blood Sampling Techniques	344
63	Blood Collection and Administration	346
64	Restraint and Handling of Foals	351
65	Biosecurity for Neonatal Units	356
66	Respiratory Therapeutics	358
67	Positive Pressure Ventilation	364
68	Tracheal Suctioning	368
69	How to Prevent the Leading Cuse of Death in Foals-Opinion	370

DRUG USE

70	Guidelines for Drug Use In Equine Neonates	374
71	Drug Formulary-Equine Neonate	381

REFERENCE VALUES

72	Hematology and Clinical Chemistry norm values-United States	405
73	Hematology and Clinical Chemistry norm values-European	410
74	Blood Gases	413
75	Immunoglubulin Concentrations	415
76	Cardiac Catheterization Pressure Measurements	417
77	Cardiopulmonary Cerebral Resuscitation	418

LIMB DEFORMITIES

78	Limb Deformities-Introduction	424
79	Flexural Deformities	427
80	Angular and Rotational Deviations-General	435

CHAPTER 1
MANAGEMENT APPROACHES TO THE NEWBORN FOAL
USE OF RISK FACTORS

Most foal deaths occur within the first week of life and often within the first 48 hrs.[1,2] The leading causes of foal problems are asphyxia, bacterial infection, starvation, exposure and dystocia. Management methods aimed at prevention of these problems may make a difference. We should use the concept of risk factors for the foal to guide our level of intervention to optimize and accelerate the detection of problems in high risk foals. This also prevents us from over-evaluating the healthy foal.

It is important to realize that newborn foals with recently acquired infection look their best shortly following birth and may first show obvious signs of problems only after illness is well established,[3] unless problems are detected early, these foals may die or require expensive and long term therapy. Newborn foals with any risk factors, including an unobserved birth in a non-clean pasture situation, should be evaluated more carefully and **immediately placed on antibiotics for 48-72 hrs duration**. (See Chapter 69)

EC - the first 16 hrs of life the neonatal gut is "open" for antibody absorption and bacteria may have enhanced opportunity for translocation and establishing bacteremia. Bacterial exposure occurs when the foal attempts to nurse (e.g. Coliforms on mare's udder, environment, etc) or has delayed nursing and the gut stays "open" longer. Antibiotics can prevent many infections when begun during the first 2-12 hrs of life. Don't wait for the foal to show signs of illness.

THREE CATEGORIES OF RISK
I. LOW RISK FOALS
   A. No maternal risk factors identified.
   B. Gestation of normal duration (Chapter 5).
   C. Events of parturition normal (Chapter 5).
      1. Stage 2 labor lasted less than 20 minutes.
      2. No significant manipulation of foal required for delivery.
      3. Foal stood by 2 hours.
      4. Foal nursed by 3 hours.

5. Placenta visually normal and < 10% of the body weight of the foal.
6. No environmental risk factors.
D. Post foaling stress score normal (Chapter 5).
E. Provide care as described for routine post foaling procedures (Chapter 7).

II. MODERATE RISK FOALS

These foals have only 1 risk factor of maternal or foal origin.

A. Place foal on antibiotics immediately post birth for 48-72 hrs.
B. Warrants a more frequent monitoring plan during the first week of life.
   1. Observe for early signs of illness (Chapter 25).
C. Laboratory evaluation for these foals (may need to serially monitor over 1 week).
   EC - Remember to use specific reference values that are age-matched and specific for neonatal foals (Chapters 72 and 73)
   1. **Complete Blood Count**
      EC - Always use differential count; a left shift may be missed if just performing a total white cell count.
   2. **Serum IgG** - Repeat determination and see if IgG is dropping from rapid consumption.
   3. **Blood chemistry** profile with electrolytes.
D. Body weight measured daily.
   1. Foals should gain 1-3 lbs (0.5-1.5 Kg) per day.

III. HIGH RISK FOALS

A. **MATERNAL CONDITIONS**[3,4,5]
   1. **Concurrent illness or fever**.
   2. **Pharmacologic** related.
      a. Sedation, tranquilizers, anesthetics may produce fetal depression.
      b. Nonsteroidal anti-inflammatory drugs.
      c. Beta-2 agonist bronchodilators may relax uterine smooth muscle.
      d. Excessive medication.
      e. In a recent study administration of **altrenogest** has not shown to alter the response to

exogenous ACTH after birth although foals had significantly lower neutrophil/lymphocyte ratio[6].
3. **Colic, endotoxemia** with or without surgery; endotoxin and bacteria may affect fetus.
4. **Vaginal discharge**.
   a. Mucopurulent exudate.
5. **Poor nutritional status**.
6. **Twins**.
   a. Twins that go to term are at risk from malposition and delivery problems.
7. Chronic lameness or incoordination.
   a. Inability of the mare to easily lie down and roll and rise so as to position foal may produce malposition.
8. **Recent transport stress**.
9. **Premature lactation ("dripping milk" before parturition) and loss of colostral proteins**.
10. **Pelvic abnormalities** from prior trauma or space occupying lesions.
11. **Maternal hyperventilation**[4]
    a. Severe pain, prolonged parturition, chronic obstruction pulmonary distress.
    b. May cause maternal respiratory alkalosis and shift hemoglobin dissociation curve. Increased affinity of maternal hemoglobin for O_2 may decrease transplacental O_2 diffusion.
12. **Prolonged gestation with oversized foal (rare).**
13. **Cesarean section**.
    a. Barbiturate anesthesia and halothane can produce fetal depression.
    b. Dorsal recumbency may compress uterine blood flow.
    c. Absence of factors which are associated with initiation of respiration in vaginally delivery.
14. **Agalactia.**
15. **History of producing a neonatal isoerythrolysis foal.**
16. **Poor mothering**- mild or complete foal rejection, extensive movements which cause foal weakness from the foal trying to follow the mare.

B. **PLACENTAL FACTORS**[2,5]
   1. **Placentitis**

2. Vasculitis and edema from systemic disease.
3. Vascular disturbances - thrombosis-infarction.

C. CONDITIONS OF LABOR OR DELIVERY[3,4,7]
1. **Any prolonged uterine contractions**.
2. **Dystocia** (Chapter 6)
    a. Leads to placental separation and decreased uterine blood flow.
    b. Aspiration of amniotic fluid, bacteria-containing fluid, or meconium can produce pneumonia and respiratory distress at birth.
3. **Partial or complete premature placental separation**.
    a. Seen as chorion protruding from vagina. Chorion has a red velvet appearance and precedes the foal during parturition.
    b. Produces foal anoxia during delivery.
    c. Correction by manual tearing of chorion and rapidly assisting delivery with immediate oxygen therapy and implementation of resuscitation protocol. (Chapter 16)
4. **Medically induced labor**.(Chapter 4)
    a. May produce premature placental separation.
5. **Parturition originating prior to 320 days gestation.**
6. **Early umbilical cord rupture** or excessive hemorrhage following severance.
    a. Controversy exists regarding amount of blood which pulses from placenta prior to separation.

D. NEONATAL CONDITIONS
1. **Congenital abnormalities** (see Chapters 41 & 42)
2. **Delayed Gut Closure** due to delay in obtaining colostrum. Normally these intestinal cells for immunoglobulin absorption are rapidly used up and a normal GI barrier is formed. Bacterial absorption across the 'open' gut leads to septicemia.[8]
    a. If foal is weak begin antibiotics immediately and treat for 48-72 hrs or longer based on signs and CBC. Weak foals have enhanced gut bacterial translocation.
3. **Failure of passive transfer**.
    a. This is usually caused by the foal being weak or by ingestion of poor quality colostrum (see Chapter 8).

b. Usually defined as less than 600-800 mg/dl of serum IgG at 16-24 hrs of age.
   c. Infection occurs principally from GI passage of bacteria across the open gut, or by umbilicus and rarely the respiratory tract.[8]
   d. Risk of low IgG (<400 mg/dl) in a low risk foal with good exam and excellent management and no delay in nursing (rapid gut closure) is minimal based on some studies.[9] Neutrophils have decreased phagocytosis and chemotaxis before colostrum ingestion.
4. **Meconium staining** around eyes and muzzle may indicate aspiration pneumonia.
5. **Prematurity**.
6. **Immature and small for gestational age**.
7. **Adverse environmental conditions**.
   a. Foaling in contaminated area.
   b. Cold and wet areas.
   c. Disrupted foaling due to over-observation.
   d. Infectious disease on the premises.
8. **Death of dam**.
   a. Administer at least 1 liter of (good quality) colostrum as soon as possible by bottle if has an excellent suck reflex; otherwise use naso-gastric tube, 8 oz at a time, every 1 hr.
9. **Foals which do not rise** and nurse by 3 hours of age.
10. **Twins**.
    a. Failure of passive transfer and septicemia are not uncommon in twins.
    b. May be small for gestational age, weak, subject to hypothermia and other problems.
11. Rejection by dam

MARE VACCINATION vaccines certified for use in pregnant mares that represent disease conditions the foal will be exposed to early in life. See http://www.vetmed.ucdavis.edu/ceh/docs/horsereport/pubs-HR23-1-bkm-sec.pdf for complete vaccination information.

Booster vaccination of mares 30 days before foaling –
   1. Botulinum toxoid, used where vaccine licensed.

2. Tetanus immunization of the newborn - Two methods
   a. Tetanus toxoid booster immunization of the mare in last 3-6 weeks before parturition preferred.
   b. Tetanus antitoxin (1500 units) within 24 hours of birth.
   c. Both methods provide 45 days of protection in the foal.[8]
3. Rotavirus- (Rotavirus vaccine-Ft Dodge)
   a. Vaccinate mare at months 8, 9 and 10 months gestation
   b. Use where rotavirus identified previously as a cause of foal diarrhea
4. Influenza – booster mares 4-6 weeks from foaling – NOTE- foals from influenza vaccinated mares do not respond to early vaccination. Begin foal vaccination from mares vaccinated at late term, at 6 months of age and use a 3 dose immunization series in the foal.
5. Equine herpes virus 1 – Rhinopneumonitis - used to prevent mare abortion due to EHV-1 –use inactivated vaccine (Pneumobort K-Ft Dodge) at 5, 7 and 9 months of gestation.
6. Equine herpes virus 4- vaccinate dam 4-6 weeks prior to foaling and start foal at 4-6 months of age using a 3 dose vaccination series.
7. West Nile Virus- Mares need to be protected from this virus in endemic areas (all of USA). Vaccination is not a risk to pregnant mare or fetus. Pregnant mares respond poorly to vaccination.

References:
1. Cohen, N.: Causes of and farm management factors associated with disease and death in foals. J Am Vet Med Assoc 204:1644-51, 1994.
2. Haas, SD, Bristol, F, Card, CE. Risk factors associated with the incidence of foal mortality in extensively managed mare herd. Can Vet J. 37:91-95, 1996.
3. Koterba A.M.: Medical management of the equine neonate. CVMA Speakers Syllabus, 96th Scientific Seminar pp 282-367, 1986.

4. Martens R.J.: Neonatal respiratory distress syndrome: A review with emphasis on the horse. Compend Cont Educ Pract Vet 4:S23-S33, 1982.
5. Valla, W.E.: Management of the high risk pregnancy; the peripartum period. Proceed Amer Coll Vet Int Med 7th ACVIM Forum, pp 417-420, 1989.
6. Neuhauser S, Palm F, Ambuehl F, Möstl E, Schwendenwein I, Aurich C. Effect of altrenogest-treatment of mares in late gestation on adrenocortical function, blood count and plasma electrolytes in their foals. Equine Vet J. 2009 Jul;41(6):572-7.
7. Sonea I.: Respiratory distress syndrome in neonatal foals. Compend Cont Educ Pract Vet 7:S462-S469, 1985.
8. Madigan, J.E.: What have colostrum deprivation models taught us about route of infection in the neonatal foal. Proceed of the Dorothy Havermeyer Workshop on Neonatal Foal Septicemia, 1995.
9. Baldwin, J.L., Cooper, W.L., Vanderwall, D.K., et al: Prevalence (treatment days) and severity of illness in hypogammaglobulinemic and normogamma-globulinemic foals. J Am Vet Med Assoc 198:423-428, 1991.
10. A guide to vaccinating your horses. CEH Horse Report. Center for Equine Health, UC Davis. Vol 23. 01/2011.

CHAPTER 2
ASSESSMENT OF FETAL WELLBEING

For many years, a rectal examination for a live, moving foal had been the extent of assessment of fetal wellbeing. Newer techniques and methods have been described and clinically utilized including placental, uterine and fetal ultrasound evaluation and blood endocrine testing which provide information on fetal growth and well being.

I. **TECHNIQUES FOR MONITORING HEALTH OF THE PREGNANT MARE**

   A. **PHYSICAL EXAM**
      1. Body weight, parasite control, immunizations, nutritional status, and prior reproductive history.
   B. **COMPLETE BLOOD COUNT AND CHEMISTRY PANEL 30-90 DAYS BEFORE FOALING**
      1. Inflammatory leukograms may represent placental or uterine problems or other maternal conditions which could adversely affect fetal health.
   C. **MATERNAL FACTORS FOR HIGH RISK FOALS**–Mare history -Chapter 1

   D. **FETAL ULTRASOUND- (See CHAPTER 52)**

II. **FETAL MONITORING TECHNIQUES** [1,9]

   A. **ENDOCRINE PARAMETER**
      1. Decreasing serum progesterone sampled in series at 2-24 hours was associated with impending abortion.[7]
      2. Single sample - Maternal serum progesterone levels are not reliable for determining fetal well being.[4]
      3. Pregnant mare blood and urine has estrone sulfate which is mainly derived from the live fetus. Fetal death causes a decline in mare estrone sulfate.
      4. Alpha Fetoprotein (AFP)-derived from the fetal liver- found to be elevated in late pregnancy in mares with twins, placentitis, premature placental separation, uterine trauma, and fetal death.[8]

6. Foal's leg movement ruptures the amniotic membrane
7. Umbilical cord ruptures within a few minutes. The amount of blood, if any, which is pumped from the placenta into the foal's circulation, is controversial.
8. If 10 minutes of Stage 2 strenuous labor produces no signs of the forelimbs or head at the vulva - the mare should be examined in a clean fashion for fetal position.
   a. If forelimbs and nose are present, allow another 10 minutes of labor.
   b. If strenuous activity fails to advance the foal - intervention is indicated - walk mare and obtain veterinary assistance.
- **C. STAGE 3** - expulsion of the placenta occurs within 3 hours of parturition.

III. IMMEDIATE POST FOALING EVALUATION - NORMAL FOALS

Evaluation of Neonatal Foal Distress*

Parameter	0	1	2
Heart rate	Absent	<60/min	≥60/min
Respiration	Absent	Slow, irregular	≥60/min Regular
Muscle tone	Limp extremities	Some flexion of limbs	Sternal
Nasal Stimulation	No response	Grimace, slight rejection	Cough or sneeze

Performed 1 minute after delivery

A total score of 7-8 indicates a normal foal, 4-6 indicates moderate depression and 0-3 indicates marked depression. Repeat evaluation in 4 minutes.

*Reproduced with permission from Martens R.J. <u>Compend Cont Educ for Pract Vet</u> 4(1):S23-S34, 1982.

b. This test is not 100% accurate but provides additional information on the time of foaling which may minimize sitting up with the mare.
   c. Another comparison study found a 53% probability that the mare would spontaneously foal within 24 hours after reaching a 4 color bar change, 20% chance of not foaling within 24 hours after 4 bar color change, and a 27% chance of foaling without reaching this cutoff level. Placental or fetal abnormalities may influence the reliability of any of these tests[3]
2. Softcheck™ Water Hardness Test Strip[b] (Determines Ca and Mg)
   a. Mammary secretions checked once daily until total hardness exceeded 120 ppm. Then mares were checked twice daily.[6]
   b. 250 ppm water hardness used as decision point (for maximal observations) along with other physical findings.[6]
   c. 72% probability of foaling within 24 hours when 250 ppm water hardness first detected in pre-foaling mammary secretions.[6]
   d. 22% chance mare would not foal in 24 hours when $\leq$ 250 ppm water hardness detected.[6]
   e. 6% chance mare would foal prior to reaching the 250 ppm water hardness.[6]
3. Titrets™ Calcium Hardness Test Kits (Determines Ca in milk only)
   a. > 250 ppm calcium carbonate content used as cut off point for ready-to-foal in one study.[6]
   b. 59% probability of foaling within 24 hours and 23% chance mare would not foal within 24 hours if > 250 ppm test result. 18% chance of foaling within 24 hr of $\leq$ 250 ppm test.
   c. Authors of study suggest using 200 ppm with this test would improve chance of foaling within 24 hours to 88%.
   d. This method considered most reliable
      EC - To use these methods, collect 1-5 ml of mammary secretion in clean plastic vial. Dilute 1:6 with double distilled water.

References:
1. Adams-Brendemuehl C., Pipers F.S.: Antepartum evaluations in the equine fetus. J Reproduction & Fertility (Suppl) 35:565,1987.
2. Colles C.M., Parks R.D.: Fetal electrocardiography in the mare. Equine Vet J 10:32-37, 1978.
3. Parkes R.D., Colles C.M.: Fetal electrocardiography in the mare as a practical aid to diagnosing singleton and twin pregnancy. Vet Res 100:25-26, 1977.
4. Pashen R.L.: Maternal and fetal endocrinology during late pregnancy and parturition in the mare. Equine Vet J 16(4):233-238, 1984.
5. Buss D.D., Asbury A.C., Chevalier, L.: Limitations in equine fetal electrocardiography. J Amer Vet Med Assoc 177:174-176, 1980.
6. Sanchii, E.: Abstract: Incidence and possible causes of abortion after colic in 105 pregnant mares. Proceed Soc Vet Parintology Cambridge, England, 1990, p 28.
7. Reef, VB, Vaala, WE, Worth, LT, et al.: Transcutaneous ultrasonographic assessment of fetal well being during late gestation: A preliminary report on development of an equine biophysical profile. Proceed. Amer Assoc Eq Pract 42:152-153, 1996.
8. Vaala, WE: Proceedings of 9th annual ACVIM forum 483-485. 1991

CHAPTER 3
DETECTION OF IMPENDING PARTURITION

An individual horse's gestation length can be extremely variable. The rate of in utero maturation of the fetus influences a particular gestation length.[1] Determination of the expected time of foaling allows appropriate observation of the foaling for detection of problems. The vast majority of mares foal at night.

I. MATERNAL PHYSICAL FACTORS

- **A. Gestation** length > 320 days.
- **B. Relaxation** of the pelvic ligaments and elongation of the vulva and relaxation of the cervix.
- **C. Waxing of teats** - small droplets of milk on the ends of nipples.
- **D. Colostrum in mammary gland**.
  EC - Must measure immunoglobulin in milk to determine if it is colostrum. Use specific gravity or glutaraldehyde test. None of these signs indicate that foaling will occur within a certain time period.

II. MAMMARY SECRETION CHANGES

- **A. Changes in electrolyte composition of mammary secretions** during late pregnancy have been used to determine fetal readiness for birth.[2,3]
- **B. Immediate prefoaling changes** are an increase in calcium to ($\geq$40 mg/dl), potassium ($\geq$35 mEq/L), and a decrease in sodium ($\leq$ 30 mEq/L).
- **C. Three field tests** [4,5,6] using a form of water hardness test strips for calcium content have indicated some practical applications.
  1. Predict A Foal ™- mare foaling predictor kit[a]
     a. 1 cc mammary section taken every evening and 5 zones on the test strip are examined.

     According to one study:[5]
1 zone or less	<1% chance of foaling within 12 hrs
4 zone	80% chance of foaling within 12 hrs
5 zone	95% chance of foaling within 12 hrs

IV. OTHER PARAMETERS OF NORMAL POST BIRTH FOALS[1,2]

A. **Time to suck** - reflex stimulated by placing a finger in the mouth - developing within 2-20 minutes.
B. **Sternal recumbency 1-2 minutes**.
C. **Time to stand** - average 60 minutes. Longer than 2 hours is considered abnormal.
D. **Time to nurse from mare** - 2 hours average. Longer than 3-4 hours is considered abnormal.
E. **Temperature** - 99-101.5.F (37.2-38.6°C) **A.M.** non-stressed value.
F. **Heart rate** - 1-5 minutes post foaling > 60 bpm; 6-60 minutes: 80-130 bpm; Day 1-5: 80-120 bpm.
G. **Respiration rate** - First 30 minutes post foaling: 60-80/min 1-12 hr: 30-40/minute.

References:

1. Rossdale, P.D.: The Practice of Equine Stud Medicine. 1st Edition, Baltimore, Williams and Wilkins, 1974.
2. Rossdale P.D.: Clinical studies on the newborn thoroughbred foal. Br Vet J 123:470-481, 1967.

CHAPTER 6
DYSTOCIA MANAGEMENT FACTORS FOR NEONATAL VIABILITY

The goal is maximum cleanliness and minor trauma to the mare (to prevent subsequent fertility problems), combined with a system for rapid correction of the dystocia or immediate referral to an experienced team if close by. Foal survival is linked to duration of time to correct the dystocia. 15 min longer duration makes a difference in number of live foals. One study showed that less than 50% of dystocias have live foals.[1] **EC** -A new technique using garden hose running water inserted into the placenta to distend the uterus and create room for manipulation has been described.

I. HISTORY

 A. Duration of the time since abdominal cramping or rupture of membranes occurred.
 B. Determine what intervention has occurred and when.
 C. Reproductive history of the mare: previous dystocia, cervicovaginitis, twins, gestational age, medication administered.
 D. If 10 minutes have elapsed after breaking water and strong abdominal contractions produce no evidence of a nose and forefeet, have qualified help assess position by vaginal exam. If feet and nose are present, allow an additional 10 minutes of labor. If 20 minutes have elapsed, have owner walk mare until veterinarian arrives.

II. DETERMINE CAUSE

 A. Abnormal presentation, position, posture, presence of twins.
 B. Incompatibility of fetal size and birth canal.
 C. Uterine inertia or other maternal factors.

III. MAKE PLAN FOR CORRECTION AND SET TIME

 A. If not making significant progress in 10-15 minutes, consider alternative approach, e.g. anesthesia or cesarean, etc.

- **B.** Epidural Block
  1. Used to prevent straining.
  2. Administer 5-6 cc 2% carbocaine hydro-chloride, or 2% lidocaine, with 4-7 cm 18 gauge spinal needle at the junction of tail hairs and caudal folds of the tail.
  3. Avoid larger volume because it may make the mare unstable in the rear quarters and complicate recovery if general anesthesia is subsequently required.
- **C.** Twitch and/or leg tied up for restraint.
- **D.** Proceed with caution because the risk to the veterinarian is high in these circumstances. Always attempt to protect yourself.
- **E.** Drugs to calm the mare.
  EC - None of the drugs listed below will make it completely safe to work with the mare.
  1. All drugs affect the fetus to a greater or lesser degree.
  2. Xylazine (0.5-1.0 mg/kg) can cause sedation. Mares can arouse from xylazine and kick violently.
     a. Causes fetal bradycardia.
  3. Xylazine (0.5-1.0 mg/kg) plus butorphanol (0.01-0.02 mg/kg).
  4. Detomidine (5-10 mg/mare; 20 ug/Kg IV) longer lasting-mare can still kick.

IV. EQUIPMENT

- **A.** Resuscitation equipment should be available (See Resuscitation Chapter 16).
- **B.** Obstetrical equipment consists of four chains (2 long, 2 short), nylon straps, two obstetrical handles, snare (calf snare or hog snare), Krey's hook, towel clamp (to grasp ear or skin), fetotome and wire, knife, sleeves, lubricant (mineral oil or methylcellulose), stomach pump and tube (to lubricate foal), stainless steel bucket.

V. TOCOLYSIS

- **A.** Agents that paralyze or reduce myometrium activity may be useful in preventing straining to repel fetus.

B. Clenbuterol hydrochloride (a Beta 2 sympathomimetic) administered at 0.4-0.5 ug/kg intra-muscularly may provide some benefit.
   1. This drug delays parturition for 5-10 hours in cattle.[3]
   2. Limited use in the horse at this time.

VI. ANESTHESIA CONSIDERATION FOR NEONATAL VIABILITY

A. Intravenous xylazine (l mg/kg) and ketamine (2 mg/kg) anesthesia can produce short term cessation of maternal straining and allow correction of many malposition problems with minimal fetal depression.
   1. Used in conjunction with a hoist (block and tackle) to raise the rear quarters, (see figure 1).
   2. If hoist is unavailable, a 3/4" thick plywood board, elevated at one end on a bale of straw, can elevate mare's rear quarters if sufficient help is present to place the mare properly.
B. General anesthesia for cesarean section.
   1. Prep ventral abdomen before anesthesia.
   2. Use local infiltrative block in ventral abdominal wall
   3. Use nonbarbiturate induction such as xylazine, diazepam/ ketamine and provide endotracheal intubation and maintenance or with low levels of isoflurane.
   4. Make all arrangements to allow the shortest time between induction and delivery of the foal.
C. Arrange for basic emergency equipment for foal resuscitation upon delivery.
   1. Have a separate group to work with foal while surgeons handle the mare.
   2. Intubate the foal before clamping umbilical cord with cesarean or complicated dystocia.
   3. Provide immediate post birth evaluation for high risk foal (Chapter 19).

References:
1. Byron, CR, Embertson, RM, Bernard, WV, et. Al. Dystocia in a referral hospital setting: Approach and results. Equine Vet J. 35:82-85, 2003
2. Hawkins, D.L.: Dystocia. Proc Amer Assoc Eq Pract 411-416,1982..
3. Smith, L.J., Schott, H.: Xylazine-induced fetal bradycardia. Abstract. Proc 2nd Int Conf on Vet Perinatology Cambridge, England p 36, 1999
4. Putnam, M.R., Rice, L.E., Wettman, R.P., et al.: Clenbuterol for the postponement of parturition and alleviation of dystocia in cattle. Proc Ann Meet Soc Theriogen 176-183, 1982
5. Luvkkanen, L, Katila, T., Koskinen, E, Same effects of multiple administration of detomidine during the last trimester of equine pregnancy. Equine Vet J. 29:400-403, 1997

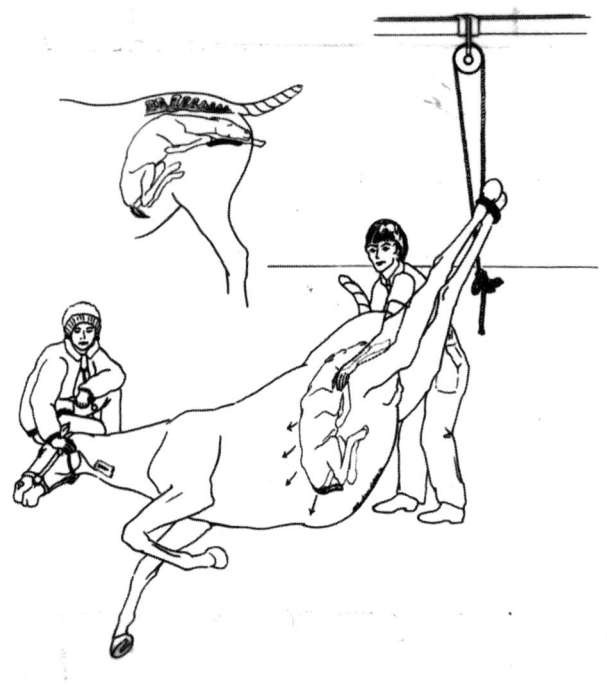

Figure 1: Short acting general anesthesia and hoist (mechanical or power) for dystocia management.

CHAPTER 7
POST FOALING PROCEDURES –ROUTINE (LOW RISK FOALS)

I. **CARE OF UMBILICUS**

   A. Allow the cord to sever on its own, unless foaling in a contaminated environment where the severed umbilicus would immediately become infected.
   B. If foaling in a contaminated area or performing a cesarean section, ligate the cord while it is constricting, with sterile umbilical tape or clamps, 1-1/2 and 2-1/2 inches from the body wall. Dip area in chlorhexidine (0.5%) solution and sever cord between ligatures. Dip exposed cord in chlorhexidine solution.
   C. Apply chlorhexidine (0.5%) (Novolsan 2% solution diluted 1 part with 3 parts sterile water) q 6 hr for 24 hr and watch for heat or swelling.
   EC - this is better than 2% iodine or betadine; don't use 7% iodine.[1]

II. **EXAMINE PLACENTA FOR INTEGRITY, WEIGHT AND SIGNS OF ABNORMALITIES**

   A. Placentas weighing >10% of the foal's body weight may be abnormal.

III. **PERFORM PHYSICAL EXAMINATION OF FOAL (See Chapter 11)**

IV. **ADMINISTER 1500 UNITS TETANUS ANTITOXIN IF DAM NOT GIVEN TOXOID BOOSTER IN LAST 4-6 WEEKS**

V. **IF IgG IS LOW DETERMINE COLOSTRUM QUALITY AND SUPPLEMENT (See Chapter 8)**

VI. **ENEMA**

   A. Many foals are given a non-irritating enema to assist with complete passage of meconium.
   B. Use fleet enemas®, soapy water (mild soaps only).

1. Use very soft tubes in the rectum. Be cautious so as to not penetrate or injure the mucosa.
2. Volume 4-6 ounces.

C. Repeated enemas may be irritating and can cause mucosal hemorrhage and edema and produce more straining.

D. Acetylcysteine (Mucomyst)® a mucolytic agent diluted in water has been effective in human infants in rapidly dissolving meconium. (See Chapter 26)

VII. COMPLETE BLOOD COUNT - optional. An in-utero problem or early infectious condition may be suggested from an abnormal CBC.

VIII. ARTERIAL BLOOD GAS - optional - can be obtained from umbilical arteries at birth.

IX. ANTIBIOTICS - Since most neonatal infections are caused by gram-negative bacteria, standard doses of penicillin or penicillin-streptomycin are unlikely to provide significant benefit. **EC** – The routine use of post birth antibiotics is controversial. With good management, cleaning the mare and rapid ingestion of colostrum antibiotics may not be needed. Routine use of antibiotics lowers incidence of septicemia in some settings.[3] Since most infections are gram negative and often mixed infections, use broad spectrum antibiotic combinations such as Procaine Penicillin 20-30,000 Units/kg intramuscularly and gentamicin 6.6 mg/kg intramuscularly once daily for 48-72 hrs. (In a 50 kg foal 5 cc of 300,000 U/ml Procaine pen and 3.3 cc of 100 mg/ml gentocin.)

X. VITAMINS

A. Selenium injections and oral vitamin E (800-1500 units) may be valuable in foals that are asphyxia cases.
EC - these foals may have elevated serum CK enzymes or have maladjustment syndrome; use in foals born to mares from selenium deficient areas not receiving selenium supplementation.

XI. DIGESTIVE TRACT INOCULUMS are not recommended, due to current lack of evidence of benefits. Liver failure and death occurred in foals following administration of a digestive tract inoculum shortly after birth; the inoculum contained excessive iron.[3]

XII. EXERCISE

A. If the foal is normal size and has normal limb conformation, it should receive paddock exercise beginning at day two.
   EC - Most foals have some valgus deformities and that is normal.[4] (see chapter on foal limbs)
B. Recent studies in New Zealand have suggested foals should have lots of exercise in the first 6 weeks of life which produces increased amounts of joint cartilage.[5]
C. Poorly ventilated, dusty stalls pose more risks to healthy foals than exposure to most outdoor environmental conditions.[6]

References:
1. Lavan, RP, Madigan, JE, Walker, R. et. Al Effects of disinfectant treatments on the bacterial flora of the umbilicus o neonatal foals. Biology of Reproduction Monographs 1:77-85.
2. Stoneham, S.: The incidence of neonatal septicemia in a selected population of Thoroughbred foals in Newmarket, England (1989-1994). Proceed. Dorothy Russel Havermeyer Foundation Neonatal Septicemia Workshop. Tufts University, N. Grafton, MA, p 13, 1994.
3. Divers, T.J., Warner, A., Vaala, W.E., et al.: Toxic hepatic failure in newborn foals. J Am Vet Med Assoc 183:1407-1413, 1983.
4. Anderson, TM, McIlwraith, CW, Douay, P. The role of conformation in musculoskeletal problems in the racing thoroughbred. Equine Vet J. 36:
5. Firth EC.: The response of bone, articular cartilage and tendon to exercise in the horse. J. Anat. 2006.Apr;208 (4):513-26
6. Ripahi, T., Koskila, P., Kotimaa, M., Koskinen, E., et al.: Serum IgG antibody concentration against environmental microbes in mares and foals during different seasons and effect of stabling practices. Am J Vet Res 51:550-555, 1990.

CHAPTER 8
COLOSTRUM - ASSESSMENT OF AND SOURCES FOR FOALS

Colostrum varies in quality (amount of IgG and type of specific antibodies) in mares. It is prudent to assess the quality of colostrum in mares at birth and have alternate sources readily available for newborn foals. Determining IgG of colostrum must be done pre-suckle and immediately postpartum. This indirectly identifies those foals which could be at high risk for failure of passive transfer. Assessment allows determination of high quality colostrum which aids adequate passive transfer immunoglobulin and/or saving some colostrum for freezing (colostrum banking).

EC - Remember that early administration of any quality colostrum which "closes" the "open" gut is also an important method of preventing infection, so feed or tube the foal with what you have initially. If you have problems with obtaining or giving colostrum always begin the foal on antibiotics and treat for 48-72 hrs.

I. ASSESSING IgG CONTENT

A. SUBJECTIVE CRITERIA
1. Thick, sticky consistency similar to liquid paraffin. Creamy yellow color.
2. Specific gravity of colostrum is correlated with IgG concentration. (See below)
3. Visual assessment not adequate to determine quality (IgG content).

B. LABORATORY ASSESSMENT OF COLOSTRUM
1. Immunoglobulin (IgG) content (Immunology Laboratory, single radial immuno-diffusion).
2. Anti-erythrocyte alloantibodies that may result in neonatal isoerythrolysis can be rapidly detected by the jaundiced foal agglutination test (JFA) (see Chapter 35).
3. Other commercial tests for IgG are available.

II. METHOD TO ASSESS COLOSTRUM[1-3]

A. COLOSTROMETER

1. This technique affords immediate results "on the farm" by determination of the specific gravity of a 5 ml aliquot of colostrum obtained immediately post foaling. i.e. pre-suckle.[4]
2. Colostral specific gravity should be > 1.060 and contain at least 3000 mg IgG/dl
3. Product name and Manufacturer: Equine Colostrometer J-281, (Jorgensen Laboratories – Loveland, Co, USA). www.jorvet.com

B. SUGAR REFRACTOMETER
1. Proven reliable for colostrum IgG- BRIX % reading
   a. Place 1 drop of colostrum on refractomer
   b. If reading is 10-15 poor IgG concentration, 15-20 borderline, 20-30% have 60g/dl of IgG in colostrum–adequate-
2. Manufacturers:
   a. Atago Sugar Refractometer, Atago Inc., Japan. www.atago.net/usa
   b. Bellingham and Stanley, Ltd. Turnbridge Wells, Kent, UK. http://www.bellinghamandstanley.com

III. PROGRAM FOR MINIMIZING FAILURE OF PASSIVE TRANSFER

A. (Using gms of IgG) Foals fed an estimated 1.5 gm of colostral IgG/kg of body weight had reasonable levels of serum IgG at 12 hrs of life.[5]
   1. Mares produced 2.3 liters ±500 ml of colostrum.[5]
   2. Foals with less than 400 mg/dl IgG at 12 hr (or foals that can't nurse) should receive 1.00-1.25 gm colostral IgG/kg of body weight. This is fed starting at 2 hr of age in volumes of 200 ml per feeding.[5]

B. (Using volumes of colostrum) If colostral IgG is normal or high, then feed foal 1-1.5 liters of colostrum starting at 1-2 hrs of age using 8 oz per feeding at 2 hr intervals. Check IgG at 12 hrs.
   1. If colostral specific gravity is 1.050 - 1.060 - supplement foal with 10-12 ounces of good quality colostrum via nasogastric tube.
   2. If colostral specific gravity is (very poor) < 1.050 - administer 24 ounces (approximately 1 liter) of good quality colostrum (sp.g. > 1.060).

C. Only pre-suckle colostrum test results can be evaluated reliably. Evaluating colostral quality after a foal has nursed 1-4 hours is of little value because the normal rate of decline in colostral quality is unknown.

IV. ALTERNATE SOURCES OF COLOSTRUM

A. Bovine colostrum has been shown to be absorbed and provides some short duration of passive transfer to foals.[6,7]
 1. It may not provide the specific antibodies needed for protection against all equine pathogens.
 2. Administer 2-4 liters (400 ml q 2 hr starting by 2 hrs of age)
 3. Use only when you don't have access to other forms of artificial or mare colostrum. Treat foal with antibiotics as well.
 4. Equi-Col Foal Colostrum™ is 100% pure natural bovine colostrum replacement in a 100g metalised sachet. This can be used as a replacement or in addition to the mare´s colostrum.
B. Commercial concentrated serum products for oral use. (Sermune™ Equine IgG) — Phone 800-552-3984;913-541-1307, www. lakeimmunogenics.com
C. Lyophilized Equine IgG
 1. (Lymphomune™) Bioqual Inc. www.bioqual.com/igG_products.asp
 2. Equine ImmunoGam™- Minigam, Equine colostrum supplement, www.bioqual.com/immuno_gam.asp
 These are derived from equine serum and are absorbed if administered in first 12 hrs of life.
 EC - I would use either product over bovine colostrum if no mare colostrum were available
D. Situation: mare has no colostrum, no source available, what to do?
 EC- Feed the foal cow's milk right from the store, feed it all it wants, and put foal on injectable antibiotics, keep in clean area, clean mares udder and rear quaters. Must close the open gut to prevent bacterial translocation. Foal needs milk within 3 hours of birth.

V. RISK FACTORS FOR MARES WITH LOW COLOSTRAL SPECIFIC GRAVITY (IgG IN MILK) [5]

A. Mares greater than 15 years of age have lower milk IgG.
B. Mares producing foals early in the year.
C. Breed: Standardbred mares have lower milk IgG.
D. Weather: mares giving birth on nice sunny days had more IgG in milk.

References:
1. Venner M, Markus RG. et. al.: Evaluation of immuno-globulin G concentration in colostrum of mares by ELISA, refractometry and colostrometry. Berl].Munch Tierarztl Wochenschr. 2008 Jan-Feb;121(1-2):66-72
2. Cash RSG. Colostral quality determined by refractometry. Equine Veterinary Education 1999;11:36-38.
3. Knottenbelt DC, Holdstock N, Madigan JE. Equine Neonatology Medicine and Surgery. Saunders, Edinburg, pp 393-394. 2005
4. LeBlanc, M.M.: Use of a modified hydrometer to assess immunoglobulin content in mare colostrum. Proceed Amer Assoc Eq Pract 152-164, 1985.
5. LeBlanc, MM, Baldwin, JL, Pritchard EL: Factors that influence passive transfer of immunoglobulins in foals. J Amer Vet Med Assoc 220:179-183, 1992.
6. Lavoie, JP, Spensley, MS, Smith, BP, Mihalyi, J.: Absorption of bovine colostral immunoglobulins G and M in newborn Foals. Am J Vet Res 50:1598-1603, 1989.
7. Holmes, MA, Lunn, DP.: A study of bovine and equine immunoglobulin levels in pony foals fed bovine colostrum. Equine vet J 23:116-118, 1991.

CHAPTER 9
ASSESSMENT OF PASSIVE IMMUNITY

The acquisition of immunoglobulins is entirely by passive transfer in foals. The speed with which this occurs following birth, the amount and types of specific antibodies in the colostrum, and the amount and types absorbed are factors in the prevention of infection. Good management may be just as important as increasing amounts of immunoglobulins in preventing infections.[1]

I. TIME FACTORS

- **A.** General Considerations
    1. Tests of serum IgG taken before 18 hours of age may indicate lower levels of IgG than will be attained at 24 hours of age, due to ongoing transport of immunoglobulins into blood via the lymphatics and continued gastrointestinal absorption.
- **B.** Early Testing of Foal Serum IgG
    1. Foal's serum IgG tested at 8-12 hr of age.
    2. IgG has been nearly completely absorbed in most foals by this time.
    3. Most foals should have at least 400 mg IgG/dl serum at this time.
    4. If IgG is < 400 mg/dl at 8-12 hours, then previously harvested colostrum can be supplemented.
    5. This minimizes the incidence of FPT, decreases the time period of immunocompromise associated with low immunoglobulin levels, and reduces the need for plasma transfusions.
- **C.** Late Testing of Foal Serum IgG
    1. 18-24 hours of age.
    2. If FPT is detected at this time plasma therapy is the only means to raise serum IgG.
    3. Delay in detecting a very low serum IgG may increase risk of acquiring infection.

II. TESTS OF SERUM IgG[2-4]
EC - Standards for the reference test of single radial immunodiffusion (SRID) vary with the SRID system. Previously the same serum sample sent to different laboratories could read

double the amount of IgG in one lab compared to another. New standards have been developed; in the meantime, several tests have proven reliable and consistent, and can be useful.

A. Single radial immuno-diffusion (SRID)
 1. IgG moves through gel to meet antibody and forms visible circles.
 2. Requires 24 hours.
 3. Measures 0-3000 mg/dl.
 4. Kits available:
    a. VMRD, Inc; P.O. Box 502, Pullman, WA 99163
       www.vmrd.com
    b. Equine-RID, Plasvacc, Inc.
       www.plasvaccusa.com
       Phone 800-654-9743.
B. Glutaraldehyde Coagulation[5]
 1. Chemical grade 25% glutaraldehyde solution.
 2. Forms insoluble complexes with basic proteins.
 3. Make 10% solution with deionized water.
 4. Use serum in test.
 5. Add 5 ml of serum plus 50 ul of glutaraldehyde and check for coagulation. Measure ≤ 400 ≥ 800 mg/dl
    a. 800 mg/dl observed in 10 minutes.
    b. Reaction in 60 minutes ≥ 400 mg/dl.
 6. Inexpensive - approx. 0.25 cents/test.
 7. Hemolysis may result in overestimated IgG.
 8. Test is reliable and accurate.[5]
 9. GAMMA-CHECK-C for colostral IgG testing commercial kit from Plasvacc Inc. (www.plasvaccusa.com).
C. Snap Test
 1. Measures <400, 400-800 and >800 mg IgG/dl.
 2. Enzyme combines with IgG for color change.
 3. Serum or plasma preferred; can use whole blood.
 4. 8-10 minutes for result.
 5. Accurate and reliable especially in lower (<400mg/dl) and higher range (>800mg/dl).[6, 7]
 6. Manufactured by Idexx Inc. www.idexx.com
D. Zinc Sulfate Turbidity[8]
 1. Method correlates well with SRID but can occasionally over-estimate amounts of immunoglobulin in the 400 mg/dl range.[9]

2. Preparation of solutions - for 1 liter: dissolve 250 mg of ZnSO4.7 H_2O granules (Sigma Chemical Co.) in 1 liter of distilled water (boiled to remove all the CO_2). Inject 6 ml of the zinc sulfate solution into a 10ml red top vacutainer tube using a syringe and small needle and preserve the vacuum in the tube. Shelf life is long if protected from air.
3. Modified zinc sulfate test for foals[10]
   a. Controls - obtain pre-suckle serum and adult serum samples and store in the freezer in small aliquots for thawing to run with a test.
   b. Bleed foals between 8 and 18 hrs of age. Separate serum.
   c. Bring zinc sulfate solution and serum to room temperature.
   d. Measure 0.1 ml (100 µl) of serum and control sample. If using a 1 cc TB syringe, fill to 0.3 and express to 0.2 and add to zinc sulfate tube.
   e. Rotate for 15 seconds.
   f. If a precipitate forms there is >400 mg/dl IgG, if hemolysis is present in serum sample results will be erroneously high.
   g. Potential problems
      i. Old solution - rapidly decomposes (max shelf life 3 months) when exposed to small amount of room air and may give false results
      ii. Temperature for test should be run at room temperature.
      iii. Hemolysis - gives false positive values.

III. DEFINITIONS OF PASSIVE TRANSFER[11]
EC - Keep in mind measurements below represent total IgG; specific antibodies against a particular pathogen may be more important than the total IgG. New levels and definitions have raised what is considered the normal IgG level.

A. < 200 mg/dl serum of IgG is complete failure of passive transfer.
B. 200-800 mg/dl is partial failure of passive transfer.
C. $\geq$ 800 mg/dl is normal or adequate passive transfer.

EC - Some confusion has occurred because 800 mg/dl has been recommended for infected foals or high risk foals. The $\geq$ 400-600 mg/dl level is still adequate for healthy low risk foals in my opinion.

IV. INTERPRETATION OF VALUES - (IgG) (Early or Late Testing)

A. $\leq$ 200 mg/dl is failure of passive transfer - recommend I.V. plasma if >18 hours old.
B. 200-800 mg/dl is partial failure of passive transfer.
   1. Treat with colostrum if <18 hours old.
   2. If <400mg/dl and >18 hours old treat with plasma or serum products.
   3. If 400-800 mg/dl, excellent management and no risk factors identified treatment is not necessary; otherwise treat with plasma and antibodies.
C. $\geq$ 800 mg/dl - normal - no treatment unless a high risk foal or sepsis is present.

V. MOST SEPTIC FOALS HAVE IgG SERUM < 400 mg/dl.[12,13]

VI. NEWBORN FOALS have reduced neutrophil function prior to ingestion of colostrum.[14]

References:
1. Baldwin, J.L., Cooper, W.L., Vanderwall, D.K., et al.: Prevalence (treatment days) and severity of illness in hypogammaglobulinemic and normogammaglobulinemic foals. JAVMA 198:423-428, 1991.
2. Metzger N, Hinchcliff KW, Hardy J, Schwarzwald CC, Wittum T.: Usefulness of a commercial equine IgG test and serum protein concentration as indicators of failure of transfer of passive immunity in hospitalized foals. J Vet Intern Med. 2006 Mar-Apr;20(2):382-7.
3. McClure JT, DeLuca JL, Lunn DP, Miller J.: Evaluation of IgG concentration and IgG subisotypes in foals with complete or partial failure of passive transfer after administration of intravenous serum or plasma. Equine Vet J. 2001 Nov;33(7):681-6.
4. Davis R, Giguère S.: Evaluation of five commercially available assays and measurement of serum total protein concentration

via refractometry for the diagnosis of failure of passive transfer of immunity in foals. J Am Vet Med Assoc. 2005 Nov 15;227(10):1640-5
5. Clabough, D.L., Conboy, S., Roberts, M.C.: Comparison of four screening techniques for the diagnosis of equine neonatal hypogammaglobulinemia. J Am Vet Med Assoc 194:1717-1720, 1989.
6. Bertone, J.J., Jones, R.L., Curtis, C.R.: Evaluation of a test kit for Pusterla N, determination of serum immunoglobulin G concentration in foals. J Vet Int Med 2:181-183, 1988.
7. Pusterla JB, Spier SJ, Puget B, Watson JL.:Evaluation of the SNAP foal IgG test for the semiquantitative measurement of immunoglobulin G in foals. Vet Rec. 2002 Aug 31;151(9):258-60.
8. Rumbaugh, G.E., Ardans, A.A., Ginno, D., Trommershausen-Smith, A.: Identification and treatment of colostrum deficient foals. J Am Vet Med Assoc 174:274-278, 1979.
9. Morris, D.D., Meirs, D.A., Merryman, G.S.: Passive transfer failure in horses: Incidence and causative factors on a breeding farm. Am J Vet Res 46:2294-2299, 1985.
10. LeBlanc, MM.: A modified zinc sulfate turbidity test for the detection of immune status in newly born foals. J EquineVet Sci 10:36-40, 1990.
11. Crisman MV, Scarratt WK. Immunodeficiency disorders in horses. Vet Clin North Am Equine Pract. 2008 Aug;24(2):299-310
12. McGuire, T.C., Crawford, T.B., Hallowell, A.L., et al: Failure of colostral immunoglobulin transfer as an explanation for most infections and deaths in neonatal foals. J Am Vet Assoc 170:1302-1304, 1977.
13. Koterba, A.M., Brewer, B.D., Tarplee, F.A.: Clinical and clinicopathological characteristics of the septicemic neonatal foal: Review of 38 cases. Eq Vet J 16:376-382, 1984.
14. Bernoco, M., Liu, I.K.M., Ehlert, C., et al: Chemotactic and phagocytic function of peripheral blood polymorphonuclear leukocytes in newborn foals. J Reprod & Fertility, Suppl 35:599-605, 1987.

CHAPTER 10
PLASMA THERAPY

Plasma has been used as preventive therapy for treatment of failure of passive transfer and therapeutically to raise antibody levels in ill foals less than 2 months of age. The majority of neonatal foals with infectious conditions such as septicemia have failure of passive transfer (IgG < 400 mg/dl). However, some studies indicate that, with good management, healthy foals with serum IgG of 200-400 mg/dl have only slight risk of acquiring illness.[1]

I. **INDICATIONS**
   EC - The controversy of which foals should receive plasma transfusions will continue until more studies on the protective and therapeutic effects of plasma are conducted.

   A. Failure of Passive Transfer
      1. At this time all foals with IgG at 18-24 hours of age < 200 should be treated with plasma
      2. Plasma transfusion is optional for healthy, low risk foals with IgG of 400-600 mg/dl at 24 hours and good post birth management.
      3. Benefit of raising the serum IgG with a plasma transfusion has limited evidence for healthy, low risk foals with IgG of 400 mg/dl at 24 hours of age and good post birth management.
   B. Infectious Conditions
      1. Foals with septicemia may benefit from plasma transfusions to raise serum IgG to the 600-800 mg/dl range.
      2. When infections are present always check IgG post plasma transfusion after 24 hrs. Levels of serum IgG post transfusion may be quite variable.
   C. For High Risk Foals
      1. Some foal conditions result in poor colostrum absorption.
         a. Prematurity
         b. Decreased gastrointestinal motility (minimal gut sounds) occurs nonspecifically in many stressed, ill foals.

2. Start plasma immediately following birth in premature foals, weak foals with poor gastrointestinal motility, and severely hypothermic and hypoglycemic foals.
3. Additional IgG from plasma transfusion in high risk foals may be beneficial.
   a. Raising levels to 600-800 mg/dl has been suggested.

   EC - Higher levels of serum IgG increase the chances of providing specific antibodies to pathogens and may be beneficial.

D. Severe disseminated intravascular coagulopathy (DIC) with life-threatening hemorrhage in conjunction with heparinization.
1. Plasma supplies antithrombin III which is the mechanism whereby heparinization produces a reduction in the hypercoagulable state.
2. Must treat the primary disorder causing the DIC.
3. Plasma administered to patients in DIC may exacerbate organ dysfunction with ongoing thrombin activation. It is important to monitor liver and kidney function and fibrin split products if using plasma in DIC.

II. TYPES OF PLASMA

A. Anti-endotoxin (J-5) Plasma
1. Made by vaccination of donors with a modified *E. coli* (J5).
2. Contains antibodies against the core lipopolysaccharide and should provide cross protection to a variety of gram negative infections.

B. Anti-endotoxin (*Salmonella typhimurium*) Plasma
1. Plasma donors vaccinated with mutant *S. typhimurium*.
2. Protection by similar mechanism as J-5. i.e. cross protection against gram negative infection with core antibodies.
3. Source – Endoserum™ - IMMVAC, Inc., Columbia, MO 65201. Telephone 800-944-7563. http://www.immvac.com/

C. Anti-*Rhodococcus equi* hyperimmune plasma (See Chapter 29)
D. Botulism - see Infections (Chapter 28)
E. Platelet rich plasma (PRP)
   1. This is used in foals with post foaling thrombocytopenia presumed associated with ingestion of antibody to the foals thrombocytes.
   2. Frozen plasma not a source of platelets
   3. Fresh harvested plasma is best - can order from plasma companies for next day delivery

III. SOURCES OF PLASMA

A. Commercial availability
   1. Use of commercial USDA approved plasma is desirable. Donors may be hyperimmunized, tested for disease conditions and plasma is free of red blood cells.
   2. Sources of plasma
      USA
      a. Plasmavacc Inc. (formerly: Veterinary Dynamics) - All types of equine plasma available.
         1535 Templeton Road, Templeton, CA 93465;
         800-654-9743
         805-434-0321
         www.plasvaccusa.com
      b. Lake Immunogenics, Inc., 348 Berg Road, Ontario, New York, 14519,
         800-648-9990, 716-265-1973.
         www.lakeimmunogenics.com
      c. MgBiologics – Ames, Iowa
         Tel: 515-769-2340. www.mgbiologics.com
      Europe
      a. Veterinary Immunogenics Ltd:
         www.veterinaryimmunogenics.com
      b. Kraeber GmbH & Co.
         www.kraeber.de
      Australia and New Zealand
      a. Plasmavacc Inc
         www.plasvacc.com

Canada
- a. Centaur Pharmaceuticals,
  503 Imperial Road Unit #3, Guelph, Ontario N1H 6T9, Phone 519-824-9570, FAX 519-824-3553. www.centaurva.com

3. Make your own plasma.

   EC - Be careful – anaphylaxis risk is much higher with untested plasma! Plasma donors need to be tested.

   a. Pre-selection of suitable blood/plasma donors on a large breeding farm or in a large practice is possible using blood typing procedures.

   b. The preferred donor is negative for A, Q, and C erythrocyte antigens and contains high level of antibody to indigenous pathogens.
      i. Contains no common anti-erythrocyte antibodies (universal donor).
      ii. Alternately, blood from the dam, a Shetland pony, or unrelated gelding with no history of transfusion, may be used if the situation warrants.

   c. Collection
      i. Plasma collected by plasmapheresis is preferred.
      ii. Centrifugation can be used but plasma may not be RBC free.

   d. Plasma can be administered immediately after collection or frozen and subsequently thawed at the time of administration. Frozen storage should not exceed 3 years.
      i. Quantitate immunoglobulin content of plasma if possible.
      ii. Assess for anti-RBC alloantibodies which could produce neonatal isoerythrolysis.

   e. Storage of non-frozen plasma increases the risk of contamination - use immediately after collection or thawing. Do not refrigerate non commercial harvested plasma longer than 12-24 hours.

IV. HOW MUCH PLASMA TO ADMINISTER

EC - It is difficult to determine exactly how much plasma is needed to raise IgG by a specific amount in an individual foal. In general, septic foals need to have more plasma administered (2-3 times the amount) to raise the IgG by 200 mg/dl compared to a healthy foal being treated for FPT.

A. Volume Determination (1 liter/45 Kg foal)
   1. A dose of 20 ml/Kg of average IgG concentration plasma results in an increase of 50-200 mg/dl serum IgG. Consequently, always check the serum IgG of the foal post treatment.
   2. Greater than 2 (4-6) liters of plasma may be needed to elevate IgG to 600-800 mg/dl in septicemic foals.
B. Milligram Amount Determination[2]
   1. A dose of 200 mg/kg of IgG in normal foals raised the serum IgG by 450 mg IgG/dl.
   2. A dose of 400 mg/Kg of IgG in normal foals raised the serum IgG by 575 mg/dl.
   3. Serum IgG decreased by 30% from day 1 to day 7 of age, post plasma transfusion.
   4. A dose of 500 mg/kg IgG has been recommended for infected patients.
C. Administration (I.V.)
   1. Experience suggests 1 liter/45 Kg healthy foal can be administered over a 15 minute period; slower if giving other fluids (maximum 2 L/hr).
   2. In sick foals or when giving greater than 2 liters, rate should not exceed 2 liters/hour.
      a. 20 ml/kg/hr delivers 1 liter/hour.
   3. Warm plasma to body temperature before administration.
      EC- must protect plasma by placing the plasma bag in a protective-sterile bag to thaw. Otherwise contamination at ports may occur.
      a. Do not thaw in very hot water or in a microwave oven; use tepid water.
      b. Use within 12-24 hours of thawing.
   4. Oral administration of plasma
      a. In foals still capable of absorbing IgG (less than 16 hours of age).

EC - This is very inefficient - better to give intravenously.
b. In foals with severe gastroenteritis may protect the bowel.

V. COMPLICATIONS

A. Plasma transfusion is believed to be generally safe. Infrequent complications include:
1. Mild reactions of tachypnea and trembling.
2. Anaphylaxis.
3. RBC destruction if the plasma has sufficient amount of antibodies to foal's erythrocytes.
4. Volume overload with subsequent hypertension
B. If a transfusion reaction develops, i.e., tachypnea, dyspnea, shaking, sweating:
1. Slow the rate of administration or stop for 5-10 minutes and restart.
2. Discontinue the administration of plasma if signs persist.
3. Epinephrine IV – 1 cc/45 kg foal of the 1:1000 for severe reactions and shock.
4. Antihistamine - IV (May produce anaphylaxis itself).
5. Prednisolone sodium succinate - 100 mg - 200 mg IV
C. Sensitization of the foal with red blood cell contamination using non commercial plasma is a potential concern although no documentation of it developing has been reported to date.
D. Serum hepatitis has not occurred in horses less than 18 months of age and does not appear to be a risk of plasma therapy in neonatal foals.

References:
1. Baldwin, J.L., Cooper, W.L., Vanderwall, D.K., et al.:Prevalence (treatment days) and severity of illness in hypogammaglobulinemic and normogammaglobulinemic foals. JAVMA 198:423-428, 1991.
2. White, S.: The use of plasma in foals with failure of passive transfer and/or sepsis. Proceed Amer Assoc Eq Pract 35th Ann Convent p 215-218, 1989.

CHAPTER 11
PHYSICAL EXAM OF THE EQUINE NEONATE

See normal post foaling parameters (Chapter 5)

I. **HISTORY**

   A. **Mare current and past pregnancy complications.**
   B. **Parturition - duration - complications.**
   C. **Post foaling times** for standing, nursing, etc.
      1. Medication or procedures performed post-birth.
      2. Umbilical care.
      3. Meconium passage.
      4. Urination observed.
   D. **Environmental factors** - infectious disease present, previous farm problems.
   E. **Short form** for neonatal post birth evaluation (example p. 46).

II. **EXAMINATION OF FOAL - RECORD ALL FINDINGS**

   A. **Observe from a distance** initially.
      1. Note degree of alertness and maternal interaction.
      2. Assess general conformation.
         a. Watch movement and gait and look for evidence of pain or lameness.
      3. Observe respiratory rate and character.
         a. Normal is 30-40 breaths/min if environmental temperatures are moderate.
         b. May be 60-80 with high environmental temperature.
         c. Small abdominal component of breathing cycle at end expiration is normal.
         d. Marked abdominal component with flared nostrils and exaggerated rib retractions or grunting is abnormal.
         e. Premature foals can exhibit abnormal paradoxical breathing pattern consisting of inward motion of the rib cage during inspiration out of phase with outward motion of abdomen.

- f. Recall metabolic acidosis and response to pain causes increased respiratory rate.
- **B. Evaluate size and maturity** with regard to stated gestational age.
- **C. Observe for "milk face"**
  1. Milk from full, non-nursed upon mammary gland may run onto foal's forehead.
- **D. Obtain temperature, pulse and respiration** of the restrained foal.
  1. Pulse normal 80-120 beats/min.
  2. Temperature 99-101.8°F (37.2-38.8°C).
     - a. High environmental temperatures can alter the foal's afternoon temperature.
     - b. A.M. temperatures are best used for daily comparisons using a temperature chart.
  3. Immediate post birth rectal temperature can fall to 98.6°F.
     - a. Shivering in cold environments is normal for 3-4 hours to generate heat.
- **E. Systems exam: Start at the head.**
- **F. Cardiovascular**
  1. Mucous membranes - normally pink and moist.
     - a. Not a good indication of degree of oxygenation of blood.
     - b. Scleral injection seen with toxemia or conjunctivitis.
     - c. Petechial hemorrhage - normal to have episcleral hemorrhages from pressure of birth canal. Abnormal on gums, tongue, palate, vulva or pinnae of the ears.
     - d. Icterus, if severe suspect neonatal isoerythrolysis or liver problem.
  2. Capillary refill time 1-2 seconds.
  3. Arterial pulse quality.
     - a. Normal is just detectable - use fingertips, check at facial, brachial and great metatarsal.
  4. Jugular pulses are abnormal.
     - a. Assess jugular distensibility, should fill up briskly if not hypovolemic.
  5. Murmurs.
     - a. Common to hear a holosytolic grade I-IV murmur at left heart base over third intercostal space for

up to one week, believed associated with ductus arteriosus.
      b. Louder murmurs with palpable thrills associated with congenital defects. See Chapter 41.
   6. Blood pressure.[1]
      a. Doppler tail method in lateral recumbency day 1 systolic 81 ± 10 mmHg, diastolic 35 ± 7 mmHg, day 7 systolic 104 ± 21 mmHg, diastolic 40 ± 14 mmHg.
   7. Distal extremities and ears should be warm with adequate circulation in a neutral thermal environment.
G. **Respiratory system**
   1. Ausculted sounds are louder than in adult.
      a. Increased rates may produce abnormally loud and harsh sounds.
      b. Inspiratory sounds louder than expiratory normally.
      c. May hear air moving over entire lung field with no wheezes or dullness and find significant abnormalities in a thoracic radiograph from interstitial disease or edema.
   2. Down lung in premature foals can become quieter and congested just from body position.
   3. Changes in respiratory rate over time may indicate increased compromise of respiratory function as well as pain, environmental temperature response, metabolic responses or transient tachypnea syndrome.
   4. Best pulmonary function test in veterinary medicine is an arterial blood gas.
      a. Oxygen levels reflect respiratory component.
      b. CO_2 levels reflect ventilation component
   5. Coughing as a symptom is not a common component of severe pulmonary problems in neonatal foals.
   6. Always evaluate patency of airway in a respiratory distress situation.
H. **Gastrointestinal System**
   1. Examine oral cavity for bite, cleft palate, and pharyngeal paralysis.
   2. Observe nursing behavior and swallowing.

3. Check medial canthus of eye and skin for meconium staining which may indicate in utero stress.
4. Gut sounds - normal to hear gurgling in four quadrants.
   a. Right and left ventral and right and left dorsal abdominal areas.
5. Observe any abdominal distension - can be associated with:
   a. Impending enteritis or ileus.
   b. Colonic torsion or volvulus if painful.
   c. Gastric distension associated with over feeding in premature foals.
   d. Obstruction from high meconium impaction or GI congenital defect.
   e. Uroperitoneum associated with ruptured bladder or urachus.
   f. Fulminating peritonitis.
6. Check for passage of meconium (dark brown to black) and patency of GI tract.
   a. Ileocolic aganglionosis, overo-overo breeding (white foals).
   b. Atresia ani or coli in any breed.

I. Genitourinary System
1. Urination usually occurs by 8.5 hours.
   a. Specific gravity low 1.001-1.015.
   b. Urethral mucous plug in some males.
      i. Attempt to urinate - improves following catheterization
   c. Persistent preputial ring in males.
      i. Inability to extend penis.
   d. Vulva and clitoris, abnormalities are enlargements possibly reflecting chromosomal problems.
   e. Check scrotum for both testicles and for scrotal hernia.

J. Umbilical region
1. Size, heat, tenderness, moisture, edema.
   a. Should learn normal appearance for age.
   b. Consider ultrasound (See Chapter 52).
2. Patent urachus.
   a. Moist hairs around navel or urine scald on inside of legs.

3. Palpate for hernia.

K. Eye - use penlight and ophthalmoscope
1. Check for ulcers or uveitis.
2. Congenital lesions - cataracts, etc. Chapter 42.
3. Pupils should be equal, large and circular in one day old foal and become small and more oval by one week of age.
4. Pupillary light response can be sluggish if foal is excited and has sympathetic override.
5. Menace response is lacking in normal foals until two weeks of age.
6. Entropion is common in ill and premature foals.

L. Musculoskeletal System
1. Conformation - avoid being over critical in first 12 hours of life.
2. Observe motion and gait.
3. Contracted tendons and weak flexor tendons often improve within a few days.
4. Angular limb deformities if not severe are best re-evaluated in a few days.
5. Check joints and physes for heat, swelling or pain.
6. Fractured ribs at birth - check closely.
7. Passive range of motion is increased along with greater fetlock drop in premature foals.
   a. May correct remarkably well if left alone and foal can nurse.
8. Wry neck and face.
   a. May correct somewhat if left alone and foal can nurse.
9. Scoliosis and kyphosis often associated with contracted limbs.

M. Neurologic System[2, 3]
1. General attitude and behavior - foals are normally "hyper", swift and "jumpy".
   a. Stands within 2 hours.
   b. Recognizes mother and mammary glands.
   c. Usually easily aroused by individuals; however, can deeply sleep and require stimulation to rise, especially after 2 weeks of age.
2. Cranial nerves.
   a. Optic nerve II.
   b. Pupils - normal unless excited.

3. Trigeminal nerve (V) foals are hypersensitive and overreact compared to adult to tactile stimuli.
   a. Palpate temporal, masseter and digastricus for symmetry.
4. Facial nerve (VII).
   a. The ear, eyelid, lip and nostril reflexes (V sensory - VII motor).
   b. Same as adult but jerky.
5. Vestibulococlear (VIII)
   a. Can hear at birth but exaggerated jerky response.
   b. Vestibular nystagmus (normal) with head movement seen at birth.
6. Glossopharyngeal (IX), vagus (X), spinal accessory (XI).
   a. Ability to swallow - check with tube.
7. Milk in nostrils may be weakness, cleft palate or temporary pharyngeal paralysis syndrome.
8. Feeding requires:[2] swallow (IX, X, XI), reflex lip movement (VII), jaw (V), and tongue (XII), and recognition - sight (II), and awareness of dam (cerebrum).
9. Hypoglossal nerve (XII)
   a. Many foals hang tongue out of mouth, normal (behavioral) if the tongue is retracted when stimulated by touch.
10. Unique reflexes of the neonatal foal.[2]
    a. Flexor or withdrawal reflex causes crossed extension of the contra lateral limb up to 3 weeks of age.
    b. Patellar reflex is brisker and more exaggerated and can be followed by clonus in neonatal foals.

References:
1. Lombard C.W., Evans M., Martin L., Tehrani J.: Blood pressure, electrocardiogram and echocardiogram measurements in the growing pony foal. Equine Vet J 16:342-346, 1984.
2. Adams R., Mayhew I.B.: Neurologic examination of newborn foals. Equine Vet J 16:306-313, 1984.
3. MacKay RJ Neurologic disorders of neonatal foals. Vet Clin North Am Equine Pract. 2005 Aug;21(2):387-406.

Chapter 11 Physical Exam of the Equine Neonate

Neonatal Post Birth Evaluation Form

Mare: _____ Date Last Bred: _____
Sire: _____ Expected Foaling Date: _____
Date Foaled:_____ Time Foaled:_____ Sex:_____Color:_____

MARE:
History of Previous Foal Problems: _____
_____
History of Problems During Pregnancy: _____
_____
Assistance Required: _____
_____

FOAL:
Time to Stand: _____ Chlorhexidine: _____
Time to Nurse: _____ Enema: _____
Meconium Passage: _____
Colostrum Absorption _____
Urination Normal: _____ PCV: _____
Colostrum Harvested: _____ CSG: _____

MARE:
Placenta Passed: _____ Temporary Vulvar Closure:_____
Placenta Condition: _____ Milk Let Down: _____
Premature Separation?: _____

FOAL EXAMINATION CONCERNS:
Laboratory Data Requested:

_____
Level of Observation Requested: _____
Recheck In: _____
DATE _____ **TIME** _____
COMMENTS _____

CHAPTER 12
ASSESSMENT OF MATURITY - PREMATURITY

EC - While there have been a greater number of successful outcomes from critical care of foals, the premature foal remains the most difficult condition to manage. Outcomes of very premature foals admitted to intensive care reveal a poor rate of survival (40-60%). Of those surviving, limb angulation, lack of calcification of bones in carpus and tarsus, and poor growth continue to cause complications. **When determining if a foal is premature, physical signs and hematology are more reliable than using gestational age.**

I. **GESTATIONAL LENGTH**

   A. **Normal range** = 320-360 days, no difference for sex, or time of year.
   B. **Less than 320 days** considered **premature**.
   C. **Gestation length** is poor indicator of individual readiness for birth.
   Terms "Immature" and "dysmature" indicate gestational age is normal, but foal has signs, behavior and physiology of a premature foal.
   D. **Foals that are small for gestational age** (term) due to in utero growth retardation.
      1. May or may not show signs of prematurity.
      2. Causes: in utero infections, twins or twin which was resorbed or mummified in early gestation, placentitis, malnutrition, other maternal uterine abnormalities.

II. **CLINICAL SIGNS OF IMMATURITY - UNREADINESS FOR BIRTH**[1]

   A. **Weaker,** take longer to rise and depressed sucking ability.
   B. **Smaller size** and reduced birth weight.
   C. **Silky hair** over back and rear quarters.
   D. **Hooves** do not dry out and separate from the "golden hoof".
   E. **Domed** forehead and soft lips.
   F. **Floppy** ears, red tongue.
   G. **Hyperextension** (hypoflexion) of fetlock joints.
   H. **Reduced tolerance** to oral feedings.

I. **Reduced body temperature** and susceptibility to hypothermia.
J. **Incomplete ossification** of carpal and tarsal bones.
 1. May predispose to angular limb deformity.
K. **Respiratory rate** may increase following birth with some evidence of respiratory distress.

III. LABORATORY FINDINGS IN UNREADINESS FOR BIRTH

A. **Adrenocortical insufficiency**.
 1. Seen as narrow neutrophil/lymphocyte ratio of 0.5-1:1 due to a neutropenia. Normal foals have a 2:1 ratio 3 hours following birth.
 2. Lymphocyte counts are higher than term foals (3500 - 5000/ul).
 3. Low plasma cortisol and no rise following administration of ACTH.
    a. Normal foals have a wider neutrophil/lymphocyte change in response to IM ACTH within 3 hours of birth.
    b. 0.01 mg cosyntropin (low dose) or 0.1 mg (high dose) (short-acting) IM total.[2,3]
    c. Foals without HPA (hypothalamic-pituitary-adrenal axis) dysfunction should have a significant rise in plasma cortisol levels 30 minutes after administration.[3]
    d. Increased plasma Vasopressin and ACTH concentrations in septic foals were associated with higher mortality in one study. Several septic foals had increased vasopressin/ACTH and ACTH/cortisol ratios, which indicates relative adenohypophyseal and adrenal insufficiency.[4]
B. **Respiratory system** compromise and blood gas abnormalities.
 1. Signs of hypoventilation - decreased PaO_2 increased $PaCO_2$.
 2. Venous pH <7.25 (normal foal >7.3) and tendency for pH to decrease.
 3. May have decreased functional surfactant and respiratory distress.
C. **Depressed blood glucose** 2 hours post foaling (<60 mg/dl; 3.3mmol/l).

- **D. Decreased absorption** of colostral immunoglobulin.
  1. Overall immune function is decreased.
- **E. Increased susceptibility to infection.**

IV. OUTCOME OF PREMATURE FOALS - BASED ON INDUCED PARTURITION MODEL[5]

- **A. Survival rates of foals** from **induced** parturition before 320 days gestation is poor.
- **B. Spontaneous births** in Thoroughbreds between 280-322 gestation have 73% survival.
  1. Fetus is prepared for delivery and final maturation processes develop
- **C. Correlation of post foaling** behavior and outcome w/o treatment.[2]
  1. If the foal does not establish righting reflexes and has weak sucking - will die.
  2. If foal becomes sternal and has good head and neck tone, strong sucking reflex, but took 2 hours to stand, will do well for 24 hours and then fade and die unless intervention provided.
  3. If foal appears viable at birth and has normal righting reflexes at delivery, can stand and suck - prognosis is better but a degree of fading still occurs in this group, 1-7 days following birth.

V. DIAGNOSTIC EVALUATION

- **A. Conduct physical exam.**
- **B. Complete blood count.**
- **C. Measure venous acid base.**
- **D. To assess respiratory maturity and function**
  1. Administer face mask oxygen (10 L/min) and measure arterial oxygen after 5 minutes. PaO_2 should be >200 mmHg. If less, have shunt or atelectasis.
- **E. Monitor serum glucose levels.**
- **F. Assess serum IgG.** Recommend giving supplemental colostrum and 1 liter plasma IV before assessment of IgG at 18 hrs because of the common finding of failure of passive transfer.

VI. TREATMENT[1]

A. **Supporting the foal** by environmental temperature control, nutrition, circulatory and respiratory support with oxygen, or ventilation may be required.
B. **Adrenal insufficiency support.**
   1. Depot long acting ACTH (Synacthen Depot®, Novartis) may provide stimulation after several days.
      a. 0.4 mg IM total dose. Repeat 6 and 12 hours with 0.2 mg IM total dose. **EC:** This is from older literature.
   2. Hydrocortisone - Sodium succinate (Cortelan® Glaxo Laboratories) or 50 mg BID Solu-Delta-Cortef® (Upjohn) has been used.
      a. Avoid pharmacological doses to prevent disruption of immune system.
      b. A short tapering course of hydrocortisone sodium succinate (Pfizer, New York) (1.3 mg/kg/day for 48h, 0.65mg/kg/d for 24h then 0.33mg/kg/d for 12h; total doses given in 6 doses as an IV bolus q4h) has potentially beneficial anti-inflammatory effects without significantly impairing innate immune function.[7]
C. **Surfactant replacement** and chemical closure of ductus arteriosus (flunixin-meglumine daily for 48 hrs) are now being attempted to increase survivability.
D. **Daily nursing care** and maintenance as per the critical foal.
   1. Watch for entropion.
   2. These foals tolerate oral feeding very poorly initially.
   3. Start total parental nutrition early.
      EC-This can greatly increase survival.
E. **Prevention and control of sepsis.**
F. **Therapy for limbs** - MUST assess by radiography the degree of ossification of carpus and tarsus. Foals body weight must be supported during early ambulation.
   1. Heel extensions taped or glued on foot have provided increased support (Chapter 76)
   2. Support wraps should not normally be used because they cause tendon relaxation.
   3. Radiograph carpus and tarsus and limit activity in foals with minimum ossification.

4. Provide optimal nutrition up to 30% of BW per day in milk while confining foal and limiting movement.
5. Many foals survive and then have damaged joints.
   a. Complete non weight bearing may be needed initially.

VII. NUTRITION SUPPORT (Chapters 23 and 24)

References:
1. Vaala, W.E.: Diagnosis and treatment of prematurity and neonatal maladjustment syndrome in newborn foals. Compend Cont Educ Pract Vet 8:S211-S222, 1986.
3. Wong DM, Vo DT, Alcott CJ, Peterson AD, Sponseller BA, Hsu WH. Baseline plasma cortisol and ACTH concentrations and response to low-dose ACTH stimulation testing in ill foals. J Am Vet Med Assoc. 2009 Jan 1;234(1):126-32.
4. Hart KA, Heusner GL, Norton NA, Barton MH.: Hypothalamic-pituitary-adrenal axis assessment in healthy term neonatal foals utilizing a paired low dose/high dose ACTH stimulation test. J. Vet Intern Med. 2009 Feb 3.
5. Leadon, D.P., Jeffcot, L.B., Rossdale, P.D.: Behavior and viability of the premature neonatal foal after induced parturition. Am J Vet Res 47:1870-1874, 1986.
6. Hurcombe SD, Toribio RE, Slovis N, Kohn CW, Refsal K, Saville W, Mudge MC: Blood arginine vasopressin, adrenocorticotropin hormone, and cortisol concentrations at admission in septic and critically ill foals and their association with survival. J Vet Intern Med. 2008 22(3):639-47.
7. Hart, KA, Barton, MH, Vandenplas, ML and Hurley DJ: Effects of low dose hydrocortisone therapy on immune function in neonatal foals. Ped Res. 2011 70 (1) 72-77.

CHAPTER 13
ASSESSMENT OF OXYGEN NEEDS

Immediate needs - Post foaling resuscitation is discussed in Chapter 16. Hypoxia in the foal which becomes ill after a seemingly normal birth is not easily detected by mucous membrane color. Cyanosis is not readily apparent until the PaO$_2$ is <40 mmHg. Hypoxia can be a component of septicemia, prematurity, neonatal maladjustment, pneumonia, atelectasis and foals that are in prolonged lateral recumbency due to any reason.

I. **METHODS OF EVALUATION WHICH MAY REVEAL NEED FOR OXYGEN**[1-3]

   A. **History** and observation of asphyxia, apnea or airway obstruction.
   B. **Auscultation and percussion** abnormalities of the chest.
      1. Limited abnormalities may be heard with diffuse diseases.
      2. There is a lack of correlation with the severity of pulmonary disease.
      3. The down lung frequently has abnormal sounds due to position.
   C. **Labored respiration** - increased amount of abdominal contraction and asynchronous rib and abdominal contractions.
   D. **Pale or cyanotic** mucous membranes.
   E. **Thoracic radiographs**
   F. **Blood gases**
      1. Arterial
         a. A hospital setting with ICU is required to effectively and safely provide long term respiratory support.
         b. Valuable in determining severity of respiratory compromise, appropriate therapy and response to therapy.
         c. PaO$_2$<80 mmHg indicates VQ mismatch, PaO$_2$<52 mmHg is life-threating and requires immediate therapy. Position of the foal and age affect the values.
         d. SaO$_2$<90% requires immediate medical attention

2. Venous
   a. Very limited value for respiratory O_2 assessment.
   b. Valuable for acid base assessment.
   c. If PvO_2<28 mmHg, may indicate need for oxygen or improved circulatory status by IV fluids or nutritional support.
   d. $PvCO_2$ >70 mmHg - arterial hypercapnia possible

G. Pulse Oximetry
1. Devices used to estimate the amount of oxygen saturation of arterial hemoglobin.
   a. The Nellcor N-200 was evaluated in studies.[4]
   b. The type of transducer attached to foal and the anatomical site is critical for accurate reading.[4]
2. Results from one study in foals.[4]
   a. Nellcor reflectance Transducer RS-10 attached to base of tail tended to underestimate the amount of arterial oxygen saturation but was very consistent and predictable.
   b. Nellcor Durasensor DS-100A (fingertip) transducer attached to the ear of foals was reliable in determining if <90% saturation or if >90% saturation. However with foals with <80% saturation it tended to overestimate O_2 saturation. When attached to lip had low sensitivity with a tendency to overestimate O_2 saturation and was not recommended for use at that site.
   c. Nellcor Oxisensor D-25 (adhesive) at the ear was judged to underestimate and be variable in readings.
   d. Clinically useful sites and transducers were fingertip transducer at the ear and tongue and reflectance transducer at base of tail. Remember that at less than 80% saturation the fingertip on the ear and tongue overestimated O_2 saturation somewhat.

   EC - We place transducer on vulva, tongue and prepuce and seem to get reliable readings.

Chapter 13 Assessment of Oxygen Needs

II. METHOD OF OBTAINING ARTERIAL SAMPLES

A. Blood Sampling Techniques, (Chapter 62).

III. CIRCUMSTANCES OF SAMPLING THAT AFFECT PaO_2 – $PaCO_2$ VALUES[5]

A. **Position of foal** - PaO_2 values during lateral recumbency are 10-40 mmHg less than if the foal is sternal or standing. Consequently sternal position is recommended in convalescing foals to improve their ability to efficiently use their lungs. Foals should be restrained in lateral recumbency for arterial sampling except when using an indwelling arterial catheter.

B. **Struggling and exertion** may alter PaO_2 and $PaCO_2$ values.

C. Inspired O_2 concentrations.

D. Degree of maturity and gestational age.
   1. Table of age related neonatal values in reference section

E. Obtaining venous blood and believing sample is arterial.
   EC - With unexpectedly low PaO_2, especially readings around 40 mmHg, always submit a venous blood gas for comparison.

IV. CONDITIONS PRODUCING HYPOXEMIA

A. **Newborns**
   1. Birth asphyxia
   2. Aspiration pneumonia - meconium.
   3. Persistent fetal circulation.
   4. Congenital heart disease.
   5. Hypoventilation - neurologic or fatigue related.
   6. Atelectasis.
   7. Surfactant deficiency.
   8. Intra-pulmonary shunts.
   9. Respiratory distress syndrome.
   10. Rib fracture

B. **Acquired after 24 hours**
   1. Septicemia.
   2. Conditions producing prolonged recumbency.

3. Respiratory distress syndrome.
4. Reversion to fetal circulation.

V. METHODS OF OXYGEN THERAPY[2]

A. If hypoxemia cannot be rapidly alleviated and the patient is ventilating adequately, oxygen therapy is indicated.

B. **Face mask** - high inspired oxygen concentrations can be attained with a face mask. The patient's nose and face should fill the mask as much as possible to reduce the dead space within the mask. Leaks allow room air to be drawn into the mask during inspiration and may be satisfactory as long as the net inspired oxygen concentration is sufficient to alleviate the hypoxemia. If not, the fresh oxygen flow could be increased or the mask could be made to form an airtight seal around the muzzle, provided expired gases are eliminated via exhaust or CO_2 absorber.

C. An oxygen insufflation catheter may be placed in the nasopharynx, through the cricothyroid membrane or intratracheally, if circumstances warrant.
   1. A soft, flexible catheter should be used for the nasopharynx.
   EC-Caudal end of nasopharyngeal catheter corresponds to level of medial canthus of eye. Don't put tube far back in pharynx; you may enter esophagus.
   2. Several holes should be present near the catheter tip to facilitate the diffusion of the oxygen into the airway and minimize its jetting against one spot on the epithelium.
   3. Oxygen flow rates of 4-6 L/min should provide a 30-40% inspired oxygen concentration. Specific flow rates should be adjusted to the needs of the individual patient.
   4. The oxygen should be bubbled through warm water so that it can be humidified prior to reaching the patient, if providing oxygen for more than 1 hour.
      a. Humidification chambers that are sterile are available to accept an O_2 line in and out.

Chapter 13 Assessment of Oxygen Needs

D. Place foal in sternal position.

E. If oxygen therapy does not alleviate the hypoxemia, endotracheal intubation and positive pressure ventilation is indicated.

F. See Respiratory Therapeutics (Chapter 66).

VI. BLOOD GAS RESPONSE TO O_2

A. Aids assessment of degree of shunting and degree of maturation.

B. Administer nasal or face mask 100% O_2 at 10 L/min for 5 minutes.
  1. PaO_2 >200 mgHg - normal degree of response.
  2. PaO_2 <160 mmHg - indicates severe shunting - requires increased monitoring and indicates more protracted illness.

VII. HYPERCAPNIA (INCREASED ARTERIAL CO_2)

A. $PaCO_2$ >60 mmHg causes:
  1. Overwhelming pneumonia.
  2. Atelectasis and edema.
  3. Hypoventilation due to brain damage, rib fracture or toxicosis (drugs, etc.).
  4. Progressive respiratory disease that leads to muscle fatigue.
  5. Apparatus dead space or insufficient fresh oxygen flow.

B. $PaCO_2$ >60 mmHg. (Treatment)
  1. Oxygen therapy will not correct - will only temporarily raise O_2 levels.
  2. Need to improve animal's ventilation.
  3. $PaCO_2$ >65 mmHg and rising with a pH <7.2 may be an indication for mechanical ventilation, or continuous positive airway pressure, or chemical stimulation of ventilation.

     EC - We have many foals with $PaCO_2$ >70 mmHg that have survived without mechanical ventilation using chemical stimulation of ventilation.
     a. Intermittent intubation and ambu bag positive pressure ventilation 2-4 times daily to expand collapsed alveoli.

- b. Doxapram hydrochloride (Dopram®) respiratory stimulant. This will increase the ventilation drive and lower $PaCO_2$ even when foal is not "drug depressed". Repeat administration may be required. (See Chapter 71) **EC**- this works for most of our hypoventilation cases. Very effective in our hands; also used to help level of alertness in dummy foals. 0.5 mg/kg iv., or 0.01-0.02mg/kg/min as a CRI.
- c. Caffeine tablets orally- 10 mg per kg initially then 2.5 mg/kg BID.
- d. Recent work indicates that doxapram significantly decreased $PaCO_2$ levels close to normal range in healthy anesthetized hypercapnic foals and in foals with HIE. Caffeine however failed to show any significant effect on $PaCO_2$ in the same studies[6,7].
- **C.** See Respiratory Therapeutics (Chapter 66).

VIII. CLINICAL SIGNS AND BLOOD GAS ABNORMALITIES[a]

- **A.** Foals showing no signs of respiratory distress or respiratory impairment with an arterial blood gas PaO_2 <52 mmHg in lateral recumbency will benefit from nasal insufflation. To raise PaO_2 to 80-100 mmHg, start with a flow rate of 2-5 liter/min and adjust rate based on blood gas values.
- **B.** Foals with signs of respiratory difficulties and PaO_2 <52mmHg will benefit from nasal insufflation of O_2 as described in (1) above.
- **C.** Foals with signs of respiratory distress with PaO_2 <52 mmHg in lateral recumbency and $PaCO_2$ >70 mmHg with a pH of ≤ 7.2 require chemical stimulation of ventilation or mechanical ventilation. (See Positive Pressure Ventilation, Chapter 51)

[a]Modified from Kosch PC, Koterba AM, Coon JJ, Webb Al: Developments in management of the newborn foal in respiratory distress: Evaluation. <u>Equine Vet J</u> 16:312-318, 1984.

IX. HOW TO DECIDE WHEN THE FOAL NO LONGER NEEDS OXYGEN

A. As the foal's respiratory condition improves with treatment and time the blood gas PaO_2 levels will increase while on the same flow of oxygen.
B. If the PaO_2 is above 80-100 mmHg, decrease the O_2 flow rate by 1/2 and recheck the arterial oxygen in about 10-15 minutes. Following this method the foal can be weaned off O_2.
C. If the PaO_2 is >52 mmHg in small for gestation age or premature foals less than 48 hours of age, >58 mmHg in term foals when on room air, discontinue O_2 therapy.
D. Continue to monitor foal and provide respiratory therapeutics.

References:
1. Kosch, P.L., Koterba, A.M., Coons, T.J., Webb, A.I.: Developments in management of the newborn foal in respiratory distress. 1: Evaluation. Eq Vet J 16:312-318, 1984.
2. Webb, A.I., Coons, T.J., Koterba, A.M., Kosch, P.L.: Developments in management of the newborn foal in respiratory distress. 2: Treatment Eq Vet J 16:319-323, 1984.
3. Sonea, I.: Respiratory distress syndrome in neonatal foals. Compend Cont Equine Pract Vet 7:S462-S469, 1985.
4. Chaffin, MK, Matthews, NS, Cohen, ND, Carter, GK.: Evaluation of pulse oximetry in anaesthetized foals using multiple combinations of transducer type and transducer attachment site. Equine Vet J 28:437-445, 1996.
5. Madigan, J.E., Thomas, W.P, Bachus, K.Q., Powell, W.E.: Arterial and mixed venous blood gases in recumbent and standing positions in newborn foals from birth to 14 days of age. Equine Vet J 24:399, 1992.
6. Giguère S, Sanchez LC, Shih A, Szabo NJ, Womble AY, Robertson SA.: Comparison of the effects of caffeine and doxapram on respiratory and cardiovascular function in foals with induced respiratory acidosis. Am J Vet Res. 2007 Dec;68(12):1407-16.

7. Giguère S, Slade JK, Sanchez LC.: Retrospective comparison of caffeine and doxapram for the treatment of hypercapnia in foals with hypoxic-ischemic encephalopathy. J Vet Intern Med. 2008. Mar-Apr;22(2):401-5.

CHAPTER 14
TRANSPORT OF THE CRITICALLY ILL EQUINE NEONATE

Proper care during transport is required for the successful outcome of the ill or premature foal that needs to be moved to a facility for constant nursing or intensive care.

I. **PROBLEMS THAT MUST BE DEALT WITH DURING TRANSPORT**[1]

   A. **Restraint and protection from trauma.**
      1. Leave the mare initially if the recumbent or weak foal cannot have a protected area in the trailer to avoid being knocked down or stepped on by the mare.
      2. Have a person ride with the foal to prevent trauma to the head, eyes, and limbs and to give medication, if necessary.
      EC - Put a very weak foal in the cab of the truck and turn on the heater. Have someone else drive!
      3. Wrap distal limb extremities.
      4. Place on protective bedding (not sawdust unless covered).
   B. **Hypoglycemia in recumbent or weak foals.**
      1. Check a dextrose strip for whole blood glucose determination.
         a. If less than 40 mg/dl (2.2 mmol/l) and the trip is long, place an IV jugular catheter and run warmed Lactated Ringers with 1% dextrose (add 20 ml of 50% dextrose into 1 liter of LR) and administer at 200 ml/hr/50 Kg.
         b. IV bolus of dextrose may produce hyperglycemia and subsequent rebound hypoglycemia.
      2. Administer 8 oz (240 ml) mare's milk (colostrum) if no gastric reflux is present.
      3. Send colostrum, if available at the farm, if the foal is less than 16 hrs of age.
   C. **Hypoxia**
      1. Administer oxygen if -
         a. Respiratory rate <30 (respiratory depression) or >80 respiratory rate and obvious respiratory distress is present.

b. Mucous membranes pale or cyanotic.
c. History of conditions which could have produced some degree of asphyxia.
2. Methods
   a. E tank O_2 will supply approximately 1 hour of oxygen at 5 liters/minute.
   b. Face mask such as 1/2 gallon jug cut in half, can be used. Allow room for exhaled air to escape.
   c. Nasopharyngeal catheter - a Harris edema flush tube or plastic IV line cut to length can be used. Tape to the nose or suture to nostril with the end of the tube positioned in nasopharynx.
   d. Rate 5-10 liter/min of 100% O_2.
   e. Provide humidification of the oxygen if used longer than 2-3 hours.
3. **Attempt to maintain sternal** recumbency for most efficient respiration. If the foal cannot be kept sternal, rotate sides every hour.
   EC - Sternal position can generally help blood oxygenation.

D. Hypothermia - Check temperature: if <99°F (37.2° C)
1. Place in warm draft free vehicle if possible.
2. Insulate area below recumbent foal.
3. Wrap in warm blankets.
4. Place down vest or sweater on the foal with front legs through the armholes or sleeves.
5. Place hot water bottles or gallon jugs adjacent to foal (insulate bottles/jugs to prevent burns).

E. Seizures
1. Administer Valium® (diazepam)(0.1- 0.2 mg/kg (5-20 mg/50 kg foal) IV slowly or Midazolam 0.1-0.2 mg/kg (start with 5 mg/50kg) to effect .
2. Recurrent seizures - place IV catheter and instruct on the administration of diazepam during transport if attendant is capable. Record medication use in log.
3. Always check blood sugar.
4. Do not use acepromazine or xylazine because they cause hypotension and depression, and acepromazine lowers threshold for seizures.

F. Consider antimicrobial therapy if delay is going to be more than a few hours to clinic.

- **G. Record vital parameters (TPR)** on paper and send foals and mares pertinent history.
- **H. Place placenta** in plastic bag and send with foal along with blood from dam in red (plain) and purple (EDTA) top tubes.
- **I. Arrange to bring the mare** to supply milk if the foal was shipped separately.

References:
1. Knottenbelt, DC: Transportation of the sick or injured foal in Knottenbelt, DC (ed.): <u>Saunders Equine Formulary</u>. 432-434. 2006. WB Saunders.

CHAPTER 15
TEMPERATURE REGULATION OF NEONATES

Hypothermia is common in ill newborn foals. They do not feed well as hypothermia greatly alters their metabolism. However, recent work suggests some hypothermia is protective as it slows down the damage from reperfusion. Consequently, re-warming the foal at a much slower rate, often just 1-2°F per hour, using a method known as permissive hypothermia is the current recommendation.

I. SOURCES OF THERMAL LOSS IN FOALS

   A. Wet newborn foals undergo rapid heat loss due to evaporation.
   B. Foals placed on cold surfaces lose heat by conduction.
   C. Foals lose heat by radiation when adjacent (without direct contact) to stall walls or windows with a negative temperature gradient across them.
   D. Foals exposed to low environmental temperatures and drafts lose heat by convection.
   E. Premature foals have 30-40% lower mean metabolic rate per surface area (mean 71W/m2) compared to healthy foals (100 W/m2) or other sick neonates (82W/m2). This will result in decreased heat production[1-3].
   F. Foals have a higher surface area to body weight ratio and a higher resting respiratory rate. These factors contribute to larger insensible fluid losses and a greater tendency to lose body heat in cool or drafty environments.

II. NEUTRAL THERMAL ENVIRONMENT

   A. **Environment** (temperature and humidity) at which foal's oxygen consumption is minimal.
   B. **A goal of the foal ICU unit**.
   C. **The optimal ambient temperature** for a newborn varies with degree of maturity and size. Smaller and premature foals need higher environmental temperatures[1].
   D. **The lower critical temperature** is the lower limit of the thermo neutral zone
      1. For 2 day old foals is 25°C (77°F)[4]

2. Normal healthy foals can be exposed to < 5°C (37°F) temperature and generate heat to maintain body temperature.[4]
3. Sick neonatal foals have lower critical temperature based on a study (average 24°C, 75°F)[1]

III. CORRECTION OF HYPOTHERMIA (<99°F; 37°C) RECTAL TEMPERATURE

A. **Hypothermia** is a severe stress which may produce a shock-like state.
B. **A sheep skin fleece** or thick blankets should be placed under the foal with an insulating pad.
C. **A man's or women's down** or nylon vest can be placed on the foal with front legs through arm holes.
D. **Blankets** such as a space blanket placed over foal will prevent heat loss but will reflect externally applied heat.
E. **Water heating pads** under the foal cannot be in direct contact or will burn the foals' skin. Hot water bottles placed adjacent to the foal are beneficial. Microwave heating gels work well.
F. Bear hugger warm air device- works well.
G. Move foal to a warm room with a temperature of 78- 80°F (25-26°C)
H. Heat lamps or infrared bulbs can be placed above the foal bed. Maintain a safe distance (3 feet, 1 m) from the foal.

IV. AVOID HYPERTHERMIA

A. **Hyperthermia** is also a severe stress and if prolonged may cause coma, stupor and convulsions with irreversible brain damage.
B. Signs are hyperventilation, sweating and agitation.
C. Rapid warming has been associated with apnea episodes.

References:
1. Ousey JC.:Thermoregulation and the energy requirement of the newborn foal, with reference to prematurity Equine Vet J Suppl.1997.Jun;(24)104-8.

2. Ousey JC, McArthur AJ, Rossdale, PD. Thermoregulation in sick foals aged less than one week. Vet J. 1997.Mar; 153(2):185-96.
3. Ousey JC.: Heat production and its clinical implications in neonates. Equine Vet J. 1990 Mar;22(2):69-72
4. Ousey, J.C., Murgatroyd, P.R., Stewart, J.H.: Thermoregulation in the neonatal foal. Proc IVPS Therm.Phys Symp. Mercer,B, ed. Elsevier Publisher. 1990, pp 653-658.

CHAPTER 16
RESUSCITATION Part 1

FOR QUICK EMERGENCY NEEDS SEE DRUG DOSES ON INSIDE COVER- CHAPTER 77 HAS CPCR STEP BY STEP.
Also see Resuscitation Part 2- Evaluation of Cardiovascular Status for Cardiac Arrest (Chapter 17).

INTRODUCTION
In general there are two different resuscitation situations in equine neonates. The first occurs immediately post birth and the second occurs more commonly in somewhat older foals suffering from anaphylaxis, traumatic, or infectious conditions. In each of these conditions differentiation of the state of asphyxia should be determined if possible. This section is a bit of background and some methods. CPCR step wise approach, drugs, etc are detailed in Chapter 77.

I. **FORMS OF APNEA**

   A. **Primary Apnea**
      1. May be preceded by exaggerated breathing efforts.
      2. Pale or blue mucous membranes.
      3. Some muscle tone.
      4. Heart rate 60-100 beats/minute.
      5. In this stage providing a patent airway will often allow the foal to breathe.
      6. See Initial Resuscitation.
   B. **Terminal Apnea**
      1. Pale or blue mucous membrane.
      2. Flaccid muscles.
      3. Heart rate less than 40.
      4. Nonresponsive.
      5. This stage requires intubation and ventilation and may require external cardiac massage. See Intensive Resuscitation.

II. **INITIAL RESUSCITATION PLAN newborn foal (primary apnea)**[1-5]

   A. **Establish Patent Airway**

1. Clear and remove amniotic membranes from nostrils.
2. Provide head-down postural drainage.
3. Strip fluids gently from nostrils with fingers.
4. Provide thoracic coupage (gentle).
5. Suction fluids (gently) from oropharynx.
   a. Provide mild suction via a tube in the pharynx on a suction device or the end of a 60 cc syringe.

B. Stimulation of Foal
1. Rub body briskly with towels.
2. Nasal tickling with straw.
3. Flex limbs (stretch receptors).
4. Put into sternal position.

C. Record Vital Signs make special note of changes in values over a time.
1. **Heart rate** - normal >60 beats/min - 1 minute after foaling; 1-2 hours of age 80-120/min.
2. **Respiratory rate** - normal >60 breaths/minute 1-5 minutes post foaling; 30-40/min 1-2 hours of age.
3. **Reflexes** - sternal positioning is normal.
4. **Mucous membranes**
   a. Color
   b. Capillary refill

D. Initiate O_2 Therapy
1. **Nasal insufflation** - 3-10 liters/min (100% O_2) - use if foal is ventilating. If foal is not making strong ventilation attempts intubate and ventilate (intensive resuscitation).
2. **Ambu Bag** - initiating "first breath" may be all that is required to establish respiration.
3. When foal does not respond with spontaneous respirations and increasing heart rate by 1-2 minutes, begin intensive resuscitation measures.

III INTENSIVE RESUSCITATION PROCEDURE[1-5]

A. Terminal Apnea
1. If foal is not making strong ventilation attempts establish an open and unobstructed airway by endotracheal intubation.

B. **Nasal (Preferred) or Oro-Tracheal Intubation**
   1. Briefly and rapidly suction nose, mouth and oropharynx.
   2. Use 7 or 9 mm Bivona nasotracheal tube. Once in place, ask is the foal moving a satisfactory tidal volume? If an open airway does not reestablish effective ventilation in the face of vigorous patient attempts, first check position of tube, auscultate, percuss the chest and perform rapid thoracic ultrasound and rule in or out a pleural space disorder, fluid in chest or pneumothorax.
C. **Connect Ambu bag with O_2** line attached (do not use Bain circuit in foals >50 kg).
   1. Hook up O_2 supply line to Ambu bag or Bain circuit
   2. Connect O_2 line to flow regulator from 100% O_2 tank.
   3. Attach 2 liter reservoir bag to Bain tubing.
   4. Adjust flow rate to 10 liter/min minimum. This flow rate is inadequate for Bain tubing circuits in foals 50 Kg or more.
D. **Begin Manual Intermittant Positive Pressure**
   1. Rate - 20-30/min.
   2. Volume delivered is approximately 500 ml/breath = 1/2 reservoir of a one liter bag.
   3. Note slight chest expansion.
      a. Do not use excessive pressure; should be no greater than 20-30 cm H_2O.
   4. Check periodically for spontaneous respiration.
   5. Once effective movement of air has been established, evaluate adequacy of oxygenation.
E. **If heartrate is below 60 Beats/Minute** See Bradycardia Chapter 17 if absent - See Resuscitation Part 2 Chapter 17 - Cardiac Arrest - Chapter 17.
F. **Provide Intermittant Postural Drainage From Nasotracheal Tube**
   1. Use gentle coupage.
G. **Place Foal On A Warm Pad** to prevent hypothermia.
H. **Place Sterile IV Catheter** surgically prep skin See fluid guidelines and drugs in Chapter 17.
I. **Re-evaluate Heart and Lungs**
J. **Obtain Blood Gas (Preferably Arterial)**

1. Immediate acid-base determination via venous blood if cannot obtain arterial sample.
2. Use pulse oximetry to measure oxygenation

K. Hypotheria Management - [99-102°F (37.2-39°C) Normal]
1. Heat lamps-be careful fire hazard- burn hazard.
2. Warm fluids.
3. Sweaters.
4. Temperature controlled room.
5. Bear hugger warm air device.

L. Obtain Blood Cultures - provide antibiotics with gram-negative spectrum if any suspicion of sepsis. Don't wait for culture results.

M. Obtain Thoracic Radiograph.

N. Evaluate Electrolytes, blood gas and acid-base and make corrections in oxygen and fluid administration.

O. Emergency Drugs and Their Doses, Etc.

III. SUPPORTIVE THERAPY POST-RESUSCITATION

A. Foals That Lack A Strong Suck Reflex should receive colostrum and milk feeding by nasogastric tube. Never <u>oral feed</u> any foal that is lying on its side or lacks a good sucking reflex (aspiration pneumonia can result). Always hold the bottle slightly lower than level of pharynx.

B. Nasogastric Tube should be placed proximal to the cardia of the stomach and sutured to the nostril. Open end should be "capped" when not feeding. Use gravity flow or "slight" pressure with syringe. Check for reflux at each feeding.

C. Heating Lights and Pads Should Be Provided. Monitor rectal temperature.

D. Keep in Sternal Position As Much As Possible.

E. Monitor Blood Gases and Acid Base Status.
1. Need arterial blood for respiratory and ventilation evaluation (O_2 and CO_2).

F. Be Clean, Wash Hands.

G. Steroid Supplementation.
1. Premature foal (50-100 mg hydrocortisone equivalent) See Chapter 12.

Chapter 16 Resuscitation Part 1

- **H. Monitor for Failure of Passive Transfer**
    1. Minimum is 400 mg/dl serum IgG.
    2. Plasma administration when indicated.
- **I. Decide if Chemical Stimulation of Ventilation or Mechanical Ventilation is Needed.**
    1. Auxiliary exams when indicated.
        a. Ultrasound
        b. ECG
        c. Special radiographic studies.
- **J. Treatment of Navel**
    1. Dip in chlorhexidine (0.5%) solution q 6 hr for 24 hrs.
- **K. Complete Daily Monitoring Checklist.**

References:
1. Martens, R.J.: Neonatal respiratory distress: A review with emphasis on the horse. Compend Cont Educ Pract Vet 4:S23-S33, 1982.
2. Goetzman, B.W.: Resuscitation of the newborn. Manual of Obstetrics. 3rd edition, Niswandir K.R. (ed). Little, Brown Publishers 1986, p 415.
3. Fielding CL, Magdesian KG: .Cardiopulmonary cerebral resuscitation in neonatal foals. Clinical techniques in Equine Practice. Vol.2. No.1. pp 9-19. 2003.
4. Palmer JE Neonatal foal resuscitation. Vet Clin North Am Equine Pract. 2007 May;23(1):159-82
5. Corley KT, Furr MO: Cardiopulmonary resuscitation on the newborn foal. Comp. Vet. Ed. 22:957-966, 2000

CHAPTER 17
RESUSCITATION Part 2
EVALUATION OF CARDIOVASCULAR STATUS

See drug doses on the inside covers and Chapter 77.
In evaluating cardiovascular status, ask five questions:

1. **Is the heart beating?** If not, go directly to cardiac arrest protocol.

2. **If the heart is beating, is the heart beating too slow, too fast or is there an arrhythmia present?** If so, go directly to discussion of bradycardia, tachycardia, or arrhythmias.

3. **If the heart is beating, is it mechanically effective** (auscultable amplitude, palpable pulse quality, **arterial blood pressure** and its proper waveform) If not, go to discussion on shock (Chapter 18).

4. **If the heart is beating, are the peripheral and visceral tissues being perfused?** If there is evidence of peripheral vasoconstriction, see Chapter 18 on shock.

5. **In the newborn is there a loud murmur** and cyanosis suggesting a congenital heart defect? (See Chapter 41)

I. **CARDIAC ARREST**

   A. **If the heart cannot be auscultated or palpated**, if peripheral pulses cannot be palpated, and if there is an absence of breathing attempts, the foal should be considered to have a cardiac arrest.
      1. **Endotracheally intubate** the foal and commence positive pressure ventilation at an airway pressure of 20-30 cm of H_2O (just enough to elevate rib cage) at a rate of 20 times per minute.
      2. **Commence external chest compression** over the heart with a strong pressure at a rate of about 60-80 times per minute.

a. **Compression technique** must be continued without interruption.
b. **Evaluate effectiveness** of compression technique by the generation of a palpable pulse with each compression and an improvement in mucous membrane color. If compression technique is not effective, change technique and proceed with pharmaceutical intervention.
3. **Insert an intravenous catheter** and rapidly administer a bolus of fluids (lactated Ringer's): 20 ml/kg (about 1 liter for a 50 kg foal), and then reassess the cardiovascular status.
4. **Administer epinephrine:**
   a. 0.01-0.02 ml/kg of 1:1000 dilution IV or intraosseally (0.5-1 ml/50kg)
   b. 0.1-0.2 ml/kg of 1:10,000 dilution intratracheally or IV (5-10ml/50kg)
   c. Can be repeated every 2-5 minutes
5. **Attach ECG electrodes** and evaluate electrical activity of heart.
   a. Flat line (asystole): administer epinephrine.
   b. Chaotic activity (ventricular fibrillation):
      Lidocaine (1-2 mg/kg)
      Amiodarone (5 mg/kg)
      Defibrillation
   c. Normal activity (cardiovascular collapse): administer a second bolus of replacement crystalloids (10-20 ml/kg).
6. **Vasopressin (ADH)**
   a. Vasopressin indicated after 2-3 attempts of failed epinephrine administration.
   b. Long half life, use only once
   c. Dose: 0.2-0.6 U/kg (10-30 U/foal)
7. **Other drugs-limited indications**
   a. **Parasympatholytics** in bradyarrhythmias, bronchoconstriction
      i. Atropine (0.01-0.02 mg/kg)
      ii. Glycopyrrolate (0.001-0.002 mg/kg)
   b. **Electrolytes**
      i. Calcium (1-10 mg/kg) to improve cardiac contractility

ii. Sodium-bicarbonate (1-2 mEq/kg) if severe acidosis present
iii. Magnesium-sulfate (14-28 mg/kg) can be useful in cases of ventricular or junctional tachyarrhythmias
   c. **Glucose** (3-5mg/kg/min) if severe hypoglycemia (<50mg/dl; <2.8mmol/l) present.
   d. **Corticosteroids- not useful** in septic, anaphylactic shock, **maybe** in suspected adrenal insufficiency of prematurity
      i. prednisolone Na-succinate 1.3 mg/kg/d (see Chapter 12).
   e. **Class III antiarrythmic drugs** if severe ventricular tachyarrhythmias unresponsive to lidocaine and magnesium sulfate
      i. Amiodarone 5mg/kg
      ii. Bretylium 5 mg/kg
B. **If external compression technique** is not judged to be effective try one of the following:
   1. Change the compression technique:
      a. Faster or slower.
      b. Harder or softer.
      c. Hold compression a little longer.
      d. Place a sand bag under chest.
   2. Administer IV:
      a. Epinephrine 0.01 mg/kg (1:1000) about 1 ml for a 50 kg foal or
      b. Norepinephrine 0.4 mg/kg or
      c. Neosynephrine® 0.2 mg/kg (phenylephrine) and/or
      d. A bolus dose of replacement crystalloids: 20 ml/kg of lactated Ringer's (about 1 liter for a 50 kg foal) and/ or a bolus of colloids at a dose of 2-10ml/kg (about 100-500 ml for a 50 kg foal).

II. BRADYCARDIA

A. If the heart is beating at a rate below 60 per minute, administer epinephrine 0.01-0.02mg/kg. (0.5- 1 ml/ 50 kg foal 1:1000) **EC:** this presumes you are ventilating the foal. Providing oxygen and breaths may allow heart rate to increase.

B. If the heart rate remains below 60, administer dobutamine (5-10 ug/kg/min) by mixing 250 mg dobutamine to 500 ml D5W, 0.9% saline, or LRS (0.5 mg/ml). Administer via minidrip (60 drops/ml) at a rate of 6-60 drops/min (for a 50 kg foal) or with infusion pump at a rate of 6-60 ml/hour using this dilution).

C. If heart rate remains below 60 or MAP<60 mmHg, increase infusion rate gradually every 15 minutes.

D. If heart rate remains below 60 or MAP<60 mmHg after a near maximum dose of dobutamine CRI, start norepinephrine at a rate of 0.1 ug/kg/min up to 1.5 ug/kg/min gradually or vasopressin at a rate of 0.25-1.5 mU/kg/min.

E. Once stabilized, monitor vitals, urine output, blood gas parameters, blood pressure frequently (every 2-4 hours).

III. TACHYCARDIA

A. **Tachycardia is a response** to an underlying stress and therapy is usually directed towards alleviating the underlying abnormality rather than the tachycardia, per se. Treat the hypovolemia, hypotension, hypoxia, hypercapnia, hyperthermia, or sympathomimetic therapy.

IV. ARRHYTHMIAS

Abnormal electrical activity is a well known phenomenon immediately after birth. Arrhythmias should not be treated in the first few hours of life, unless they manifest in clinical signs (cyanosis, respiratory distress, pulmonary edema, fatigue).

A. **Atrial fibrillation** in newborn foals.[1]
 1. Irregular heart rate without pulse deficits.
 2. Pale or cyanotic mucous membrane.
 3. Detected at birth and lasting more than 3 hours.
 4. Foals are depressed, unable to rise, respiratory distress.
 5. May spontaneously disappear.
 6. Treatment with 300 mg Procainamide IV.[1]

B. Although there is a wide variety of arrhythmias which may manifest themselves, aside from sinus bradycardia and tachycardia, and atrioventricular conduction block (same causes and treatment as bradycardia), premature atrial (PAC) and ventricular (PVC) pacemaker activity and bundle branch blocks (BBB)[2] are the most common. In general, they should be considered to be a sign of an underlying disease process and should not be treated specifically. Premature ventricular contractions may progress in severity (frequency, multifocal) and predispose to ventricular tachycardia and fibrillation, and may at some point require specific therapy. The salient questions to answer from the electrocardiogram are:

1. **Is the rate too slow or too fast?**
2. **Is the rhythm regular or irregular?**
3. **Is the PQRST waveform consistently present and/or approximately normal in size and shape?**
4. **Is there synchrony between the ECG and the palpated pulse? Are all of the pulses of equal quality?** Pulse deficits may be caused by:
   a. Premature atrial contractions.
   b. Premature ventricular contractions.
   c. Variable diastolic ventricular filling, especially with high heart rates.
   d. Electromechanical dissociation (correct fluid and electrolyte abnormalities; calcium, magnesium and glucocorticosteroids may be beneficial).
5. **Is there a P wave prior to each QRS or is the P-R interval shortened?** Absence of a P wave differentiates VPCs from right BBB and right ventricular hypertrophy.
6. **Is there a compensatory pause after the PQRST waveform in question?** (Premature atrial and ventricular contractions are usually followed by a pause.)
7. **Is the S-T segment in the isoelectric line?** S-T segment depression is usually attributed to myocardial hypoxia or potassium or calcium abnormalities but may commonly occur with no other demonstrable cardiopulmonary problems.

8. **Are the T waves abnormally large?** (normally less than 25% of the height of the R waves; be sure to measure the actual height since small R waves may make the T wave appear to be tall).
   a. T waves may normally be a positive or a negative deflection or may be biphasic.
   b. Abnormally tall tented T waves may be due to hyperkalemia, hypoxia or atrial dilatation (excessive venous return) and tachycardia.
9. **Is there any artifact or unexpected wave on ECG?** Poor quality electrocardiograms will result if the electrode-patient contact has high impedance. Usually this is minimized by using an electrolyte gel such as commercial ECG paste, Phisohex® soap, ultrasound coupling gel or alcohol (which dries fast and is not recommended). Skin resistance can be reduced by defatting the skin with acetone and de-epithelializing it by scrubbing.

References:
1. Machida, W., Yasuda, J., Too, K.: Three cases of paroxysmal atrial fibrillation in the thoroughbred newborn foal. Equine Vet J 21:66-68, 1989
2. Bonagura JD, Miller MS: Junctional and ventricular arrhythmias, J Equine Vet Sci 5:347, 1985.
8. Stewart JH, Rose RJ, Barko AM: Echocardiography in foals from birth to three months old, Equine Vet J 16:332,1984.

CHAPTER 18
SHOCK (SIRS)

Shock has different terminologies in modern critical care. Systemic Inflammatory Response Syndrome (SIRS) and other acronyms are used. For the purpose of this manual it refers to the manifestation of inadequate tissue oxygenation most often caused by decreased perfusion. It is characterized by the loss of homeostasis attributable to breakdown of hemodynamic control mechanisms that produces decreases in cardiac output and effective circulating volume, which results in an inadequate tissue perfusion.

Based on the etiology there are 6 different types of shock
1. **Hypovolemic**
   - Hemorrhage
   - Fluid deficits
2. **Distributive**
   - Sepsis
   - Anaphylaxis
   - Neurogenic
3. **Cardiogenic**
   - Heart failure
4. **Obstructive**
   - Pulmonary emboli
   - Cardiac tamponade
5. **Hypoxic**
   - Severe hypoxemia
   - Inability to utilize oxygen
6. **Metabolic**
   - Severe hypoglycemia
   - Adrenal dysfunction

Signs of impending arrest:
- **Bradycardia or asystole**
  <40-60 bpm or irregular HR
- **Irregular to absent RR**
  < 10 bpm, gasping
- **Mydriasis**
  Sluggish or nonresponsive papillary response
- **Marked hypotension**
  No pulse pressure
  MAP≤ 40 mmHg
- **Monitoring**
  Sudden decrease in end tidal (ET) CO_2 indicates cardiac output is low

Two main causes of arrest in foals
1. Peripartum asphyxia - HYPOXEMIA
   Focus: oxygenate and ventilate
   Prognosis good if intervention is early

2. Secondary to metabolic derangements /septic causes
   Focus: traditional ABC approach
   Prognosis poor (severely ill foal)

These are managed slightly differently, and carry a different prognosis

Which foals are candidates for CPR?
- Those with potentially reversible disease processes
- Peripartum asphyxia
- Otherwise healthy foal – dystocia, C-section etc

Foals with metabolic diseases that are potentially treatable
- HYPP
- Uroperitoneum
- Hypovolemic shock

I. **BASIC HAEMODYNAMIC MONITORING**

  A. **Physical Exam** (See Chapter 11)
  1. Mentation
  2. Heart rate
  3. Pulse pressure and temperature of the extremities
  4. Mucous membranes
  5. Other signs: respiratory rate, skin turgor, sunken eyes.
  B. **CBC/Chemistry/IgG/Fibrinogen/Lactate/Clotting Profile**. (See normal values at Chapter 72, 73)
  C. **Arterial Blood Gases,** Capnography, Pulsoximetry (See Chapter 74).
  D. **Urine Output**[1] is an important indicator of renal blood flow and glomerular filtration rate. Hemodynamic interventions that are increasing urinary output are likely to be beneficial. Minimum output should be 2-4 ml/kg/h. Normal urinary output is 6 ml/kg/h.

E. **Arterial Blood Pressure** (ABP) and Central Venous Pressure (CVP).[2-5]
   1. **Arterial blood pressure (ABP)** can be fairly accurately measured with *indirect* measurements using a #4 neonatal cuff. Doppler measurements can also be performed.

      Direct measurements using an intra-arterial catheter connected to a pressure transducer are the most accurate; however they require advanced maintenance. Reported mean arterial values (MAP) for healthy foals are 84±3.7mmHg at birth and 101.3±4.4 mmHg at 2 weeks of age, when using the direct measurement and 95±13 when using the indirect technique. Mean ABP should always be maintained above 60 mmHg and is both an important target and an indicator of the therapy. Decreased ABP can occur during decreased cardiac output as well as decreased vascular resistance (vasodilatation).
   2. **Central Venous Pressure (CVP)** is the intraluminal pressure within the cranial vena cava. It is regulated by
      a. central venous blood volume
      b. venomotor tone
      c. cardiac function

   The optimal central venous pressure in foals is approximately 2-10 cmH$_2$0. Normal CVP is the end point of the fluid resuscitation. Measurements require 20 cm catheter (double or triple lumen). CVP is measured as the mean of the a-wave (pressure change during atrial contraction).

   Persistent elevation of CVP increases the risk for edema formation and should be avoided.

F. **Cardiac Output, Stroke Volume, Systemic Vascular Resistance**
   1. These measurements are advanced and time-consuming although they can be performed in animals with no financial constraints or special conditions.

II. TREATMENT OF SHOCK

A. *Fluid replacement* (**resuscitation**[6]) If the CVP is low, administer an IV bolus of fluids (See Chapter 22).
   a. Replacement fluid therapy: LRS, Plasma-lyte 148, Normosol R: 10-20 ml/kg then reassess.
   b. Colloid therapy
      i. Plasma: 10-25 ml/kg
      ii. Hetastarch: 2-10 ml/kg

B. *Inotropic and Vasopressor* therapy[6-8]

   Fluid therapy acts to increase stroke volume by increasing end diastolic volume of the ventricle, whereas inotropic drugs decrease end-systolic volume by increasing myocardial contractions and therefore increasing stroke volume. Neonates require inotropic drugs if they are unresponsive to proper fluid therapy or exhibit normal or elevated CVPs while having impaired peripheral oxygenation.

   a. **Dobutamine** is a synthetic sympathomimetic drug (adrenergic agonist) that has a high affinity to β1-adrenoceptrors and weak affinity to α-adrenergic receptors. It increases cardiac stroke volume and improves splanchnic perfusion presumably through its action on β2 receptors. It should be diluted in D5W or LRS and given as a continuous rate of infusion a dose starting at 1-5ug/kg/min.

   Vasopressor agents act through the stimulation of vascular smooth muscle tone, therefore have an important role of redistributing the circulating blood volume and increasing the peripheral vascular resistance (PVR).

   b. **Norepinephrine** is a strong α-adrenergic stimulant and has some affinity to β1-adrenoceptors. It is useful to restore organ perfusion in vasodilatory shock. It also improves cardiac output as a result of its effect on β1-adrenoceptors. It may be used in combination with dobutamine at a starting dose of 0.1ug/kg/min to a maximum dose of 1.5 ug/kg/min[9,10]

   c. **Epinephrine** is a potent non-selective α- and β-adrenergic stimulant. Although it is a potent vasopressor it has been shown to have detrimental effect on splanchnic circulation, therefore is **not** recommended as a first line vasopressor. Starting dose of epinephrine is 0.1 ug/kg/min.

d. **Phenylephrine** has been shown to decrease stroke volume in healthy anesthetized horses. Therefore its use is not recommended in equine patients.

e. **Dopamine** in recent human studies **failed to** demonstrate beneficial effect of dopamine on splanchnic circulation; it may actually have detrimental effect on organ perfusion. In addition dopamine suppresses the production of anterior pituitary hormones except for ACTH in humans.
EC – Don't use in foals.

f. **Vasopressin** also known as antidiuretic hormone (ADH)
   i. Healthy anesthetized foals had increased mean arterial pressure (MAP) after administration of vasopressin.
   ii. Vasopressin has been shown to be potent in cases of sepsis or endotoxemia. It restores vasoconstrictor effects of catecholamines and is also a highly powerful vasoconstrictor alone. This effect may reduce cardiac output, and **therefore it is recommended to administer in conjunction with an inotropic drug.** The major side effect of the drug is the dose dependent decrease on splanchnic perfusion. Suggested dose in foals is 0.25-1.5 mU/kg/min.

g. **Methylene Blue** limited information. The proposed effect is the inhibition of NOS, a nitric oxide producing enzyme, and therefore decreasing the vasodilation and increasing the myocardial contractility. Side effects include methemoglobinemia, staining of the skin and the urine. Further investigations are needed before the introduction of this drug in the equine neonatal medicine.

In Summary inotropic and vasopressor therapy must always be addressed to the individual animal. Response to treatment should always be closely monitored. One should restore circulating blood volume first by administering iv crytalloids and/or colloids, because combination of hypovolemia and vasopressor therapy has detrimental effects on stroke volume and on organ perfusion. Current evidence suggests that the first choice inotrope is **dobutamine** in the equine neonate. If the animal remains hypotensive, vasopressor therapy is also indicated (**norepinephrine, vasopressin**).[11]

EC - Never try to use vasopressors, norepinephrine or vasopressin by drawing up in a syringe and giving slowly – always dilute and use fluid pumps! And any outside the vein wall causes a major slough.

C. *Corticosteroids:* The use of corticosteroids in shock remains controversial[12]. Administration of low dose corticosteroids shorten the periods of shock but it does not improve survival rates[11]. If given, physiological doses of short acting steroids should be used only (50 mg prednisolone sodium succinate IV). Larger doses should always be avoided.

D. *NSAIDs:* Low dose flunixin meglumine (Banamine®) 0.25 mg/kg QID has been shown to lessen manifestations of endotoxemia when administered early but it may contribute to gastric ulceration, decrease renal perfusion and cause medullary crest necrosis .

E. *Pentoxyfilline* is a rheological agent, which has a phosphodiesterase antagonist effect as well as TNF-α blocking properties. It is used in horses for the treatment of endotoxemia, sepsis and for prevention of laminitis. It can be administered in a dose of 7.5 mg/kg iv diluted in fluids or orally every 8-12 hours.

F. *Polymyxin-B* is an antibiotic that has endotoxin-binding properties. It is likely beneficial in endotoxic and septicemic patients. Administration is associated with nephro and neurotoxicity. Dose is 1000-6000 U/kg/12 h iv.

G. *Antioxidants* **and** *Vitamins* may be added to combat against increased free radical production. DMSO can be given at a dose of 0.1-1 g/kg IV BID. Others have used allopurinol 40mg/kg PO, vitamin C at a dose of 50mg/kg IV SID and Vitamin E 10-40 U/kg PO SID. **EC**- Don't give any of these during period of "open gut" (<12 hrs of age).

H. *Hyperimmune plasma* (J5) (See Chapter 10) may have the additional benefit of containing anti-endotoxin

I. **Antibiotics** (see Chapter 70) are an essential part of the therapy during bacterial septic shock. A recent study has demonstrated that the administration of B-lactam antibiotics further increases the concentration of endotoxin in circulation due to destruction of the bacterial wall components. Therefore anti-endotoxic therapy may be considered in conjunction with antimicrobial therapy.

J. **Anti-coagulants** have been used widely in equine medicine to decrease the incidence of coagulopathies during procoagulant stages. *Unfractionated heparin* acts as a potent cofactor of ATIII, although it can cause aggregation of red blood cells and a reversible decrease in PCV. The dose is 20-100 U/kg TID. *Low molecular weight heparin* (dalteparin, enoxaparin) binds to factor X and V, and has less effect on ATIII. The dose of dalteparin is 50 U/kg SID. The dose of enoxaparin is 40 U/kg SID.

K. **Parenteral nutrition**. Foals with shock or sepsis usually are not able to tolerate enteral nutrition. See Chapter 23 for details.

L. **Insulin therapy** maybe indicated in foals with shock or sepsis. A recent study has shown decreased survival rates in foals with persistent hyperglycemia or hypoglyycemia[13].

References:

1. McAuliffe, S. B: Neonatal examination, clinical procedures and nursing care in McAuliffe, S. B, Slovis, N. M.: Color Atlas of Diseases and Disorders of the foal. 43-78. WB Saunders. St. Louis. 2008.
2. Corley KT, Donaldson LL, Furr MO.:Arterial lactate concentration, hospital survival, sepsis and SIRS in critically ill neonatal foals. Equine Vet J. 2005;37 (1):53-9.
3. Thomas WP, Madigan JE, Backus KQ, Powell WE: Systemic and pulmonary haemodynamics in normal neonatal foals. J Reprod Fertil Suppl. 1987;35:623-8.
4. Fielding CL, Magdesian KG, Carlson GP, Rhodes DM, Ruby: Application of the sodium dilution principle to calculate extracellular fluid volume changes in horses during

dehydration and rehydration. <u>Am J Vet Res</u>. 2008;69(11):1506-11.
5. Magdesian KG: Blood lactate levels in neonatal foals normal values and temporal effects in the post-partum period, <u>J Vet Emerg Crit Care</u> 13:174, 2003.
6. Magdesian, KG.: Crtical care and Fluid therapy for horses in Smith BP.(ed.) <u>Large Animal Internal Medicine.</u> 4th edition. 1487-1505. WB. Saunders. 2008.
7. Corley KT.:Inotropes and vasopressors in adults and foals. <u>Vet Clin North Am Equine Pract.</u> 2004;20(1):77-106.
8. Corley KT.: Cardiovascular monitoring and therapy. <u>Proc. of Rossdale and Partners Foal Care Course</u> 2008;83-90.
9. Hollis AR, Ousey JC, Palmer L, Stephen JO, Stoneham SJ, Boston RC, Corley KT: Effects of norepinephrine and combined norepinephrine and fenoldopam infusion on systemic hemodynamics and indices of renal function in normotensive neonatal foals. <u>J Vet Intern Med</u>. 2008;22(5):1210-1215.
10. Hollis AR, Ousey JC, Palmer L, Stoneham SJ, Corley KT: Effects of norepinephrine and a combined norepinephrine and dobutamine infusion on systemic hemodynamics and indices of renal function in normotensive neonatal thoroughbred foals. <u>J Vet Intern Med</u>. 2006;20(6):1437-42.
11. Corley KT, Axon JE.:Resuscitation and emergency management for neonatal foals.<u>Vet Clin North Am Equine Pract</u>. 2005;21(2):431-55.
12. Sprung CL,Briegel J, et al.:Hydrocortisone therapy for patients with septic shock. <u>N Engl J Med.</u> 2008;358(2):111-124.
13. Hollis AR, Furr MO, Magdesian KG, Axon JE, Ludlow V,Boston RC, Corley KT. Blood glucose concentrations in critically ill neonatal foals. <u>J Vet Intern Med</u>. 2008;22(5):1223-7.

CHAPTER 19
INITIAL EVALUATION AND MINIMUM DATA BASE

Foals with severe illness always look their best shortly after birth. Early clinical signs of depression or slow to start nursing, etc., may be significant and if economically feasible should be worked up with the same data base as an obviously ill foal.

Any foal that is collapsed, hypothermic, hypotensive and unresponsive needs immediate resuscitation to avoid irreversible cardiopulmonary failure (See Chapter 16-18).

I. **EVALUATION OF FOALS NOT REQUIRING INITIAL RESUSCITATION**[1-3].

   A. Observe the foal from a distance and note the level of alertness, rate and pattern of respiration, degree of effort, gait, etc.
   B. Place the foal in a suitable, warm, protected environment, close to the mare for initial evaluation.
   C. Check mucous membranes and use oxygen during evaluation if indicated.
   D. Perform brief overview exam noting any obvious problems such as trauma (cracked ribs, congenital anomalies, hernias, swellings, etc.)
   E. Check rectal temperature.
      1. If < 100°F (37.8°C) and if foal is recumbent, place on insulating pad, wrap in blankets, raise environmental temperature, apply heat lamps.
   F. Obtain blood culture (use good technique to preserve vein).
   G. Place IV catheter.
   H. Draw EDTA, heparin and clotted tubes from IV catheter or jugular or peripheral vein.
      1. Complete blood count STAT (perform differential and determine immature neutrophil count (bands, etc) and examine cells for signs of toxicity)
      2. Venous blood gas and Na^+, K^+, Cl^-, and creatinine STAT
      3. Submit chemistry panel
      4. Lactate determination stat

Chapter 19 Initial Evaluation and Minimum Database

    5. Colloid oncotic pressure determination

I. STAT blood glucose; spin heparinized blood and use dextrose strip, or glucometer on plasma. Minimum dextrose requirement is 4-5mg/kg/min (250 cc 5% dextrose/hour for 50 kg foal)[1,2].

    1. If glucose is < 60 mg/dl (3 mmol/l) start 1-2% dextrose (make 1% dextrose by adding 20 cc of 50% dextrose to 1 liter replacement fluids and administer it in 30-60 minutes).

    2. Some foals may require additional dextrose after fluid replacement. If maintenance 2.5% or 5% dextrose fluid rates does not meet the needs, up to 10% dextrose can be administered, although it is hyperosmotic and requires careful titration with a fluid pump.

    3. One may switch to parenteral nutrition in foals that remain hypoglycaemic for extended periods of time (>6 hours) (See Chapter 23).

    4. Start prewarmed IV replacement fluids with 1% dextrose in (LRS, Normosol-R, Plasmalyte-148) in foals that are normoglycaemic.

J. Assess serum IgG STAT -

    1. If obtain a high value and foal's serum protein is < 4.5 g/dl repeat test with control sample.

K. Measure blood pressure in recumbent foals (doppler on tail).

L. Obtain blood gas or determine oxygen saturation with pulse oximetry (see Chapter 13).

M. Assess maturity - <u>Radiograph carpus and tarsus</u> if suspect premature of dysmature.

N. Weigh foal.

O. Perform standard post foaling care (chlorhexidine 0.5% to navel, tetanus prophylaxis, enema if indicated).

P. Obtain a thoracic radiograph.

Q. Ultrasound umbilicus and check size of bladder
EC - a lot of sick foals don't 'feel' a big bladder and will rupture; monitor for this frequently

R. Complete comprehensive physical exam and record findings.

S. Evaluate physical findings and laboratory data, compute sepsis score[2], and initiate therapy. (See Chapter 28 for sepsis score).

1. If your history, examination and instinct suggest sepsis is a possibility, repeat blood culture if 1 hour has passed and **start foal on IV antibiotics and consider plasma administration**.

References:
1. Koterba, A.M.: Identification and early management of the high risk neonatal foal: averting disasters. Equine Vet Educ 1:9-14, 1989.
2. Brewer, B.D., Koterba, A.M.: The development of a scoring system for the early diagnosis of equine neonatal sepsis. Equine Vet J 20:18-22, 1988.
3. Magdesian KG, Fielding CL, Madigan JE : Volume Replacement in the Neonatal ICU: Crystalloids and Colloids. Clinical techniques in Equine Practice. 2:1,20-30, 2003.

CHAPTER 20
DAILY PLAN AND MONITORING OF THE CRITICAL CARE PATIENT

I. MONITOR, RECORD AND INTERPRET VITAL SIGNS

Frequency of monitoring depends on the patient's condition. Vital signs including mentation, heart rate, respiratory rate, temperature, GI motility and comments on tubes, catheters, surgery sites and fecal output should be recorded at least every 4-6 hours.

II. ARTERIAL BLOOD PRESSURE AND URINE OUTPUT

These parameters are critical to measure and document in recumbent patients. Mean arterial blood pressure should be kept above 60mmHg. Although neonates do not produce significant amount of urine within the first 12-24 hours of life, after that minimum production should be 2-4 ml/kg/h if hydration is adequate.

III. WEIGH DAILY

A. **Interpret daily** weight change for growth which is 1-3 lbs/day ($\approx$1 kg/day) for most foals.
B. Very sick foals may lose weight within the first 24-48 hours of life. **EC-** weight loss will then produce extreme weakness.
C. Foals which gain more than expected in a 24 hr period are having fluid retention (maybe inappropriate ADH). Slow fluids down and monitor urine output.

IV. ORAL FEEDINGS - FREQUENCY AND AMOUNT

A. **Amounts of colostrum or milk;** and type of milk - goat's milk, mare's milk or milk replacer and frequency of feedings which is usually 1-2 hours.
  1. Bottle feeding is recommended **only** if a strong suck reflex is present and always keep bottle below level of the pharynx to prevent aspiration, otherwise use a stomach tube.

2. Strictly keep the time intervals between feedings (1-2 hrs) to avoid colic, gastric distention or enteritis.

V. PARENTERAL FEEDING.

- **A. Deduct** the amount of volume given this route from the total fluids determined for the day. Always mark new bags of TPN when started.
- **B. Dedicate** one injection port solely to the parenteral nutrition.
- **C. Aseptic technique** is critically important with the administration and catheter care with patients receiving parenteral nutrition.
- **D. Long term** (polyurethane or silicone) catheters **only** should be used for this purpose.
- **E. Check** liver enzymes, triglycerides daily.

VI. INTRAVENOUS FLUIDS
– Record type, flow rate and total daily volume of fluids. Always calculate volumes with all types of fluids given to prevent overhydration or interstitial edema (crystalloids, colloids, parenteral nutrition, enteral nutrition, medications diluted in larger amounts of IV fluids). Additives should be labeled on the fluids as well as noted on records.

VII. FREQUENCY OF CHEMISTRY AND HEMATOLOGY PROFILES

- **A. Daily recheck of CBC and chemistry profiles is recommended in hospitalized neonates.**
- **B. Check glucose** and acid base every 4-6 hours if prior hypoglycemia or receiving glucose containing fluids.
- **C. Check lactate** levels every 6 -12 hours in foals with poor perfusion or hypotension.
- **D. Check PCV/TP** every 6-12 hours in foals high risk for immune-mediated hemolytic anemia.
- **E. Check electrolytes and acid base balance** in patients with severe acidosis, electrolyte derangements, or diarrhea every 6-12 hours.
- **F. Check creatinine/BUN/electrolytes** more than once a day if renal compromise is suspected.
- **G. Check bile acids, ammonia, and bilirubin** daily in foals with hepatic failure or hepatoencephalopathy.

H. **Check fibrinogen** every 24-48 hours in foals with suspected bacterial infection.
I. **Check Clotting** profile (PT, APTT, FDP, ATIII, platelets) as indicated in septic foals or in foals with high risk of coagulopathies.
J. **Measure** central venous pressure (CVP) and colloid oncotic pressure (COP) in critical patients once a day.

VIII. PLASMA AMOUNTS AND FLOW RATE

A. **Always check** the foal's serum IgG post transfusion and monitor serially.

IX. OXYGEN FLOW RATES

A. **Maintain PaO_2** 80-100 mmHg when on supplemental O_2.
B. **PaO_2 >58 mmHg** without supplemental oxygen may be acceptable in small foals in **lateral recumbency and < 36 hours of age**. Arterial blood gas should be collected when recumbent foals are in sternal position.
C. **Determine PaO_2/FIO_2 ratio** and change the inspired O_2 according to the results.
   1. Normal is 500 (100mmHg PaO_2 /0.21 inspired oxygen percentage).
   2. <300 indicates acute lung injury (<60mmHg PaO_2) without O_2 supplementation
   3. <200 indicates Acute Respiratory Distress Syndrome (<40mmHg PaO_2) without O_2 supplementation
D. **Remember** CO_2 does not have diffusion limitation properties like O_2. Normal or decreased $PaCO_2$ with low PaO_2 most likely reflects a diffusion problem (cardiopulmonary disease; increase FIO_2), whereas high $PaCO_2$ with normal or low PaO_2 reflects inadequate ventilation (HIE, botulism, musculoskeletal diseases, CNS problems. Use respiratory stimulant or mechanical ventilation in these cases).

X. FREQUENCY OF ARTERIAL BLOOD GAS

A. **Twice daily** minimum if on O_2 insufflation.
B. **4-6 times** daily if on a ventilator.

XI. **DOSE AND FREQUENCY** of antibiotics, sedatives or anticonvulsants (if seizuring), antipyretics, analgesics or other medications.

XII. **CHANGE THE LEVEL AND INTENSITY** of care gradually. As the patient improves do not discontinue all the treatments at the same time targeted to the same organ system (fluids and diuretics or bronchodilators and nebulization)

XIII. **RECHECK** abdominal ultrasound for size of bladder; monitor gut motility and distension, etc.

XIV. **REDO COMPLETE PHYSICAL EXAMINATION ONCE DAILY AND RECORD.**

XV. **DETERMINE REST PERIODS WHEN FOAL CAN SLEEP**

    A. **After oral feedings** - 1 hour of rest is desirable.
    B. **Turn lights down** and be quiet.

XVI. **DAILY CONVEY PROGRESS** to owner and referring veterinarian and keep appraised of current costs.

References:
The authors used their own experiences based on the NICU Protocol of UC Davis and other Critical Care Clinics.

CHAPTER 21
DAILY NURSING CARE

I. **INTRAVENOUS CATHETERS** (See Chapter 61)

  A. **Placement of catheters** should be sterile and aseptic.
  B. **Change dressing**, clean and inspect site and catheter daily.
  C. **Change catheter** depending on the catheter type
   1. teflon catheters may be used up to 48-72 hours
   2. polyurethane catheters may last up to 2-3 weeks
   3. silicone catheters can be used for up to a month

II. **FLUID ADMINISTRATION SETS AND FLUIDS**

  A. **Change administration sets** daily if glucose containing fluids are given or if IV line must be broken frequently, change every 48 hours if line remains intact.
  B. **For ambulatory foals** use a coiled extension set and secure it to the fluid harness.
  C. **Change all fluid containers** (including PN) hanging longer than 24 hours.

III. **OXYGEN ADMINISTRATION EQUIPMENT**

  A. **Change O_2 insufflation** lines and humidifiers every 24-48 hours.
  B. **Change or inspect nasal** insufflation catheter 2-3 times daily to see if holes are plugged.
  C. **Check** frequently for fluid accumulation in the lines which may occlude O_2 flow.
  D. **Monitor** pressure if using a cylinder.

IV. **BODY POSITION AND EXERCISE**

  A. **Sternal** or semi-sternal position with thorax upright allows best ventilation and perfusion of the lungs.
  B. **Body position** should be changed every 2-4 hours. If possible, assist the foal to stand for about 5 minutes as often as possible, but at least turn and stand the foal every 4 hours.

C. **In term foals**, passive range-of-motion exercises performed several times each day may help to stimulate circulation and prevent tendon contractures.
  D. **Premature foals** with incomplete ossification of the cuboidal bones (carpus, tarsus) should not be encouraged to stand in the first several days.
  E. **Recumbent foals with fractured ribs** should be moved very carefully with the assistance of two people.
  F. **'Sling assisted outdoor experience'** appears beneficial. This is taking the foal 'for a walk' but essentially exposes the foal to the outdoor environment. Subjectively appears to improve foal demeanor and mentation.

V. BEDDING

  A. Foals with their dams should be bedded on straw rather than shavings which get into the eyes, nose and mouth.
  B. Critical foals (usually removed from the mare) should be placed on a soft mattress with a readily cleaned surface. Ideally the mattress should be contoured so that urine and other fluids pool away from the foal. Warm, dry, clean blankets should be used under the foal as well as on top of the foal.
  C. If the foal has limb problems, have minimal bedding to allow foot support on flat surface.

VI. UMBILICUS

  A. **Treat umbilical stump** with (0.5%) chlorhexidine solution 3-4 times during the first three days of life.
  B. **Inspect stump daily** for signs of infection or patent urachus.
  C. **Ultrasound** if any concern.

VII. EYES

  A. **Inspect** frequently for evidence of corneal abrasion from trauma or entropion. A head protector may be used to reduce trauma to the eyes in struggling patients.
  B. **Use artificial tears**, Lacrilube ointment® or antibiotic ointment at least 4-6 times daily to prevent corneal desiccation

VIII. PERINEUM AND SHEATH

A. **Clean and apply petroleum** jelly or Desitin® ointment as necessary to prevent scalding from urine and diarrhea.
B. **Urinary catheters** should be used only when medically necessary. Human colostomy bags may be modified for urine collection without catheterization.

IX. REST - DON'T FORGET TO ALLOW QUIET TIME FOR FOALS TO SLEEP!

References:
1. The authors used their own experiences in this chapter based on the protocols at UC Davis.

CHAPTER 22
FLUID AND ELECTROLYTE BALANCE

Due to the neonates unique fluid spaces, maintenance of proper fluid balance and frequent monitoring are essential. The 4 decisions that have to be made in neonatal fluid therapy are: the type of fluids, the rate of administration, the goals of the therapy and the limits of specific fluid therapies. **EC- For an emergency fluid resuscitation protocol go directly to the end of the chapter**.

I. GUIDELINES FOR FLUID THERAPY:

EC- remember this take home point: Results of studies suggest that administration of an isotonic electrolyte fluid containing a physiologic concentration of sodium may not be appropriate for use in neonatal foals that require maintenance fluid therapy.[1,2]

A. Neonatal Charactistics
1. Increased risk of infection requires absolute adherence to strict asepsis protocols for intravenous catheterization and fluids.
2. Fluid and energy intake are directly linked on the normal all milk diet.
3. Any medical or physical disorder which impairs nursing or milk availability will have immediate and profound effects on energy and fluid balance.
4. In normal foals urine output is very high and fecal output is low.
5. Body fluid compartments differ. Relative to body weight total body water, plasma volume and extracellular fluid volume (ECF) are much larger in foals. Compared to adults, water content of the body is 10% higher (75-80% vs. 65-70%). The extracellular and intracellular ratio is 50%-50% in neonates compared to 40%-60% in adults. 75% of the extracellular fluids are within the interstitium. The colloid oncotic pressure of the plasma is lower than in adults (20mmHg vs. 25 mmHg), therefore increased hydrostatic pressure can lead to interstitial edema more rapidly than in adults (overhydration) [3,4].
6. Premature animals may have even larger body fluid compartments relative to body weight.

7. Foals have a higher surface area to body weight ratio and a higher resting respiratory rate. These factors contribute to larger insensible fluid losses and a greater tendency to lose body heat in cool or drafty environments.

B. **Fluid Intake**
1. Fluid intake as milk in the newborn nursing foal approaches 80 to 100 ml/kg/day (4 to 5 L/day in a 50 kg-foal) taken as small frequent feedings which may range from 100 to 300 ml every hour or two. Milk intake may approach 150-250 ml/kg/day in slightly older foals!! This large fluid intake is necessary to provide adequate energy from the all milk diet and to maintain appropriate digestive processes. Normal urine output is high, (5-10 ml/kg/h), and specific gravity is low (<1010 g/l).

C. **Fluid Therapy**
1. The first goal is adequate transfer and absorption of colostral immunoglobulins (Chapter 8).
2. Route of fluids: Several categories with regard to route of administration for fluid therapy requirements.
   a. **Orphan foal**, bright, alert, standing, good suck reflexes, no serious medical problems.
      - **Bottle or bucket feeding**
      - **Nurse mare**
   b. **Weak or ill foal, suck reflex present but weak**, able to maintain sternal position for part of the time, no obvious gastrointestinal abnormality, gestational age >320 days.
      - **Feeding via naso-gastric tube.**
   c. **Weak or ill foals with weak to no suck reflex.** Dehydrated, hypoglycemic, recumbent foals with obvious gastrointestinal disease, or major fluid deficits due to diarrhea, evaporative losses.
      - **Intravenous fluids.**
      - **Parenteral feeding.**

D. **Guidelines For Initial Fluid**
It is absolutely essential that the initial body weight be measured and subsequently recorded at regular time intervals.
1. **Types of Fluids**
   a. **Crystalloids**

i. isotonic: Lactated Ringer's, Normosol R, Plasmalyte 148, 0.9% sodium chloride, isotonic bicarbonate) (EC- use this for replacement of deficits and NOT maintenance.
ii. **hypertonic:** (5% bicarbonate, 7.2% saline, 0.9 % sodium chloride with 5% dextrose)
iii. **hypotonic:** (Plasmalyte 56, Normosol M, 0.45% Saline, 2.5% Dextrose)
EC - use these for maintenance fluids.
b. **Colloids:**
i. protein based: plasma, whole blood, hemoglobin products, albumin
ii. polysaccharide based: hetastarch, pentastarch, dextran.

2. **Distribution of Fluids**

Isotonic fluids distribute within the EC according to volume (75% interstitium, 25% plasma). Hypertonic fluids remain in the EC space and draw fluid from IC space. Hypotonic fluids distribute in the EC and IC evenly until osmotic forces equalize. Colloids distribute within the EC plasma space only (unless capillary leak is present).

3. **Maintenance – Intravenous Fluids**

EC- Studies have shown that giving normal neonatal foals isotonic fluids produces Na retention and other adverse problems. Use hypotonic fluids for maintenance and use isotonic for initial replacement.

These recommendations provide the maintenance requirements of the weak or recumbent foal that requires intravenous therapy but is not severely dehydrated, hypotensive or in shock.

EC- In foals with birth hypoxia do not overhydrate.

a. **Fluids:**
i. Plasmalyte 56, Normosol M: These fluids are hypotonic (110 mEq/l osmalarity). They contain less sodium (40 mEq/l), more potassium (13 mEq/l). They also contain magnesium instead of calcium. Acetate (16 mEq/l) is the only alkalinizing part in these fluids. Chloride to sodium ration is 1:1,

which is a disadvantage for patients with hyperchloremic acidosis.

    ii. <u>Sodium chloride 2.5% and dextrose 2.5%.</u> The solution lacks potassium or other electrolytes as well as alkalinizing agents. Ideal for patients with hyperkalemia.

    iii. <u>Dextrose in water (5%).</u> Isotonic as a solution, but as glucose is metabolized it is then a source of free water. It should not be utilized in replacing fluid deficits or hypovolemia. It provides 170 kcal/l energy and lacks electrolytes.

b. **Volume**
  i. 80 to 120 ml/kg/day (4-6 L in a 50-kg foal)
  ii. Palmer's estimate is 100ml/kg for the first 10 kg bodyweight, 50ml/kg for the second 10 kg bodyweight and 25 ml/kg for the remainder of the body weight[5].
  iii. Warm fluids to body temperature and best if administered as continuous IV infusion (flow rate 3-5 ml/kg/hr).
  iv. As foals gain strength oral administration of liquid nutrients (milk or milk replacer) should supplement and eventually supplant IV therapy.

c. **Monitoring** maintenance fluid therapy. The most critical component of the plan for fluid therapy is the clinical and laboratory assessment of response to therapy and resulting adjustments in the volume, rate or composition of administered fluids.
  i. <u>Glucose</u>
    - Q4H or more often.
    - Adjust flow to maintain glucose between 80-160 mg/dl (4.5-9mmol/l).
  ii. <u>PCV and TPP</u> – SID-BID. Normal range for foals is broad. Increasing PCV and TPP or developing signs of hypovolemia are indications for more sodium containing fluid.
  iii. <u>Plasma electrolytes</u>, bicarbonate – SID. Monitor more frequently if status changes.

iv. <u>Body weight.</u> Record body weight at least BID. Foals on maintenance fluids should have small daily weight gain. Significant weight loss indicates inadequate, inappropriate therapy, or excessive fluid losses and the cause should be determined. Large, rapid and continued weight gain suggests fluid accumulation and the cause should be determined.
v. <u>Urine output.</u> Urine output should be high- 6 ml/kg/h. Oliguria or anuria in the face of fluid therapy indicates a serious problem and the cause must be promptly and fully determined.

   EC- if the foal's urine is concentrated and output is low and the foal is gaining too much weight from fluid retention-- may have inappropriate ADH syndrome and have to lower rate and amounts of fluid.

II. ESTIMATION OF FLUID DEFICITS

A. Clinical markers
   1. Clinical markers in <u>hypovolemia</u>
      - mentation
      - heart rate
      - pulse quality
      - extremity temperature
      - CRT
      - mucous membrane color
      - jugular refill
      - urine production
   2. Clinical markers of <u>dehydration</u>
      - tacky mucous membrane
      - dry cornea
      - reduced skin turgor
      - sunken eyes
   3. Classification of dehydration
      a. Mild: 5% of body weight
      b. Moderate: 10% of body weight
      c. Severe: 15% of body weight

Chapter 22 Fluid and Electrolyte Balance

B. Clinicopathologic and biochemical markers
1. <u>Serial PCV and TP</u>: Clinical evidence of hypovolemia or marked increase in PCV and TP are grounds for continued administration of sodium-containing replacement fluids.
2. <u>Lactate</u>: End product of anaerobic metabolism; will increase in shock due to inadequate oxygen delivery to the tissues. Obtaining a normal lactate is the end-point of fluid resuscitation. Monitor lactate during fluid replacement
   <u>Causes for increased lactate are:</u> tissue hypoxia (hypovolemia, seizures, exercise) enhanced glycolysis (SIRS, cathecholamines, thiamine deficiency, alkalosis, salycilates, B2- agonists, theophylline) and reduced clearance due to liver or renal dysfunction[6].
3. <u>Serum creatinine</u>: might be increased after parturition due to placental compromise, and decreased oxygen delivery. Elevated levels should normalize within 24-48 hours after birth with a gradual decrease.
4. <u>Hyponatremia</u> (i.e., Na <130 mEq/L) represents a "relative water excess". It may indicate excessive loss of sodium and potassium as with <u>diarrhea</u>, adrenal insufficiency, excessive administration and/or <u>retention of free water</u> which also results in increased body weight, <u>ruptured bladder</u> with third space fluid accumulation in the abdomen, false hyponatremia due to hyperlipemia, hyperglycemia, and/or hyperproteinemia.
5. <u>Hypernatremia</u> (i.e., Na >146 mEq/L) represents relative water deficit.
6. <u>Hyperkalemia</u> (i.e., K >5.5 mEq/L) is commonly associated with volume depletion, metabolic acidosis, renal compromise, and ruptured bladder. Correction of hyperkalemia depends on restoration of effective circulating blood volume to assure adequate renal function. Administration of glucose at rates sufficient to produce hyperglycemia will tend to drive potassium into the cells. Avoid potassium containing fluids.
7. <u>Hypokalemia</u> (i.e., K <3 mEq/L) may develop following correction of a metabolic acidosis or as the

result of potassium depletion if potassium is not provided. If renal function is normal, hypokalemic patients can tolerate 10 to 40 mEq/L of potassium in IV fluids given at a moderate to slow rate (max rate 0.5 mEq/kg/h).

8. Hypoglycemia and hyperglycemia is a common and continuing problem for the neonatal foal. Maintenance of energy reserves may require parenteral nutrition as detailed in Chapter 23.

9. Metabolic acidosis if sufficiently severe to require bicarbonate administration necessitates close monitoring of acid-base balance (initially every 30 to 60 minutes). Arterial samples are absolutely critical in foals with compromised respiratory function especially if assisted ventilation is required. Venous blood gases are adequate to assess metabolic acid-base abnormalities but should be relied upon only when respiratory function is normal. After the initial administration the objective should be the gradual and progressive correction of metabolic acidosis over a 12- to 24- hour period. Excessive, rapid bicarbonate administration may cause respiratory depression and CO_2 retention or hypokalemia. Mixed acid-base abnormalities occur frequently in foals.

C. Other monitoring tools (See Chapter 20)
1. Mean arterial blood pressure (MAP)
2. Central venous pressure (CVP)
3. Urine output and characteristics

III. RESUSCITATION and REPLACEMENT

Resuscitation procedures will vary with the primary cause. The following approach will apply to the resuscitation of the premature foal, the dehydrated, volume depleted foal with diarrhea, intestinal obstruction, sepsis or shock. Careful monitoring of response to therapy should be performed at short time intervals with therapy adjusted, according to the monitored response and determination of the primary causal factors.

Chapter 22 Fluid and Electrolyte Balance

A. **Principal problems.**
1. Plasma volume depletion -Sodium-containing replacement fluid (Ringer, Lactated Ringer's Normosol R, Plasmalyte 148, 0.9% saline).
2. Hyperglycemia.
3. Metabolic acidosis: restoration of blood volume may ameliorate an acidosis and prompt fluid replacement may be all that is required. Sodium bicarbonate should only be given cautiously, if necessary (i.e. severe metabolic acidosis base deficit >8-10mEq/L) preferably as an isotonic fluid. Blood gases must be closely monitored (i.e., every 60 minutes at first) particularly in patients requiring oxygen or assisted ventilation. Persistence of a base deficit greater than 6mEq/L in the face of volume replacement provides grounds for bicarbonate administration.
Calculation of bicarbonate required:
HCO_3 (mEq) = Body weight (Kg) X 0.4 (L/Kg) X base deficit (mEq/L). The rate of bicarbonate administration will vary with degree of acidosis and primary disease process.
With a severe metabolic acidosis up to one half of the calculated bicarbonate requirement can be administered in the first hour. The remaining bicarbonate is given over the subsequent hours as indicated by monitoring of acid-base balance. Rapid complete or excessive correction of acid-base abnormalities can have severe adverse CNS repercussions. Isotonic bicarbonate is better than hypertonic (5%, 8.4%). **To make isotonic bicarbonate add 150 mEq (mmol) Sodium-bicarbonate ($NaHCO_3$) to 1 L sterile water**.

B. **Resuscitation** - Intravenous fluids[7].
1. Crystalloids
   a. Lactated Ringers: first line fluid in resuscitation. It may be disadvantageous in patients with hyperchloremic metabolic acidosis and with hyperkalemia.
   b. Normosol R, Plasmalyte 148: these are similar to LRS with few notable differences. They contain magnesium instead of calcium; therefore can be administered with plasma or

whole blood. They contain acetate and gluconate instead of lactate. This can be an advantage in patients with liver failure. They contain less chloride and more sodium, therefore the strong ion difference is larger (SID=47 mEq/l)
   c. <u>0.9% sodium chloride</u>: can only be used in special situations due to the 0 potassium content (uroperitoneum, acute renal failure, HYPP crisis). Due to high chloride content, saline is not recommended in metabolic acidosis.
   d. <u>Isotonic Bicarbonate</u>: best indications are inorganic metabolic acidosis, uroperitoneum. One has to monitor these patients for hypokalemia, metabolic acidosis, hypocalcemia. Bicarbonate administration should be performed cautiously in foals with hypoventilation.
2. Colloids
   a. <u>Biologic colloid solutions</u>:
      1. <u>Plasma</u> is an excellent colloid for neonates. The administration of large doses of plasma (20-40 ml/kg) is not cost prohibitive. The COP of plasma is approximately 20-25 Hgmm. In addition to oncotic effects, it also serves as a carrier for hormones, drugs and is a good source of clotting factors. Foals should be monitored for adverse reactions.
      2. <u>Whole blood</u> may be indicated as a colloid in cases of hemorrhagic shock. Complications associated with transfusion are due to incompatible red blood cells and transferred leukocytes. Citrate toxicity and hypocalcemia are potential side effects too.
   b. <u>Synthetic colloids:</u>
      1. <u>Hydroxyethyl starch (hetastarch)</u> is the most commonly used colloid in equine medicine in the USA. The COP is approx. 30mmHg, so it is a more cost effective colloid than plasma[7,9]. The primary side effects are coagulopathies through reductions in clotting factor VIII and vWF. Platelet count may be altered too.

Recommended dose in adult horses is 8-10 ml/kg.
2. Pentastarch: medium molecular weight colloid, the COP is 40 Hgmm. Other advantage is the larger volume expansion compared to other synthetic colloids.
3. Dextrans and Polygelatins are also used for the treatment of hypoproteinemia and decreased colloid oncotic pressure, but allergic reactions and coagulation disturbances appear to be more common in horses.
4. Synthetic oxygen carrying substances like Oxyglobin® (Biopure, Cambridge, MA) contain polymerized bovine hemoglobin. Hemoglobin also provides oncotic effect.

3. **Volume**
   a. 10-20 ml/kg for crytalloids initially
   b. 2-10 ml/kg for colloids
   c. Reassess for the additional needs (pulse quality, CRT, lactate, arterial blood pressure, CVP, monitor for signs of pulmonary edema, SQ edema)
   d. Initial crystalloid doses may have to be repeated 1-4 times.
   e. It is nearly impossible to accurately predict the fluid requirements of these patients. Initial estimates can be made and then adjustments made based on response to therapy. As a general rule: the more critical the patient, the shorter interval for assessment and re-evaluation of therapy.

IV. CASE BASED APPROACH

Obtunded, recumbent, 12 hour old, 45kg thoroughbred foal. T=95F, R=24, P=84, MM: pale, CRT:4.5 sec, cold extremities, ileus. Marked hypovolemia, lactate=7.8 mEq/l, glucose=54mg/dl (3mmol/l), IgG<200 mg/dl, MAP=44 mmHg,

Initial management:
Intranasal oxygen therapy

Sternal recumbency
Broad spectrum antimicrobials
Slow warming (1-2°F/hour)

Fluid therapy:
1. 20 ml/kg (1L) replacement crystalloid (LRS, Normosol-R, or Plasmalyte-148) with 20 cc 50% Dextrose added - give over 30 minutes

Reassessed clinical parameters:
Obtunded, R=28, P=80, T=94.5°F, lactate=6.9mEq/l, glucose=92 mg/dl , MAP=56mmHg

2. Give another 20ml/kg (1L) replacement crystalloid (LRS, Normosol, or Plasmalyte) with 20cc 50% Dextrose over 30 minutes
3. Give 20ml/kg (1L) Hi-gamma Plasma over 1 hour

Reassessed clinical parameters:
Holding the head, moderate suckle reflex, R=36, P=92, T=97.5°F, lactate=3.8 mEq/l, glucose=135 mg/dl (7.5mmol/l), MAP=74mmHg

Now swtich to maintenance fluids: Continue fluid therapy at lower rate of 4-5 ml/kg/h (1L fluid q4-6 hours.)
Continue monitoring (Physical exam, MAP, Lactate, Electrolytes, Blood gas etc)

4. If still no marked improvement with fluid resuscitation and the foal is rehydrated, then proceed to inotropic therapy (dobutamine, See chapter 17 & 18). If inotropic therapy fails add vasopressor as well (norepinephrine, vasopressin).

Chapter 22 Fluid and Electrolyte Balance

Table 1. List of the most commonly used replacement and maintenance crystalloids and their electrolyte contents available in the United States.

Electr. content Crystalloid type	Na^+	K^+	Cl^-	Ca^{2+}	Mg^{2+}	Osm mEq	Organic anions
Replacement							
LRS	130	4	109	3	0	272	28 lactate
Saline	154	0	154	0	0	308	0
Ringers	148	4	156	4.5	0	310	0
P-lyte 148	140	5	98	0	3	294	27 acetate, 23 gluconate
Norm R	140	5	98	0	3	294	27 acetate 23 gluconate
Maintenance							
P-lyte 56	40	13	40	0	3	111	16 Acetate
Norm-M	40	13	40	0	3	110	16 Acetate
0.45% Saline+ 2.5% dextrose	77	0	77	0	0	280	0
5% dextrose	0	0	0	0	0	252	0

References:
- Dr. Gary Magdesian's Neonatal Medicine class notes and resident lecture notes were used extensively in this chapter.
1. Spensley, M.S., Carlson, G.P., Harrold, D.: Plasma, red blood cells total blood, and extracellular fluid volumes in healthy horse foals during growth. Am J Vet Res 48:1703-1707, 1987.
2. Fielding CL, Magdesian KG, Elliott DA, et al: Use of multifrequency bioelectrical impedance analysis for estimation of total body water and extracellular and intracellular fluid volumes in horses. Am J Vet Res 65:320, 2004.

3. Runk DT, Madigan JE, Rahal CJ, et al: Measurement of plasma colloid osmotic pressure in normal thoroughbred neonatal foals. J Vet Intern Med 14:475, 2000.
4. Magdesian KG, Fielding CL, Madigan JE, et al: Measurement of plasma colloid pressure in neonatal foals under intensive care: comparison of direct and indirect methods and the association of COP with selected clinical and clinicopathologic variables. J Vet Emerg Crit Care 14:108, 2004.
5. Palmer JE: Fluid therapy in the neonate: not your mother's fluid space, Vet Clin North Am Equine Pract 20:63, 2004.
6. Magdesian KG: Blood lactate levels in neonatal foals: normal values and temporal effects in the post-partum period, J Vet Emerg Crit Care 13:174, 2003.
7. Jones PA, Tomasic M, Gentry PA: Oncotic, hemodilutional, and hemostatic effects of isotonic saline and hydroxyethyl starch solutions in clinically normal ponies, Am J Vet Res 58:541, 1997.
8. Magdesian KG, Fielding CL, Madigan JE : Volume Replacement in the Neonatal ICU: Crystalloids and Colloids. Clinical techniques in Equine Practice. 2:1 20-30, 2003.
9. Jones PA, Bain FT, Byars DT, et al: Effect of hydroxyethyl starch infusion on colloid oncotic pressure in hypoproteinemic horses, J Am Vet Med Assoc 218:1130, 2001.

CHAPTER 23
PARENTERAL NUTRITION

Partial or total parenteral nutrition is routinely used and is an integral part of neonatal intensive care. Advances in delivery systems and development of long-term, double or triple lumen intravenous catheters have allowed greater utilization of parenteral nutrition. In contrast to human infants, foals should gain a significant amount of weight daily (1-3 lbs, ≈ 1 kg) following birth. **EC-For quick start of formula used at UC Davis see TPN Straight Talk - simple set up (p. 114).**

I. INDICATIONS

A. Neonatal foals that have not been able to consume at least 10% of their body weight in milk for a 48-72 hour period.

B. Neonatal foals that have daily weight loss (even just 1 pound) for 24-48 hours and cannot consume at least 10% of their body weight in milk during next 24 hrs.

C. Premature foals or critically ill foals with gastric reflux and minimal gut motility on day 1 or 2 of life. **EC** Don't wait for weight loss, start TPN and feed only when GI motility returns

D. All neonatal foals that are not gaining daily weight while receiving maximal tolerated amounts of enteral nutrition.
   1. Base line, maintenance caloric requirements are 100-150 Kcal/kg/day.[1]
   2. Resting caloric requirements are (premature or recumbent foal) lower because of the low activity level (50Kcal/kg/day).

E. Conditions which may require TPN.
   1. Prematurity.
   2. Severe, persistent diarrhea.
   3. Septicemia with secondary ileus.
   4. Respiratory distress with secondary ileus.
   5. Post-gastrointestinal surgery
   6. Persistent gastric obstruction.

F. Effects of protein malnutrition.
   1. Decreased immune function.
   2. Weakness - depression - incoordination.
   3. Decubital sores.

Chapter 23 Parenteral Nutrition

4. Angular limb deformities.
5. Failure to grow.

II. GENERAL PRINCIPLES OF PARENTERAL NUTRITION

- **A.** Dextrose alone won't meet energy demands.
    1. Dextrose provides 3.4 Kcal/gm.[1]
        a. 5% dextrose contains 170 Kcal/L.
    2. Since **resting** caloric requirements in a 50 kg foal are approx. 2500 Kcal/day, and 5% dextrose contains 170 Kcal/liter it would take 15 liters of 5% dextrose/day IV to meet this energy demand.
    3. Dextrose solutions ≥10% can be irritating to veins. Other problems with hypertonic glucose are hyperglycemia, glucosuria, and fatty liver.
- **B.** Lipids provide 9.0 Kcal/g and essential fatty acids.[1]
- **C.** Amino acid solutions can be used as protein source.[1]
    1. Amino acids in "veterinary jugs" have grossly inadequate levels of amino acids for TPN.[1]
    2. Use an 8.5% amino acid solution.
    3. Must balance ratio of nitrogen with energy; non protein calories per gm of nitrogen should be 100-200.[1]
- **D.** Solutions of dextrose, protein and lipid can be combined for 'all in 1 bag' administration and meet energy and protein requirements for maintenance and growth.
- **E.** Parenteral nutrition requires minimum of 1 day to get started, 1 day on, and 1 day to wean off.
- **F.** Fluid (water) requirements will not be met with these solutions. Foals need approximately 100-120 ml/kg of fluid a day.
- **G.** Always try to feed small amounts enterally if possible while using parenteral nutrition.

III. ADMINISTRATION[2]

- **A.** **A dedicated IV port** that is not used for giving any other medications or drawing blood samples is required to prevent infection.
    1. If medication must be administered through this line, stop TPN solution, wipe injection port with alcohol

and 2% iodine and flush with heparinized saline before and after medication administration.
- B. **Jugular Catheter (See Chapter 61)**
    1. **Teflon** catheters are not recommended and should be avoided for TPN administration. This catheter coupled with a hyperosmotic fluid like TPN carry high risk for thrombosis and catheter-induced sepsis.
    2. **Polyurethane** Single, double or triple lumen Mila®, Arrow®, Cook®, Jorvet® IV catheters with a guidewire or peel away introducers can be used in a size of 4-7FR X 5-10" (12-25cm).
    EC- Our NICU uses this type preferably triple or at least double lumen catheters.
    3 **Silicone elastomer** catheters (Mila®, Braun®, Arrow®, Cook®) with single or double lumen (60cm X 5-7Fr) have minimal thrombogenicity and can be left in a central vein for up to 30+ days.
- C. **Rate of Administration** needs to be carefully controlled.
    1. A constant flow rate is required.
    2. Infusion pumps are essential.
    3. A buretral system without pump can be employed but not recommended for extended periods.
    4. Target rate should be calculated to meet resting requirements (50 Kcal/kg/day)
    5. Start at 25% of the goal rate to allow the physiology to adjust, then gradually increase every 4-6 hours while monitoring blood glucose levels every 4-6 hrs.
    6. Solutions are generally increased in volume over 24 hours to reach the target level.
    7. Once the target level is tolerated, the rate can be increased to provide 75 Kcal/kg/day.
- D. **Change all IV lines associated with the TPN solution** once daily.
- E. **Change hanging solutions** once daily.

IV. SOLUTIONS AND ADMINISTRATION[2-4]

Parenteral nutrition solutions should be mixed under a hood, wearing sterile gloves and mask. Alternatively with the Baxter All in One Bag® solutions can be mixed on a disinfected counter in a draft free environment.

Chapter 23 Parenteral Nutrition

- **A.** Partial parenteral nutrition formula.
  1. 500 ml of 50% dextrose – energy.
  2. 500 ml 8.5% amino acid solution, 100 ml contains 14.3 gm nitrogen.
  3. Provides 1 Kcal/ml.
  4. Start at 25 ml/hr and work up to 100 ml/hr over a 24 hour period.
  5. Withdraw over 12-24 hours to avoid sudden hypoglycemia.
  6. Monitor.
     a. Serum glucose BID
     b. Urine glucose frequently.
     c. Serum K^+; watch for hypokalemia.
     d. BUN once daily - to assess tolerance to nitrogen.
- **B.** All in one parenteral nutrition – amino acids, glucose
  1. Energy from: 1000 ml of 50% dextrose
  2. 500 ml of 20% lipid emulsion.
  3. Nitrogen from 1500 ml of 8.5% amino acid solutions.
  4. **Mix** dextrose and amino acids **first**; then add lipid when using Baxter All in One Bag; or can piggyback lipid solution on Dextrose-AA line.
     a. All in One Bag has 3 leads for plugging into each stock solution of amino acids, dextrose and lipids.
  5. Start at 25 ml/hr and work up to 100 ml/hr over 24 hours. It provides 1.07 Kcal/ml.
- **C.** **Electrolytes** can be added to the solutions.
  1. I prefer **not** to add the electrolytes, but drip a KCl solution in another vein and add Na^+ and other electrolytes as needed. Severe hypernatremia has developed with adding recommended electrolytes to the TPN.
- **D.** **Vitamins** and **Minerals** need to be added to the PN formula

V. TPN STRAIGHT TALK- SIMPLE SET UP:
(Gary Magdesian's favorite TPN recipe)

1 L of 50 % dextrose
1.5 L of 8.5 % amino acids
0.5 L of 20 % lipids

Total volume: 3.0 L of PN. Caloric content is approximately 1.13 kcal/ml. Put it all in one bag.

To provide 50 kcal/kg to a 50 kg foal, approximately 2200 ml are required per day, equating to 91 ml/h. As this is tolerated the PN can be increased to provide approximately 75 kcal/kg/day, or 140 ml/h.

If the animal has lipid derangements, then I leave out the lipids and do:

> *1 L of 50 % dextrose*
> *1 L of 8.5 % amino acids*
> *This has an energy content of 1.02 kcal/ml*

I also supplement vitamins and minerals – B- complex in fluids and a commercial human TPN vitamin mineral mix in the PN solution.

Potassium and calcium and phosphorus can be added as needed. I usually supplement Mg through the use of Mg-containing fluids at a maintenance rate. Plasmalyte and Normosol have 4 meq/l of Mg.
> *Potassium is added to fluids (or PN) at 20-30meq/l.*
> *Phosphorus can be added at 0.01 mmol/kg/L for an 8-12 h period per day.*

VI. COMMON PROBLEMS – COMPLICATIONS[4]

A. Hyperglycemia[1]
1. During the initial 24 hour adaptation, elevated blood sugars of < 200 mg/dl (11 mmol/l) are tolerated.
2. Prolonged hyperglycemia (glucose > 180 mg/dl; 10 mmol/l) can cause fluid loss and other problems.
   a. Glucose becomes converted to fat within liver.
3. With severe infection such as septicemia, glucose may not be metabolized at normal rates.
   a. Decrease infusion rate of TPN.
   b. Initiate insulin therapy.
4. May increase metabolism of glucose and cause increased production of CO_2 and increase work of breathing.

B. Hyperlipidemia[1]
1. May be observed as gross lipemia.
2. Serum triglyceride (>200 mg/dl; 2.3 mmol/l) and cholesterol may increase.
3. Slow rate and concentration of lipid emulsion from 20% to 10%.

C. Metabolic Acidosis
1. Principal cause is excess chloride in electrolyte solution. As chloride anion increases, HCO_3^- anion decreases and have base deficit.
2. Lower chloride in supplemental fluids.
3. If acidosis severe - correct as described (Chapter 22).

D. Hypokalemia
1. Associated with hyperglycemia (K^+ moves intracellularly), or with losses from diarrhea.
2. Supplement with potassium chloride solution in 10-30 mEq/L KCl solutions.
3. Do not exceed flow rates of 0.5 mEq/kg of potassium/hour.

E. Infection
1. Catheter associated or solution contamination.
2. With careful attention to detail this is infrequent.

References:
1. Spurlock, S.L., Spurlock, G.H., Parker, G., et al.: Long term jugular vein catheterization in horses. JAVMA 196:425-430, 1990.
2. Magdesian KG. Parenteral nutrition in foals. Personal Communication and Teaching material. UC Davis. 2010.
3. Magdesian KG., Wilkins, PA.: Neonatology in Orsini, Divers (eds):Equine emergencies. Treatment and Procedures. Third Edition. Saunders. Philadelphia. 2008. 486-543.
4. Myers CJ, Magdesian KG, Kass PH, Madigan JE, Rhodes DM, Marks SL. Parenteral nutrition in neonatal foals: Clinical description, complications and outcome in 53 foals (1995-2005).Vet J. 2008 Apr 25.

CHAPTER 24
ENTERAL NUTRITION

Milk provides nutrients, cells, enzymes, hormones, protective and trophic factors, minerals and electrolytes. It is thought that many of these factors contribute to development and maturation of the gastrointestinal tract.[1] Therefore, every attempt should be made to provide colostrum and mare milk to the foal.

I. GENERAL CONSIDERATIONS

- **A. Ill foals** should be kept as close to the mare as possible.
    1. Maintain bonding - prevent foal rejection.
    2. Stimulate lactation.
    3. Severely ill foals in special rooms for care should have intermittent mare visits.
- **B. Routes of Administration**
    1. **Assisted nursing** –If foal has a strong suckle, help the foal to stand next to mare
    2. Nasogastric tube
        a. Use small size tubes (see Chapter 58)
        b. If feeding frequently, place small tube in stomach and feed slowly.
        c. A tube can be left in place and the foal can nurse the mare and still be tube-fed to supplement.
    3. Bottle
        a. Use lamb nipple.
        b. Never bottle feed a foal with a weak suck reflex - aspiration pneumonia and/or inadequate nutrition may develop.
    4. Bucket
        a. This is easier in healthy orphans than ill foals.

II. NORMAL FOALS WITHOUT ILLNESS

- **A. Healthy foal** with mare
    1. Nurses up to 7 times/hour.[2]
    2. Consumes 16-28% of BW/day or approximately 155 ml/kg/day.[2]
    3. Mare's milk production is approximately 15ml/kg/day.
    4. Foal energy metabolism is approximately 5.5 Kcal/hr.

Chapter 24 Enteral Nutrition

5. Gains 1-3 lbs (approximately 0.5-1.5 kg)/day.

B. Orphan foal
1. Provide adequate colostrum during first 24 hours of life (see Chapters 8 & 9).
2. Bucket feed foal starting day 2.[3]
   a. Let foal suck on finger and move bucket up to foal's mouth.
   b. Feed 5 equal feedings of up to 25% of body weight/day.
   c. Feed 4 equal feedings/day in week 2 and 3 feedings/day in weeks 3-8.[3]
   d. Offer creep ration approximately 1 lb/day. At week 2 feed 1 lb/month of age consisting of 16% protein ration.
3. Nurse mare - has many advantages.

C. Colostrum feeding
1. Feed 1-1.5 liters (32-48 ounces) of good quality colostrum (see Chapter 8).
   a. Give 8 oz (240 ml) approximately every hour for the first 8-10 hours of life.
   b. Feed by nasogastric tube unless has **excellent** suck reflex.
2. Check serum IgG in foal.

D. Agalactia Management
1. Most commonly associated with mare consuming fescue infected with *Acremonium coenophialum* fungus.
2. If exposed to fescue, treat pregnant mare 30 day prior to foaling with domperidone at 0.55mg/kg per day orally[4]. Treat into lactation period.

   If mare has poor udder development post foaling treat with domperidone at 1.1 mg/kg per day orally to stimulate prolactin for milk production[4].

   Sulpiride, a dopamine (D2) receptor antagonist, increases prolactin levels and therefore milk production. 0.5 mg/kg administered IM. Twice a day has shown to be effective by different studies[1,2].

III INDUCTION OF LACTATION IN NON-LACTATING MARES

Daels et al [5], were the first to describe induction of lactation in non-foaling mares. The protocol used to induce lactation in 24 "dry" mares was as follows:

1. Mares delivered and nursed at least one foal.
2. Days 1 - 7: placement of a vaginal sponge containing 500 mg altrenogest and 50 mg estradiol benzoate.
3. Days 8 - 14: the first sponge was replaced with a second vaginal sponge containing 500 mg altrenogest and 50 mg estradiol benzoate.
4. Day 8: administer estradiol benzoate (50 mg, IM) and prostaglandin (5 mg dinoprost®, IM).
5. Days 8 - 14: administer sulpiride (1 mg/kg, IM) twice daily.
6. Day 9: begin milking mares. The mare was milked five times per day using a milking machine designed for goats. Oxytocin (5 IU, IM) administered ≈2 min before milking.
7. A modification of the above system as been described - available via IVIS on web at no cost: http://www.ivis.org/proceedings/aaep/2006/steiner/chapter.asp?LA=1

IV. MILK REPLACERS

A. **The best** milk replacer is real mare milk.
B. Mare's milk substitutes.
   1. Foal-Lac™ (Pet-Ag: www.petag.com)
      a. Recently reformulated, easy to mix and better tolerated
   2. Mare's Match (Land O Lakes, Webster City, IA) www.lolmilkreplacer.com
      a. 15% fat, 22-25% protein.
      b. Powder formula in cans, 5 or 20 lb bags.
      c. Feed as a 10% solution.[3]
      d. Foals scour for average of 2-3 days with formula.[3]
      e. Feed 25% of body weight/day.
   3. Acidified cold ad libitum formula (Buckeye Mare's Milk Plus, Buckeye Feeds, Dalton, Ohio; 800/321-0412).
      www.buckeyenutrition.com

                a. Designed to be feed free choice via bucket.
                b. No antibiotics or preservatives but stays fresh and can change at 12 hr intervals. Considered ideal for orphans and bucket feeding.
                c. Well tolerated by foals and palatable.[2]
                d. Inexpensive.
         4. Goat's milk
                a. Foals seem to like it.
                b. Causes firm stools and may lead to significant impaction.
                      i. May need 1/2 - 1 oz of mineral oil once or twice daily
                c. Fresh goat milk is expensive.
                d. Report of metabolic acidosis when feeding goat's milk to some foals.
                   EC- I have seen this in one foal and acidosis was severe and corrected with change to mare's milk replacer. Foals present as lethargic and not eating with tCO_2 on panel low (pH 7.0) and often a high serum chloride associated with low serum bicarbonate level. Make your own: 24 oz cow milk, 12 oz saturated lime water, 4 tsp dextrose (not table sugar), 4 oz evaporated milk, 4 oz warm water, 1 tsp white corn syrup. Or simply 8 oz 2% cow's milk, 1 tsp white corn syrup.

V. FEEDING ILL AND CONVALESCING FOALS

A. Even with knowledge of the nutritional requirements, the feeding regimen for the individual sick or convalescing foal must be tailored to that animal. Prior problems of diarrhea, infections, ileus, etc., must all be taken into account. Two needs must be met 1) hydration and 2) caloric balance. For example, a recumbent, unable to stand 3 day old foal with sepsis will not often tolerate the amounts of milk to provide the caloric intake a healthy 3 day old orphan foal will consume.

B. Sick Foals
   1. Foals that are ill from a variety of problems often develop an ileus and may bloat, or reflux with tube feeding.

2. Our approach is to start the severely sick foal with small amounts (50 - 100 ml) of milk. If well tolerated, we work up to 10% of BW intake by feeding q 1 hr. Can check the tube for residual milk in the stomach by aspirating on tube. If milk is still in the stomach we wait 1 hour and check again. If the foal is bloated or has persistent reflux or profuse nonresponsive diarrhea, consider intravenous nutrition.

C. Convalescent Foals
1. When the foal becomes stabilized and can begin to stand for a few minutes and becomes more alert and hungry, we can begin to approach the 20-30% of BW/day milk intake required for growth and development. Normal and convalescing foals gain 1-3 lbs/day.
2. Simply diluting the milk in an animal that is **not** dehydrated will often not soften the stool. Increasing the sugar content of the milk with syrup or giving 1/2 - 1 oz of mineral oil orally once daily will often solve the problem. Weigh the foal daily to determine how well your feedings are doing. A bathroom scale that weighs you and the foal will work well.

D. Other Recommendations
1. **Warm the milk before feeding.**
2. **Use clean equipment** – bottles, nipples, tubes.
3. **Make milk replacer** twice daily and keep refrigerated until used.
4. **If digestive upsets develop** on a particular milk replacer, try another or try goat's milk.
5. **Attempt to teach foal bucket feeding.**
6. **Add good quality roughage** and foal pellets, approximately 16% protein beginning at 10-14 days of age.

Table I. **Ill Foals - Approximate Volumes and Feeding Intervals -Mare's Milk, Milk Replacer, Goat's Milk**[3] (If the foal is hungry and having no digestive upset, increase the amount fed gradually - **these are the minimum.**)

Age (days)	Feeding Interval (hours)	Feeding Volume (ml)	Total Volume per day (L)	Milk intake total % of body weight
1	0.75	150	5	10
2	1	250	6	12
3-5	1	333	8	15
6-8	1-1.5	550	10	18
9-11	1.5	750	12	20
12-14	2	1000	12-14	20-22
>15	3	1500-2000	12-16	20-25

VI. TREATMENT OF FOAL REJECTION

A. **Recent work suggests that prostaglandin administration** may be useful in overcoming rejection of the foal by the mare. Mare must have had a foal at least once and have raised the foal in a satisfactory/normal way. Give mare sulpiride twice a day for 4-8 days and then 3 ml of Estrumate IM about 10 min before introduction of the foal (longer is ok but shorter is not recommended)[6].

References:
1. Wilson, J.H.: Plasma amino acid concentration in neonatal foals fed defined enteral formulae or goat's milk. Abstract. Proceed International Soc of Vet Perinat. Cambridge, England, 1990.
2. Wilson, J.H.: Feeding considerations for neonatal foals. Proceed Amer Assoc Eq Pract 1988, pp 823-829.

3. King, S.S., Nequin, L.G.: An artificial rearing method to produce optimum growth in orphaned foals. <u>Equine Vet Sci</u> 9:319-322, 1989.
4. Redmond, LM, Cross, DL, Strickland, JR, et al.: Efficacy of domperiodone and sulpiride as treatments for fescue toxicosis in horses. <u>Amer J Vet Res</u> 55:722-729, 1994.
5. Daels PF, Duchamp G, Massoni S, et al. Induction of lactation in non-foaling mares and growth of foals raised by mares with induced lactation. In: <u>Proceedings of the Eight International Symposium on Equine Reproduction</u> 2002; 859-8616.
6. Daels PF. Induction of lactation and adoption of an orphan foal. <u>Proceedings of Belgian Equine Practitioners Meeting</u> 2009, 28-33.

CHAPTER 25
CLINICAL SIGNS OBSERVED IN THE SICK EQUINE NEONATE CONSIDERED NORMAL AT BIRTH

I. **SOME FOALS may be normal at birth and develop any of these signs** within the first few days of life. These signs are not specific for any particular disease or infection but represent a need for evaluation.

   A. **Depression** - mild.
   B. **Change in behavior.**
   C. **Loss of suck reflex or affinity for mare.**
   D. **Diarrhea** with mild depression with or without colic is of special concern in foals less than 6 days of age.
   E. **Seizures** - (Chapter 31)
      1. Early or "mild" seizures in foals seen as staring and blinking frequently and an unawareness of the environment.
      2. Grand mal
      3. Post seizure depression and blindness may be all that is noted in some foals. May only observe evidence of trauma from seizure and recumbency
   F. **Petechial hemorrhages** - ears and mucous membranes. Normal birth trauma can produce episcleral hemorrhages.
   G. **Fever** - (not present in 50% of septicemias).
   H. **Any lameness in a foal less than 4 weeks of age.** Never assume the mare stepped on the foal - rule out infection always.
   I. **Swollen, hot or painful joint.**
   J. **Injected, substantially icteric** or blue mucous membranes.
      1. Mild icterus seen in some normal foals with no other clinical signs.
   K. **Jugular pulses, palpable thoracic thrill.**
   L. **Labored respiration.**
      1. A cough is uncommon even with severe respiratory disease in equine neonates.
   M. **Colic - constipation or abdominal distension.**
   N. **Dysuria, stranguria.**

O. **Milk in nostrils may be caused by a cleft palate or weakness.**
   1. Differentiate from temporary pharyngeal paresis; a syndrome seen which self-corrects within several days. Feed by tube initially.
P. **Ocular abnormalities** - hyphema, hypopion, corneal ulcers.
Q. **Umbilical abnormalities**
   1. Increase size, presence of drainage, moisture, swelling or heat.
   2. Patent urachus.

CHAPTER 26
MECONIUM RETENTION

Meconium consists of digested amniotic fluid, glandular secretions, mucus, bile and epithelial cells, is greenish black to light brown, has little odor and has a tarry consistency. It is usually first seen to be evacuated from the foal within 3 hours after birth.

I. **ETIOLOGY**

   A. **High prevalence** in males suggests a narrowed pelvis plays a role.
   B. **Meconium** is retained in the large colon (high retention) or in the rectum - near the pelvic inlet (low retention).
   C. **Time of passage** is not the determinate of the condition but rather the difficulty or discomfort associated with attempts at passage.

II. **CLINICAL SIGNS**

   A. **Develops** 6-24 hours following birth.
   B. **Restlessness**, attempts to defecate, swishing or 'flagging' of the tail, walking around the stall, tail elevation and straining.
   C. **Advanced signs are** colic pain, lying down and getting up, rolling, and lying upside down. These signs are usually associated with a high retention.
   D. **May appear** to be attempting to urinate frequently.

III. **DIAGNOSIS** is based on clinical signs and, with a low impaction, by manual palpation of a firm mass via a well lubricated finger in the rectum of an adequately restrained foal.

   A. Persistent signs of recurrent pain with lack of passage of the lighter color milk stool in a less than 36 hour foal are suggestive.
      1. Persistent, unrelenting pain should be investigated with an abdominal ultrasound, abdominal paracentesis, hemogram and abdominal radiography. (See Chapter 50)

2. Differentials include colon torsion, intussusception, volvulus of the small intestine, enteritis, atresia coli, lethal white syndrome, diaphragmatic hernias with bowel strangulation, enteritis, ruptured bladder and cystitis.

IV. TREATMENT

EC - For years authors have referred to low and high meconium retention syndromes. Our recent work with treating severe colic due to meconium retention with acetyl-cysteine solution enemas[1] suggests to me that "high" meconium retention is not a syndrome and most of the problem is at the pelvic inlet. We have not performed a single meconium surgery at UC Davis since using the acetyl-cysteine formula in 1990. Similar results were also reported in a referral practice.[2]

A. Meconium retention
1. Responds to one or two pints of warm soapy water administered per rectum through a soft, flexible tube by gravity flow.
    a. Use caution to avoid mucosal trauma with a tube in the rectum.
    b. Forceps or firm metal instruments to grasp the meconium is **not** recommended by the authors due to risk of trauma and mucosal penetration.
    c. Repeated enemas of 3 or more are often not rewarding.
2. **4% Acetyl-cysteine**[1-3]
    a. The acetyl-cysteine breaks down the mucoid component of meconium. Works best at pH 7-8.
    b. Medical treatment for refractory meconium retention has been very successful in our hands.[1]
    c. Can use the sterile Mucomyst™ (Bristol Laboratories, Evansville, IN 47721) or powdered N-Acetyl-L-Cysteine if available.
    d. Solution preparation from powder: add 1.5 level tablespoons (20 gm) of baking soda ($NaCO_3$) powder to 200 ml of water and then add 8 gms of acetyl-cysteine (1 packed tablespoon). It makes a pH 7.6 solution. **EC-**watch out for

hypernatremia with the baking soda in some sick foals (**EC**: thanks Jon P).
   e. Solution preparation from Mucomyst™ - add 40 ml of the 20% solution (10 ml vials) to 160 ml of water to make the 4% solution.
      i. This costs approximately $30.00.
      ii. Solution is pH balanced.
      EC I prefer this over making out of powdered acetyl cysteine.
   f. **Administration**
      i. Restrain foal; ± sedation.
      ii. Insert a size 30 French Foley™ catheter with 30cc balloon (Argyle-Division of Sherwood Medical, St. Louis, MO 63103), into the rectum approximately 1-2 inches.
      iii. Inflate balloon on end of catheter - slowly.
      iv. Administer 4-8 oz (120-240 ml) of 4% acetyl-cysteine slowly.
      v. The Foley™ catheter allows retention of the enema - keep in for up to 45 minutes, then deflate balloon, remove catheter.
      vi. May repeat enema in 1 hour.
      vii. May require 1-3 hours to soften meconium and pass stool.
3. **Still a problem,** the two acetyl-cysteine enemas have not worked now what?

Use a plastic 'weed wacker' (strimmer) wire (smooth, not serrated) the kind used to cut weeds on a machine (Figure 1). Cut the 'plastic wire' about 14 inches in length. Bend it to form a loop at one end. Insert the bent part of the loop into the rectum and pass so it goes through the pelvic inlet and then the loop expands around the meconium. Pull it back and a big wad of meconium will be on the end within the loop (Figure 2). Repeat as needed. Use lube. If the foal's rectum becomes very swollen may need one dose (2 mg) dexamethasone and use antibiotics because bacteria may translocate across the inflamed gut. Use flunixin for pain.

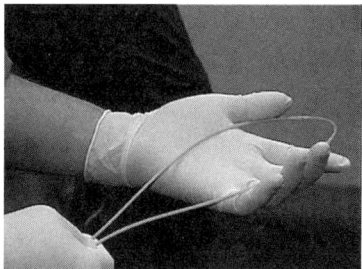

Figure 1: Weed wacker (strimmer) wire bent for use in meconium retention enema evacuation.

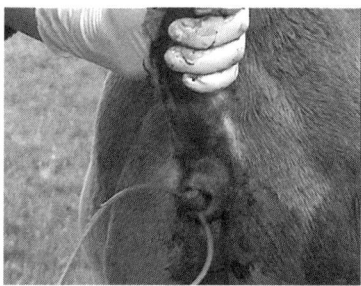

Figure 2: Evacuation of meconium using weed wacker (strimmer) wire.

B. High meconium retentions

EC -Try the acetyl-cysteine +/- loop even if you think you have one of these. In my experience, they are always low.

1. Others have suggested administration, via nasogastric tube, of either mineral oil (8 oz; 240 ml), milk of magnesia (4 oz; 120 ml) or castor oil (2 oz; 60 ml).

    EC- see low retention therapy

    a. Intravenous fluid therapy for hydration or to increase fluid in the colonic lumen can be beneficial.

    1-2 liters of warmed lactated Ringer's IV.

    b. Pain control can be attempted with butorphanol or, if necessary, flunixin (Banamine®, Schering) at 1.1 mg/kg once daily.

2. Foals with persistent low grade pain and lack of improvement with medical treatment may require surgery in a low percentage of cases.

V. PREVENTION

A. Early post birth administration of a small enema such as Fleet® (C.B. Fleet) will often soften the first passed stool but have no effect on a high meconium retention or subsequent accumulation of meconium in the pelvic inlet.
B. Allow early exercise
C. CAUTION -
  1. Large volumes of **any** solution used as an enema can produce severe electrolyte imbalance.
  2. Water intoxication with severe hyponatremia and neurologic signs has been observed with large volume water enemas.
  3. Fatal hyperphosphatemia has occurred in human infants with phosphate retention enemas.

References:
1. Madigan, J.E., Goetzman, B.W.: Use of an acetylcysteine solution enema for meconium retention in the neonatal foal. Proceed Am Assoc Eq Pract 1990:117-118.
2. Hughes, FE, Moll, KH, Slone, DE. Outcome of surgical correction of meconium impactions in 8 foals. J Equine Vet Sci 16:172-175, 1996.
3. Pusterla N, Magdesian KG, Maleski K, Spier SJ, Madigan JE.:Retrospective evaluation of the use of acetylcysteine enemas in the treatment of meconium retention in foals: 44 cases (1987-2002). Equine Veterinary Education 16:133-136, 2004.

CHAPTER 27
NEONATAL MALADJUSTMENT SYNDROME

This is a descriptive term for a set of symptoms. Foals may show signs of being a "dummy foal" associated with septicemia, bacterial meningitis (rare), hypoxic encephalopathy from unobserved birth asphyxia, brain edema or hemorrhage, **reversion to fetal cortical status**, or congenital lesions in the CNS (hydrocephalus). **EC:** It is impossible for most clinicians to perform a full battery of tests to sort these etiologies out and some treatment must be administered without a conclusive diagnosis. Always treat concurrently for infection until absolutely proven otherwise. While the cause has previously been considered to be hypoxic encephalopathy, our studies suggest it is caused by a reversion or persistence of fetal cortical status - this is when the biochemistry required to keep the foal sedated and quiet in utero persists and at birth the 'wake up' call does not occur.[1] Watch for new treatments to come forth soon.

I. CLINICAL SIGNS

   A. May or may not be associated with an apparently normal birth. Signs develop within 72 hours of birth.
   B. Loss of awareness of environment, recumbency, inability to stand, disorientation, struggling randomly, loss of affinity for mare and nursing, poor suck reflex, blindness, seizures, opisthotonus, airway origin bark ("Wander-barker") may be heard in some foals although this is rare.
   C. Duration of symptoms last 1 day in most cases (with early treatment) and up to 5 days or more in others.

II. SUSPECTED ORIGINATING FACTORS[2]

   A. **Hypoxic encephalopathy** suspected in 92% of cases in earlier study.[2]
      1. Placental problems 55%, gestational problems 21%, premature placental separation 34%, dystocia 30%.
      2. Overall 59% had delivery that included dystocia or premature placental separation.

Chapter 27 Neonatal Maladjustment Syndrome

- **B. Septicemia**
  1. Earlier studies indicated up to 50% develop a component of bacterial infection if no antibiotic treatment.
  2. Recent studies all incorporated aggressive antimicrobial treatment and reported good outcomes with supportive care.
- **C.** Meningitis (rare cause) (See Infections; Chapter 28).
- **D.** Congenital lesions - hydrocephalus most common.
- **E. Reversion to fetal cortical status- EC-** This is a term I have used to describe the brain activity of these compromised foals. We have the hypothesis that signals that "wake" the foal up from an in utero or "fetal cortical state" have failed in some of these foals and neuropharmacological modulation may provide some benefit (See treatment).
- **F.** CNS hemorrhage or edema.
- **G.** Metabolic insults - hypoglycemia, electrolyte alterations, acidosis, hypothermia.
- **H.** Endotoxins.
- **I.** In utero infection.

III. PROGNOSIS

- **A.** Excellent prognosis (80% survival) reported with intensive care and lack of significant bacterial component.[2]
- **B.** Older study reported if any one of the following, only 30% survival.[3]
  1. Positive blood culture.
  2. <400 mg serum IgG.
  3. Diarrhea.
  4. Occult blood in feces or gastric reflux.
  5. Abnormal thoracic radiographs.
  6. Abnormal behavior at birth.
- **C.** After 5 days, if no improvement, prognosis is poor; after 6 days even worse in one study.[3]
- **D.** If they recover, "are they going to be normal?" a farm manager or owner often asks.

  EC- Best guess answer is 'Yes' with example being Kentucky derby winner Strike The Gold who was a "dummy" foal.

IV. DIAGNOSTIC WORKUP

- **A.** Work up as described in Chapter 19.
- **B.** Serum creatinine kinase elevated in 61%, which may reflect birth hypoxia and muscle damage.[2]
- **C.** **Serum Creatinine elevated in 32%.**[2]
  This is not due to kidney damage but reflects difficult birth and entry of fetal kidney waste products found in allantoic and fluids into foal circulation. **EC-** Check urine to be sure. If there is significant kidney disease you will usually find abnormalities with increased blood or glucose or casts etc. Remember normal foals have proteinuria in first 36-48 hrs.

V. THERAPY

- **A.** **Don't over-hydrate** and contribute to CNS edema- be careful with fluid volumes (Chapter 22).
- **B.** **Antimicrobials** always because of open gut and high risk of infection. (Chapter 70).
- **C.** **Nutrition:** Tube feed with colostrum and milk. Parenteral nutrition if needed and nursing care (Chapters 23, 24).
- **D.** **Oxygen insufflation**, **respiratory stimulants** if needed (Chapter 66).
- **E.** **CNS treatment** to stimulate "I have been born" signal (<u>**EC these are experimental - not a recommendation but a sharing of what some have used and had some improvement, or none at all**</u>)
  1. Pergolide (0.5 mg-1.0 mg once daily orally for 48 hrs).
  2. Naloxone 5 mg IV once **EC** - See References 4 and 5.
  3. **EC** Pregnenolone pathway inhibitors - (check new literature in the next year or two).
  4. Apply 'Madigan squeeze method'[6].
- **F.** Apply 20 min of thoracic squeezing (See foal restraint and reference 6).
- **G.** **Treat for cerebral edema**
  1. 10% DMSO solution intravenously at 0.5 - 1 gm/kg (for 50 kg foal add 45 ml of 90% DMSO solution into 500 ml of 5% dextrose).

2. Mannitol - 0.25 gm/kg IV q 6-8 hrs for 24 hr. **EC-** This drug does **not** enhance brain hemorrhage and we use it in many NMS foals.
3. Flunixin meglumine 0.5-1.0 mg/kg q 12 h for 24 hr.

H. Treat seizures (Chapter 31).
I. Inotropes and vasopressors (Chapter 18).
J. Ileus, colic, gastrointestinal ulcers (Chapter 34).

References:
1. Madigan, JE, Haggett, EF, Pickles, KJ, Conley, A, Stanley, S, Moeller, B, Toth, B, Aleman, M. Allopregnanolone infusion induced neurobehavioral alterations in the neonatal foal: I is this a clue to the pathogenesis of neonatal maladjustment syndrome? Equine Vet J. 44 S41 109-112, 2012.
2. Bernard, WV, Reimer, JM, Cudd, T, Hewlett, AA. Historical Factors, Clinicopathologic Findings, Clinical Features, and Outcome of Equine Neonates Presenting, with or Developing Signs of Central Nervous System Disease. Proceed Amer Assoc Eq Pract 41:222-223, 1995.
3. Clement, S.F.: Behavioral alterations and Neonatal Maladjustment Syndrome in the foal. Proced 31st Amer Assoc Eq Pract 145-148, 1985.
4. Ting, P, Pan, Y. The effects of Naloxone on post-asphyxic cerebral pathophysiology of newborn lambs. Neurol Res 16:359-364, 1994.
5. Milligan, C, Webster, L, Piros, ET. et al. Induction of Opioid Receptor-Mediated Macrophage Chemotactic Activity After Neonatal Brain Injury. J of Immunology. 154:6571-6581, 1995.
6. Toth, B, Aleman, MA, Brosnan, RJ, Dickinson, PJ, Conley, AJ, Stanley, SD, Nogardi, N, Williams, DC and Madigan JE. Evaluation of squeeze induced somnolence in neonatal foals. Am J Vet Res 73(12)1881-9, 2012.

CHAPTER 28
INFECTIONS

Epidemiologic studies of disease and death in foals up to six months of age indicate that the risk of disease is greatest in neonatal foals (first 7 days of life).[1] The leading cause of death in this group is septicemia (blood borne bacterial infection). In most papers, failure of passive transfer is listed as the leading cause of these infections. The practice of assessing passive immunity was associated with decreased morbidity due to septicemia.[1]

EC - Many (>25%) of confirmed septicemia foals have greater than 800 mg/dl IgG. Additionally, many foals with low IgG are sick at birth and have poor vigor and vitality. It is my opinion that this high rate of infection in this age group is best explained by delayed gut closure and bacterial invasion across the "open" gut rather than low IgG. (Chapter 69).

I. **SEPTICEMIA**[1-3] - The most common cause of death in foals admitted for intensive care.

   A. **Causative agents** - US and British studies indicate majority have a gram-negative component. E. coli, Actinobacillus spp, Klebsiella spp, Enterobacter spp, Pseudomonas spp were most common.
      1. Streptococcal infection does occur but is usually in conjunction with a gram-negative.
   B. **Onset within 3-4 days of age**.
      1. Some infections develop in utero and will be present at birth.
      2. Foals frequently show first physical signs after infection has already been established for a considerable period of time.
   C. **Predisposing conditions**.
      EC - What all these conditions have in common is exposure to pathogens prior to colostrum ingestion
      1. Prematurity.
      2. Delayed access to colostrum.
      3. Failure to ingest adequate quantity of colostrum and specific antibody.
      4. Maternal risk factors - (Chapter 1).

5. Maladjustment syndrome (NMS, Chapter 27).
6. Twins.
7. Adverse environmental conditions.

D. **Clinical signs** - often cannot differentiate from neonatal maladjustment syndrome.
   1. Early signs may be depression, lethargy, decreased mammary sucking and a behavior change.
      a. Fever (>102°F, 39°C) occurs in less than 50% of cases.
      b. Hypothermia <100°F (37.8°C) not uncommon.
   2. Advanced
      a. Petechiation - pinnae of ears, mucous membranes of oral cavity, vulva, (episcleral hemorrhages are common after normal foaling from birth canal pressure).
      b. Anterior uveitis.
      c. Diarrhea.
      d. Coma, convulsions.
      e. Respiratory distress.
      f. Dehydration.
      g. Poor pulse quality.
      h. Swollen joints.

E. **Clinical pathology of septic foals**[2] - obtain Stat.
   1. < 400 mg/dl serum IgG is common; some are within the 400-800 mg IgG range.
   2. Complete blood count finding - always do a WBC differential count.
      a. Neutropenia < 4000/ul. (Remember premature non-infected foals have neutropenia.)
      b. Neutrophilia > 12,000/ul.
      c. > 50 band-neutrophils.
      d. Toxic cells - Dohle bodies, toxic granulation or vacuolization in neutrophils.
      e. Fibrinogen > 400 mg/dl.
      f. Hypoglycemia - 50% of cases have glucose < 80 mg/dl (4.4 mmol/l).
      g. Arterial oxygen < 70 mmHg in 40% of cases.
      h. Acid-base status indicating a mild to severe acidosis is common.

F. **Blood culture** is indicated in any suspected case of sepsis (See Chapter 59).

1. Required of all foals entering intensive care unit.
2. Take before antibiotics or at trough periods before next administration.
3. Do not delay antimicrobial treatment of suspected septicemia to complete a "series" of cultures at 2 hour intervals.
   a. Take 1 set initially upon admission -provide workup and repeat in 1-2 hours and then begin antimicrobials intravenously if laboratory work does not **rule out** sepsis.
4. Negative in 50% of cases with septicemia.

G. **Sepsis Score** - A method of attempting to predict infection based on history, physical exam and clinical pathology designed by Brewer et al.[4] Table 1

H. **Therapy**
   1. Antimicrobial.
      a. Based on a review of UCD equine neonatal septicemia isolates from field and in-house cases, the probability for antimicrobial susceptibility:

100%	Imipenem
90-99%	Ciprofloxacin, Ceftazidime
80-89%	Ceftriaxone, Amikacin, Netilmicin, Cefaperazone, Ceftizoxime
70-79%	Aztreonam, Gentamicin
60-69%	Ceftiofur, Chloramphenicol, Ticarcillin/Clavulanate, Trimethoprim/sulfamethoxazole, Ipericillin, Azlocillin
50-59	Amoxicillin/clavulanate, Ampicillin/sublactam, Tetracycline, Cephalothin
40-49%	Ticarcillin
20-39%	Ampicillin, Penicillin G, Sulfamethazine
< 20%	Rifampin, Oxacillin, Erythromycin, Tylosin

      b. See antimicrobial therapy - Chapters 70 and 71.
      c. **EC**–The choice of starting antimicrobial therapy is a clinician's choice. One popular combination is Cefitiofur 10 mg/kg IV slowly BID and

Amikacin 21 mg/kg IV or IM once daily. This is based on our studies, with isolates we have found, and may vary geographically.
2. Plasma therapy to increase IgG (Chapter 10).
3. Fluid therapy (Chapter 22).
   a. Correct any hypoglycemia.
   b. Correct any acidosis and dehydration.
   c. Maintain renal perfusion.
   d. Shock and dehydration treatment (Chapters 18, 22).
4. Nutritional Support (Chapters 23 and 24).
   Prognosis is guarded with blood culture positive foals; mortality may be 50% even with intensive care. When presented collapsed in semi coma - prognosis very poor.

K. **Complicating potential sequelae** to septicemia.

Osteomyelitis	Corneal lesions
Pneumonia	Patent urachus
Arthritis	Joint infections
Gastric ulcers	

II. PNEUMONIA

A. **Pneumonia Is present** in some cases of septicemia. Can be acquired in utero or develop following bacteremia and is also a complication of many compromised foals.
   1. **Auscultation** not well correlated with pulmonic disease. A change in resting respiratory rate may be an indicator of developing pneumonia.
   2. **Pneumonia** in neonatal foals is complicated by a lack of significant coughing as a symptom and defense mechanism.
   3. **Meconium aspiration** is seen as a greenish staining of the medial canthus of the eye or nares.

B. **Viral**
   1. Equine herpes 1-congenital.
   2. Adenovirus produces anorexia, polypnea, nasal and ocular discharge. Foals recover unless immunosuppressed. Diagnosis is by inclusion body on post mortem of lung.

C. Differentiate pneumonia from:
 1. **Respiratory distress syndrome** by radiographs, tracheal wash - negative, blood culture negative. Often prematurity, dysmaturity associated.
 2. **Transient tachypnea** has normal chest sounds, radiographs, and CBC, blood culture negative, acid base, and glucose normal but temperature may be increased Possible lack of central control mechanism for thermoregulation. Foals are bright, alert, nursing. May last > 14 days.
 3. Birth asphyxia or hypoxia.
    a. History of foaling problems or maternal risk factors.
D. Assessment
 1. **Chest radiographs.**
 2. **Blood gases - arterial.**
 3. **Physical exam**
    a. Increase in resting respiratory rate.
    b. Auscultation variable.
    c. Neonates frequently lack cough with severe pneumonia.
E. Therapy
 1. **Appropriate antimicrobial** therapy for an adequate duration - often 2-3 weeks.
 2. **Physical therapy** consisting of nebulization, coupage, airway hygiene.
    a. Sternal recumbency, oxygen, bronchial dilators.
    b. Early ambulation.

III. MISCELLANEOUS INFECTIOUS CONDITIONS

A. Equine Herpes I
 1. May be born fully mature and dead.
 2. May have normal birth and become weak within hours, fail to rise, and may clinically resemble septicemia cases, often with neurologic signs.
 3. Susceptible to secondary bacterial infection which can complicate diagnosis.
 4. Immunosupression, neutropenia, lymphopenia, (WBC <2000/µL), hyperplasia or necrosis of thymus or spleen.
 5. Interstitial pneumonia.

6. Diagnosis: PCR for EHV-1 on blood and nasal swab; postmortem lung tissue.
7. Inclusion bodies in lungs (histopathology) and postmortem PCR sensitivity found to be highest in the lungs[5].
8. Infected foals which have not nursed may have low serum neutralized antibody to EHV-1 from in utero infection and immunological response.
9. Acyclovir/Valacyclovir has been tried with unconfirmed success.
10. See Chapter 1 for vaccination protocol.

B. Botulism[6,7] - Shaker foal syndrome - causative organism is *Clostridium botulinum*, usually type B or C.

1. **Clinical Signs**
   a. Onset may be gradual over 2-4 days or rapid over 12-36 hours.
   b. Dysphagia.
   c. Dribbling milk, inability to swallow.
   d. Age: birth - 8 months, most common under 8 weeks of age.
   e. Dilated pupils - slowly responsive.
   f. Muscle weakness
   g. Eyelid and tail tone decreased.
   h. Muscle fasciculations after standing or walking.
   i. Ultimately collapse and respiratory failure and aspiration pneumonia.

2. **Differential Diagnosis**
   a. Hypocalcemia, hypoglycemia
   b. Septicemia
   c. White muscle disease

3. **Diagnosis**
   a. Toxin demonstration in serum not reliable in horses due to low amounts which cause disease.
   b. *Clostridium botulinum* spores in intestine not diagnostic but present in 80% of foals with Botulism.
   c. Toxin isolation from intestines.
   d. CSF is normal.
   e. Electromyography may aid diagnosis.

4. **Treatment**
    a. Polyvalent equine antitoxin - early in disease 200 ml dose - expensive. (See plasma chapter 10)
    b. Penicillin - IV QID.
    c. Nursing care.
    d. TPN or tube feeding.
    e. Aminoglycosides, 3, 4 diaminopyridine, aminopyridine, are all <u>contraindicated</u>.
    f. Limit movement.
    g. Provide ventilatory support if respiratory compromise develops.
5. **Prevention**
    a. Botulism type B toxoid to pregnant mares three times before parturition with last dose 2-3 weeks before foaling.

C. **Tetanus**
1. **Etiology**
    a. *Clostridium tetani* organism. It may develop within 7 days of birth, most common secondary to umbilical infections.
2. **Clinical Signs**
    a. Dysphagia
    b. Prolapse of 3rd eyelid
    c. Stiff, reluctant to move
    d. Tetanic muscle spasms - triggered by noise and touch
    e. Nostrils flared, ears held back, tail partially elevated
    f. Normal sensorium with convulsive type spasms
    g. Opisthotonus
3. **Differential Diagnosis**
    a. Hypocalcemia
    b. Hypoglycemia
    c. Meningitis has abnormal CSF, normal in tetanus.
    d. Strychnine poisoning
    e. White muscle disease
    f. Hyperkalemic periodic paralysis
4. **Diagnosis**
    a. No laboratory tests to diagnose

b. Clinical signs, vaccination history and rule out other causes
c. Condition of umbilicus, or puncture wound to feet or body

5. **Treatment**
   a. Penicillin IV QID
   b. Tetanus antitoxin - 5000 units. (Binds toxin outside CNS only. Will not reverse toxin)
   c. Sedation, muscle relaxants
   d. Rest, quiet, nursing care, nutritional support
   e. Ventilatory support - if indicated
   f. Duration 20-30 days, prognosis poor

6. **Prevention**
   a. Vaccination of mare with tetanus toxoid 3-4 weeks before foaling
   b. <u>Foals of unvaccinated dams should receive 1500 units tetanus antitoxin at birth</u>
   c. Provides 45 days of protection

D. **Meningitis**
   1. Most commonly secondary to septicemia
   2. Clinical signs initially are non-specific including depression, anorexia, weakness
      a. May be followed by neurologic signs of twitching, hyperesthesia, ataxia, hypermetria, strabismus, nystagmus, anisocoria, head tilt, opisthotonus, blindness, ear and eyelid droop, intention tremor, recumbency.[8]
   3. **Diagnosis** - CSF tap (see Chapter 60)
      a. Protein increase - greater than 150 mg/dl.
      b. WBC - mainly neutrophils > 20 cells/ul.
      c. Bacteria in Gram stain intracellularly.
      d. Glucose < 80% of blood glucose - may not be valid in foals.
      e. Negative findings do not rule out meningitis.
   4. **Treatment**
      a. Systemic antimicrobials with good CNS penetration and gram-negative spectrum.
      b. Trimethoprim sulfa - limited spectrum.
      c. Cefotaxime 25-40 mg/kg q 6-12 hr - penetrates CNS, good for bacterial infections of CSF.[9]

      d. Other antibiotics may also penetrate an inflamed CNS.
      e. Anticonvulsants
      f. Supportive care
      g. Ceftiofur does not penetrate the non inflamed CNS and probably is not a good choice in foals.
      h. Human studies indicate dexamethasone (0.15 mg/kg) prior to antimicrobial therapy and for 4 days improves survival and decreases morbidity when used with 3rd generation cephalosporin that penetrates CNS.
  5. **Prognosis**
      a. Guarded to poor depending on duration and immune status of foal.

E. **Tyzzer's Hepatitis (*Clostridium piliformis* infection)**
  1. <u>Age 9-42 days</u>, found dead or present with seizures, marked depression or coma, head-pressing, with noticeable icterus.
  1. <u>Usually a well fleshed foal</u>; occur as individual cases.
  3. Laboratory work reveals severe <u>hypoglycemia</u>, acidosis and elevated liver enzymes.
  4. <u>Palpate painful enlarged liver</u> after i/v infusion of dextrose and bicarbonate - biopsy liver to confirm.
  5. Most foals die; however, recent works suggest some foals may survive with intensive care treatment consisting of antibiotics, fluids and total parenteral nutrition for 5-7 days.[10,11]
  6. In Arabian foals, check for SCID with this disease.

F. **Candidiasis** (systemic) - Seen in foals treated in intensive care with multiple antibiotics, venous catheters, urinary catheters, and endotracheal tubes.[12]
  1. Localized infection may occur on the tongue, nasal passages and intestinal tract.
  2. Systemic infection produces fever, septicemia, joint infections, panophthalmitis, glossitis.
  3. Treatment with amphotericin B; or fluconazole 4 or 5 mg/kg PO q 24 hrs for minimum of 4-6 weeks.

G. **Listeria monocytogenes** septicemia has been reported in a 21 day old foal.[13]

Table 1: Modified Sepsis Score

From: Brewer, B.D., Koterba, A.M.: <u>Equine Vet J</u> 20:18-22, 1988. Used with permission.

Localized or generalized sepsis is likely if score > 12. **The sepsis score should be repeated daily in the following instances:**
1. The score is in the questionable range on day 1 (11-14)
2. The foal's zinc sulfate test registers under 800 or the globulins are less than 1.5 g/dl
3. The foal's clinical condition has not improved at all by day 2 or is deteriorating

Findings	Number of points to assign				
	4	3	2	1	0
Placentitis, vulvar discharge, high risk foaling		yes			no
Premature gestational age (days)		<300	300-310	310-330	>330
Petechiation, scleral injection		severe	moderate	mild	none
Fever			>102	<100	
Hypotonia, depression, coma, seizures			marked	mild	normal
Uveitis, diarrhea, respiratory distress, swollen joints, wounds		yes			no
Neutrophil count (/µl)		<2000	2000-4000	4000-8000	normal
Band neutrophils (/µl)		>200	50-200	>50	none
Toxic changes	marked	moderate	mild		none
Fibrinogen (mg/dl)			>600	400-600	<400
Blood glucose (mg/dl)			<50, >200	50-80	80-180
IgG (mg/dl)	<200	200-400	400-800		>800

References:
1. Cohen, ND: Causes of and farm management factors associated with disease and death in foals. J Am Vet Med Assoc 204:1644-1651, 1994.
2. Koterba A.M., Brewer B.D., Tarplee F.A.: Clinical and clinicopathological characteristics of the septicemic neonatal foal: Review of 38 cases. Equine Vet J 16:376-383,1984.
3. Corley KT, Pearce G, Magdesian KG, Wilson WD: Bacteremia in neonatal foals: clinicopathological differences between Gram-positive and Gram-negative infections, and single organism and mixed infections Equine Vet J. 39(1):84-9, 2007.
4. Brewer, B.D., Koterba, A.M.: Development of a scoring system for the early diagnosis of equine neonatal sepsis. Equine Vet J 20:18-22, 1988.
5. Hornyák A, Bakonyi T, Kulik M, Kecskeméti S, Rusvai M.: Application of polymerase chain reaction and virus isolation techniques for the detection of viruses in aborted and newborn foals. Acta Vet Hung. 54(2):271-9, 2006.
6. Whitlock R.H.: Botulism in large animals. Proc of Amer Coll Vet Int Med 1986.
7. Moore BR: Bacterial meningitis in foals. Comp Cont Educ 1995, p 1417-1420.
8. Wilkins PA, Palmer JE: Botulism in foals less than 6 months of age: 30 cases (1989-2002). J Vet Intern Med. 17(5):702-7, 2003.
9. Ringger, NC, Pearson, EG, Gronwall, R, et al.: Pharmacokinetics of ceftriazone in healthy horses. Equine Vet J 28:476-479, 1996.
10. Byars, TD, Rueve, E, Peek, SF.: Neonatal hepatic frailure in a Thoroughbred foal: successful treatment of a case of presumptive Tyzzer's disease. Equine Vet Educ 6; 6:307-309, 1994.
11. Borchers A, Magdesian KG, Halland S, Pusterla N, Wilson WD. Successful treatment and polymerase chain reaction (PCR) confirmation of Tyzzer's disease in a foal and clinical and pathologic characteristics of 6 additional foals (1986-2005). J Vet Intern Med.20(5):1212-8, 2006.
12. Reilly, LK, Palmer, JE.: Systemic candidiasis in four foals. J Am Vet Med Assoc 205:464-466, 1994.
13. Wallace, SS, Hathcock, TL: *Listeria monocytogenes* septicemia in a foal. J Am Vet Med Assoc 207:1325-1326, 1995.

CHAPTER 29
RHODOCOCCUS EQUI DIAGNOSIS, PREVENTION AND TREATMENT

Rhodococcus equi continues to present a major problem for foals world wide. Earlier work indicated the pathogenic strains of *R. equi* have a unique 15-17 kd antigen that is plasmid mediated.[1,2] This is thought to be why some farms have a lot of *R. equi* and others do not. All studies using vaccines directed against these 15-17 kd virulence factors as of 2012 are yet to be proven effective.

I. CLINICAL PRESENTATIONS OF *R. EQUI* INFECTION (3 weeks to 6 months of age)

- **A.** Subclinical
    1. Foals are not observed to be ill but have lung abscesses that resolve on their own. Radiographs reveal abscesses, serology positive and transtracheal wash are positive.
- **B.** Pneumonia
    1. May be bronchial, broncho-interstial or lung abscesses.
- **C.** Osteomyelitis
    1. Can be in any bone but 3 reports of vertebral osteomyelitis in male Quarter horses.[3]
- **D.** Septicemia - Uveitis
    1. Present with severe acute uveitis.
- **E.** Gastrointestinal
    1. Abscesses in mesentery and gut wall.

II. DIAGNOSIS

- **A.** Transtracheal wash
    1. *R. equi* usually cultured if it is there.[4]
    2. A high percentage of foals on an endemic farm may culture positive at some time.[4]
    3. Use gram stain and culture - often have mixed infections with *Strep* spp.
- **B.** Ultrasonography[2] (Chapter 53)
- **C.** Radiography

D. Polymerase Chain Reaction
   E. Blood culture
      1. May be positive in some disseminated infections and with osteomyelitis.
   F. Aspirate of bone or abscess
   G. Serology
      1. A positive ELISA indicates exposure and not necessarily clinical disease.
      2. AGID test touted to indicate active infection when positive.
      EC - In my opinion this test is positive with exposure and clinical infection. It lagged behind tracheal wash in picking up early infection in our studies.

III. **TREATMENT**
EC- Because of problems with diarrhea associated antimicrobial therapy, new approaches have been suggested.

   A. Azithromycin 10 mg/kg once daily orally[1]
      1. Alone or used with rifampin in combination
   B. Clarithromycin- 7.5 mg/kg q 12 hrs orally
      1. It can reach greater concentrations in lung
      2. When used in combination with rifampin was superior to erythromycin-rifampin and azithromycin-rifampin[1]
   C. Erythromycin (25 mg/kg TID) orally has been used for several years, although it is mostly replaced by azithromycin and clarithromycin due to less side effects and better efficacy.
   D. Antibiotic resistance is being detected.

Duration of treatment is difficult to determine - minimum of 3 weeks (up to 2 months) and use ultrasound ± radiographs if possible to determine resolution of infection.

IV. **EARLY ANTIBIOTIC TREATMENT PROPHYLAXIS**

   A. Azithromycin orally daily for the first 2 weeks of life[5]
      1. Study showed a decreased incidence of clinical R. equi using 10 mg/kg azithromycin orally every 48 hrs during the first week of life. **EC-** Don't give anything orally in the first 12 hrs because of risk of enhanced

absorption of the open gut. This approach may increase antibiotic resistance.

V. IMMUNOPROPHYLAXIS

- **A.** Hyperimmune Plasma Sources
  1. Vaccination of adult horses
     a. Donor selection-horses must be tested negative for EIA and anti-erythrocyte antibodies.
     b. Administer *R. equi* bacterin intramuscularly 3 times at 3 week intervals
     c. Test serum before and at 3 weeks following last bacterin injection for *R. equi* titer via ELISA or AGID specific for *R. equi* antibody. To be an adequate donor *R. equi* ELISA titer should be > 90 units. Serum total IgG levels do not correlate with specific *R. equi* antibody levels.
     d. Collect plasma via plasmapheresis, store frozen in 1 liter bags.
  2. Commercial plasma sources
     a. Several companies that manufacture and sell plasma have hyperimmunized donors with *R. equi* bacterin. (See Chapter 10)

VI. ADMINISTRATION OF HYPERIMMUNE PLASMA[6,7]

- **A. Timing** of administration
  1. Proper timing of administration is paramount to success of the prevention program.
  2. Plasma must be given **prior** to significant *R. equi* exposure. It is **not** effective as a treatment.
     a. If a foal is incubating a subclinical infection, plasma will not stop the progression.
  3. Determine from previous farm history and weather conditions when foals first develop *R. equi* in your area.
  4. Foals born early in the year (January and February) in our area are not transfused until spring because *R. equi* is not a problem until that time. Do **not** start plasma too late.

5. After the onset of spring or in areas with immediate post birth exposure to *R. equi*, administer plasma within 48 hours of birth.
6. Plasma may need to be repeated in 4-6 weeks. Measure *R. equi* ELISA titer at 2 week intervals in some foals to determine trend for decline of antibody. Repeat if levels go below 20 ELISA units.
7. Levels of *R. equi* ELISA antibodies rise from natural exposure at 6-12 weeks.
8. A high level of ELISA antibody indicates either immunity or active infection and late ineffective production of antibody.

B. **Method** of administration
   1. Restrain foal and place jugular 14 ga. catheter
   2. Administer 1 liter of plasma IV over approx. 15 minutes. (Chapter 10)

C. **Mare vaccination with *R. equi***
   1. Our experiments indicate colostrum derived antibody from *R. equi* vaccinated mares is not protective against *R. equi* pneumonia
   2. If mares are vaccinated we still recommend administration of hyperimmune *R.equi* plasma to the foal.

References:
1. Prescott, JF, Fernandez, AS, Nicholson, VM, et al.: Use of a virulence associated protein based enzyme-linked immunosorbent assay for *Rhodococcus equi* serology in horses. Eq Vet J 28:344-349, 1996.
2. Slovis NM, McCracken JL, Mundy G. How to use thoracic ultrasound to screen foals for *Rhodococcus equi* at affected farms. In *Proceedings. Am Assoc Equine Pract* 51:274-278, 2005.
3. Guiguere S, Lavoie JP.: *Rhodococcus equi* vertebral osteomyelitis in 3 quarter horse colts. Equine vet J 26:74-77, 1994.
4. Ardans, AA, Hietala, SK, et al.: Studies of naturally occurring and experimental *Rhodococcus equi* pneumonia in foals. Am J Vet Res 129-144, 1986.

5. M. K. Chaffin, N.D. Cohen and R.J. Martens Chemoprophylactic Effects of Azithromycin against Rhodococcus equi Pneumonia among Foals at Endemic Equine Breeding Farms, 53rd Annual Convention of the American Association of Equine Practitioners 2007, Orlando, FL, USA, P8134.1207
6. Madigan, J.E., Hietala, S., Muller, N.: Protection against naturally acquired *R. equi* pneumonia with administration of hyperimmune anti-*R. equi* plasma. J Reprod & Fertility (Suppl) 44:571-578, 1991.
7. Martens, R., Martens, J.G., Fiske, R.A.: Rhodococcus equi foal pneumonia: Protective effects of immunoplasma in experimental foals. Equine Vet J 21:249-255, 1987.

CHAPTER 30
NEONATAL SALMONELLOSIS

Studies from the past decades indicate that certain *Salmonella* serotypes can be carried asymptomatically by the mare in feces and expose the foal at birth and cause clinical salmonellosis in the foal within 12-72 hours of age.[1-3]

I. **CLINICAL PRESENTATION**[1-3]

  A. **History**
   1. Apparently healthy mare
   2. Normal pregnancy and parturition
   3. Post birth normal parameters, exam and adequate serum IgG.
   4. May have multiple cases of diarrhea developing at 12-72 hr of age
  B. **Clinical signs-foal**
   1. Scleral injection
   2. Depression
   3. Fever
   4. Watery diarrhea ± mild colic
   5. Mild limb edema ± joint swelling
   6. Death
  C. **Clinical Pathology**
   1. Initial CBC may be normal
   2. Leukopenia- toxic cells, left shift
   3. Hyperfibrinogenemia
   4. Positive blood culture for *Salmonella spp*
   5. Fecal culture positive for *Salmonella spp*
   6. Necropsy enterocolitis, nephritis, endocarditis, Salmonella cultured from multiple organs
   7. PCR can be performed from feces and blood.
  D. **Epidemiology**
   1. Mares shed *Salmonella spp* at time of parturition. They may be fecal culture negative prior to stress of parturition.
   2. Mares may ingest a *Salmonella spp* in feed that is not pathogenic to adult horses but capable of causing disease in neonates.

May need to culture mares 5-10 times to detect shedding.
3. Mare defecation at stage 2 labor contaminates perineum and provides source of *Salmonella spp* to foal during udder sucking and contaminates environment.

II. CONTROL MEASURES[1]

A. Foals
1. Keep foal from back end of mare until mare washed
2. Feed colostrum milked from mare before foal rises
3. Antibiotic IV starting at 12 hours and continued for 3 days
   a. **Choose** antibiotic based on culture and sensitivity.
   b. **Aminoglycosides** (gentamicin, amikacin) are effective against some Salmonella strains.
   c. **3rd and 4th generation cephalosporins** (cefotaxime, ceftazidime, cefquinome, and cefepime) have excellent efficacy against most Salmonella strains.
   d. **Fluroquinolones** (enrofloxacin) are even more effective against resistant strains, but they can cause cartilage damage. Client consent is recommended before using this.
   e. **Carbepenems** (imipenem) are the most potent antibiotics available however they are very costly ($200/day for 50 kg foal) and should be used very cautiously due to bacterial resistance concerns.
4. Administer anti-endotoxin plasma IV within 12-24 hrs (See Chapter 10).
5. Blood culture foal prior to antibiotics and every day for 3 days post antibiotics (Chapter 59)
6. Additional treatments and prevention for sepsis, shock, endotoxemia. (Chapter 18, 22, 69, 70)

B. Mares
1. Attempts to identify asymptomatic Salmonella shedders based on fecal culture is difficult.[4]

2. Mares shed Salmonella intermittently and may shed only at stress of parturition.
3. Prior to expulsion of afterbirth, wrap placenta in plastic sack to minimize contamination of perineum.
4. Complete bathing of mares post-foaling.
   a. Hose mare down while standing outside foaling stalls immediately post birth.
   b. Betadine scrub bath and towel dry.
   c. Keep mare's head in door of stall to observe foal.
   d. Completely dry mare and milk out colostrum.

C. Environment
1. Determine level of foaling area contamination by multiple (40 +) cultures of area.
   a. Swab a premoistened (dip in enrichment broth) culture tip on cement, walls, corners, stocks, under stall mats, etc.
   b. Culture all feed sources, especially those containing animal byproducts (fat, bone meal, etc).
2. Isolate foaling area, use foot baths, hand washing, and/or latex gloves, separate coveralls, limit movement of horses.
3. Disinfect entire area and disinfect stalls post foaling.
4. Pasture track all foals that are fecal culture positive for salmonella to one set of pastures and negative foals to another set of pastures.
5. Fecal shedding should stop after several weeks (monitor a small group of foals for this).

III. ADDITIONAL CONTROL MEASURES

A. *Salmonella* bacterin
1. Prepare from pure culture of isolate.
2. Test bacterin on research horses.
3. Vaccinate mares with owner permission.

B. Vaccinate plasma donor horses with *Salmonella* bacterin
1. Test antibody response.
2. Harvest plasma by plasmapheresis and administer to newborn foals.

References:
1. Madigan, J.E., Walker, R., Hird, D.W., et al.: Equine neonatal salmonellosis: clinical observations and control measures. Proc Amer Assoc Equine Pract 1:371-375, 1990.
2. Walker, RL, dePeralta, TL, Villanueva, MR, Snipes, KP, Madigan, JE, Hird, DW, Kasten, RW.: Genotypic and phenotypic analysis of *Salmonella* strains associated with an outbreak of equine neonatal salmonellosis. Vet Microbio 43:143-150, 1995.
3. Walker, RL, Madigan, JE, Hird, DW, et al.: An outbreak of equine neonatal salmonellosis. J Vet Diag Invest 3:223-227, 1991.
4. Pusterla N, Byrne BA, Hodzic E, Mapes S, Jang SS, Gary Magdesian K.: Use of quantitative real-time PCR for the detection of Salmonella spp. in fecal samples from horses at a veterinary teaching hospital. Vet J. Sep 2009.

CHAPTER 31
NEONATAL SEIZURES

While seizures are uncommon in adult horses, the foal may seizure associated with a variety of problems. Prompt therapy to stop the seizure in progress, providing therapy to raise the seizure threshold, and attempting to determine the cause is the appropriate management protocol.

I. SIGNS AND SYMPTOMS

   A. **Subtle signs** are blinking, staring, unaware of environment, lip smacking, drooling, abdominal breathing patterns.
   B. **Generalized convulsions** or seizures seen as violent, involuntary muscle movements, opisthotonus, limb paddling and extensor rigidity.

II. DIFFERENTIAL DIAGNOSIS

   A. Apnea - usually secondary symptom of trauma, birth asphyxia, encephalitis, overwhelming infection, prematurity or mechanical airway obstruction.
   B. **Hypocalcemia**
      1. Documented case in an equine neonate associated with very low serum calcium (< 6.0 mg/dl) and seizures.
   C. **Terminal stages of acute overwhelming** conditions.

III. CAUSES [1]

   A. Hypoxia
      1. Associated with asphyxia.
   B. **Cranial Trauma**[2,3]
      1. Cerebral syndrome consists of blindness, depression, wandering toward the side of the lesion.
      2. Midbrain syndrome
         a. Hemorrhage or compression secondary to cerebral edema.

b. Depression, sluggish pupil response, strabismus, nystagmus, ataxia or extensor rigidity.
3. Brainstem - trauma to poll.
   a. Fracture of occipital and petrosal bones.
   b. Cranial nerves damaged - head tilt, facial nerve damage.
   c. Optic nerve dysfunction, nystagmus, depression.
   d. Dilated or non-responsive pupils associated with poor prognosis.

C. Metabolic
1. Electrolyte abnormality - Hypocalcemia as a cause in 1 foal.
   a. Mg^{++}, Na^+ abnormalities associated in infants.
2. Hypoglycemia - Paddling, recumbency, loss of cranial nerve function, blindness.
   a. Can cause permanent neuron cell death if prolonged.
3. Lysosomal storage disease in a foal with seizures.

D. Infection[3]
1. Seizures can occur as a symptom associated with septicemia without meningitis
2. Bacterial meningoencephalitis[3]
   a. Organisms cultured from CSF of foals include *E. coli, Klebsiella, Streptococcus, Staphylococcus aureus, Actinobacillus.*
3. Viral - congenital and acquired.

E. Idiopathic epilepsy of Arabian foals[4].
1. Starts at weanling age and can often be controlled with medication.

F. Neonatal maladjustment syndrome (Chapter 27).

G. Congenital anomalies[5]
1. Dandy-Walker Syndrome with corpus callosum missing.
2. Confirm with contrast CT or MRI.

IV. EVALUATION

A. History of foaling events to determine possible birth asphyxia or stress.

- B. **Physical exam**, complete blood count with differential.
- C. **Serum measurements** of glucose, calcium, sodium, magnesium, bicarbonate, creatinine and ammonia.
- D. **Arterial blood gases** to determine any hypoxemia and acid-base disturbance.
- E. **Lumbar puncture** to analyze CSF for protein, WBC, glucose levels and bacterial or viral culture. See section on CSF tap methods and interpretation.
- F. **CT scan**, if available and problem is severe, recurrent, and nonresponsive.
- G. **Skull radiographs** if suspect direct trauma.
- H. **Electroencephalogram (EEG).**
    1. Abnormalities seen in idiopathic epilepsy of Arabians[4].
    2. May document cause as primary neurologic origin.
    3. May be performed standing with xylazine butorphanol sedation in some foals.

V. TREATMENT[1]

- A. **Correct primary cause if possible.**
- B. **Maintain patent airway and administer oxygen if indicated.**
- C. **Avoid cerebral edema** - brain herniation from cerebral edema associated with equine neonatal seizures has occurred.
    1. Restrict IV fluids unless severely hypovolemic.
    2. Correct decreased serum Na+ if present.
    3. IV DMSO (non-label use, inform clients), administer 1 gm/kg in 20% solution (Domoso-Diamond) - slowly I.V.[for 50Kg foal using 90% DMSO (mix 55 cc DMSO in 1 liter of 5% dextrose) give once daily for 3-4 days].
    4. If suspect possible increased intracranial pressure - opisthotonus, anisocoria, deep abdominal breathing: Give mannitol I.V. 0.25 gm/kg slowly up to q2hrs.
- D. **Correct metabolic imbalances**
    1. Glucose - in the absence of any availability of blood chemistries - Administer 5-10% dextrose 50 cc rapidly IV and 200-300 ml for next hour of glucose containing fluid (1% or 2.5% solution) and observe

for improvement. If serum glucose documented to be low (<40 mg/dl; 2.2 mmol/l) give 10% dextrose I.V. (add 100 ml of 50% dextrose to 400 ml sterile water) at 120 ml/hr/50 kg. Monitor for increases in serum glucose.
   2. Calcium, 2 ml/kg of 23% calcium gluconate slowly IV - over 30 minutes monitor heart rate for bradycardia or arrhythmia - use with caution - cardiac arrhythmias can develop.
   3. Acid-base and electrolytes.
E. **Use antibiotic therapy if infection present.**
   1. Seizures associated with septicemia not uncommon. Does not necessarily indicate meningitis or brain infection.
   2. I.V. Penicillin with gentamicin or amikacin does not penetrate non-inflamed CNS.
   3. If CSF tap indicates infection (bacteria on GM stain, protein >150 mg/dl and WBC > 6/ul with neutrophils) use antibiotic which penetrates CNS.
      a. Trimethroprim-Sulfa - 5 mg/kg (based on trimethroprim content) given IV TID; however, very limited spectrum for organisms implicated.
      b. Cefotaxime, ceftazidime, cefquinom, cefepime (3rd and 4th generation) cephalosporins reach a high concentration in the CNS, and have wide spectrum activity.
      c. Chloramphenicol - lipophilic penetrates most tissues.
      d. Other antibiotics such as Penicillin G and ampicillin may cross into CNS when meninges inflamed.
F. **Monitor body temperature** - prevent hyperthermia or hypothermia.
G. **Anticonvulsant Therapy**
   1. Stopping seizure in progress.
      a. **Diazepam (Valium)** - give 5-15 mg slowly I.V. - take several minutes before increasing at 5 mg increments; has short half-life and may need to be repeated.
      b. **Midazolam**. - 0.1 to 0.2 mg/kg for seizures or sedation - it has some advantages over

diazepam: accumulate less due to water solubility, found to be more effective and safer in human neonates. It can be used as a CRI for seizuring foals because it does not accumulate to the same degree as diazepam. It is cardiovascularly safer than phenobarbital, plus can be discontinued any time. It can be used at a dose of 0.04-0.16 mg/kg/h with good success for as long as 48-72 hr.

    c. **Phenobarbital** for prolonged and recurrent seizure
        i. Anesthesia and respiratory depression can occur at doses of 20-30 mg/kg.
    d. **Bromide (potassium or sodium salt)** used in combination with phenobarbital to aid refractive seizures - recommended dose 20-40 mg/kg, PO, sid, or bid in divided doses (potassium salt) or 17-30 mg/kg PO, sid or bid in divided doses (sodium salt). Bromide is generally well tolerated but side effects include gastric irritation, polyuria, sedation, ataxia. Bromide toxicosis (bromism) is characterized by neurologic signs of lethargy, disorientation, delirium, and ataxia. Bromide should not be used with renal dysfunction. Bromide intoxication should be treated with an IV infusion of normal saline to promote renal excretion.
    e. **Xylazine or phenothiazine tranquilizers are contraindicated since they decrease the seizure threshold.**

2. Prevention - Goal is to increase seizure threshold.
    a. Recommended if more than 1 seizure/day has occurred.
    b. Phenobarbital -
        i. Loading dose - 20 mg/kg diluted in 30 ml saline and given IV over 30 minutes. **EC-This dose causes severe depression.**
        ii. Maintenance dose 2-9 mg/kg TID IM or IV. **EC-**May be adequate without loading dose.

       iii. Determine blood levels - therapeutic range 15-40 ug/ml in humans.
   c. Primidone has been used in foals at 2 gm/50kg orally initially and maintenance at 0.75 gm/50kg BID orally[7].
   d. Always wean off therapy over several weeks by gradually lowering the daily dose. Abrupt withdrawal may produce seizures.

VI. PROGNOSIS

  A. Neonatal maladjustment syndrome when not associated with infectious process has a good survival rate[8]
  B. Associated w/septicemia - Nowadays survival rates are as high as 60-80% in advanced NICU settings.
  C. Associated w/hypoglycemia - dependent on underlying cause of hypoglycemia.
  D. Trauma - observe for trends.[2,3]
    1. Improvement in mentation and cranial nerves - favorable sign.
    2. Progressive loss of cranial nerves - poor prognosis.
    3. Miotic pupils initially and then become dilated and nonresponsive - poor prognosis.
    4. Coma for 36 hrs - prognosis very poor.

References:
1. Koterba A.M.: Medical problems in neonatal foals. Calif Vet Med Assoc Speakers Syllabus 282-366, 1986.
2. Mayhew I.G., MacKay R.J.: The nervous system. Equine Med. and Surgery, 3rd Edition. 1159-1241, 1982.
3. Adams R., Mayhew I.G.: Neurologic disease. Symposium on Neonatal Equine Disease. W.B. Saunders 209-234, 1985.
4. Aleman M, Gray LC, Williams DC, Holliday TA, Madigan JE, LeCouteur RA, Magdesian KG.: Juvenile idiopathic epilepsy in Egyptian Arabian foals: 22 cases (1985-2005). J Vet Intern Med. 20(6):1443-9, 2006.
5. Cudd, T.A., Mayhew, I.G., Cottrell, C.M.: Agenesis of the corpus callosum with cerebellar vermian hypoplasia in a foal resembling the Dandy-Walker syndrome: pre-mortem diagnosis

by clinical evaluation and CT scanner. Equine Vet J 2:378-381, 1989.
6. Blythe L.L., Craig, A.M., Appell, L.H., et al: Intravenous use of Dimethyl Sulfoxide (DMSO) in horses: Clinical and physiologic effects. Proceed Amer Assoc Eq Pract 32nd Meeting, p. 441-446, 1986.
7. May C.J., Greenwood RE.S.: Recurrent convulsions in a thoroughbred foal: Management and treatment. Vet Rec 101:76-77, 1977.
8. Clement S.F.: Behavioral alterations and neonatal maladjustment syndrome. Proc of Am Assoc Equine Pract 145-149, 1985.

CHAPTER 32
IMMUNODEFICIENCIES

Several specific immunodeficiency syndromes occur in the foal and may be manifest in the neonatal period or later in life.

I. CLINICAL SIGNS OF AN IMMUNODEFICIENCY[1,2]

   A. Onset of infections early in life.
   B. Repeat infections that are poorly responsive to therapy.
   C. Infections caused by commensal organisms or organisms of low pathogenicity.
   D. Disease resulting from use of attenuated live vaccines.
   E. Failure to respond to vaccination.

II. SEVERE COMBINED IMMUNODEFICIENCY OF ARABIANS[3-5]

   A. **Autosomal recessive (Chromosome 9)** requiring carrier to carrier breeding. Primarily Arabian, but Appaloosa and crosses have been reported.
   B. **Illness from 2 days to 4-1/2 months** of age but usually when the colostral IgG begin dropping.
      1. Adenovirus is a significant pathogen in SCID foals
      2. Other pathogens associated with SCID are *Pneumocystis carinii, Cryptosporidium parvum, R. equi*, Influenza virus and *E. coli*.
      3. Affected foals rarely survive beyond 5 months of age.
   C. **Presuckle SCID screening test.**
      1. Serum IgM: absent in SCID foals, low level of IgM is found in normal foals.
      2. Lymphopenia <1000/ul.
   D. **Diagnosis requires multiple factors**
      1. Lymphopenia <1000/ul (usually less than 500/ul).
      2. Decreased levels of immunoglobulins (IgM and IgG) after 6-8 weeks of age and declining with age.
      3. Lack of lymphocyte response to mitogens.
      4. Lymphoid hypoplasia, thymus, lymph nodes, spleen on post mortem.
      5. γ-interferon deficiency

     6. Genetic testing is also available.
        www.vgl.ucdavis.edu/services/scid.php
  E. **Treatment and prevention**
     1. No practical treatment
     2. Genetic testing of the breeding animals

III. **SELECTIVE IgM DEFICIENCY**[4,5]

  A. Most common in **Arabians** and **Quarter horses**.
  B. **Increased susceptibility to infection** – 2 clinical syndromes.
     1. Foals or weanlings less than 1 year of age. Typical signs of immunodeficiency present (persistent or recurring infections) which responds to antimicrobials but recurs.
     2. Older horses (2-5 years of age) which have long history of recurring infections and some of these horses also have evidence of lymphosarcoma.
  C. **Diagnosis** after colostral antibody declines.
  D. **Serum IgM** more than twice the standard deviation lower than age-matched controls with normal or elevated levels of IgG, IgA.
  E. **Peripherial lymphocyte** count is normal.
  F. **Adult horses** with selective IgM deficiency should have further investigation to assess if lymphoproliferative neoplasia is present.

IV. **AGAMMAGLOBULINEMIA**

  A. **Described** in Standardbred, Thoroughbred and Quarter horses.
  B. **Rare**; inability to produce B lymphocytes, seen only in males.
  C. **Recurrent infections** in first year of life.
  D. **Diagnosis** - older foal (>3 months) with normal lymphocyte count but no detectable B-lymphocytes, no IgA or IgM, and very low or absent IgG.
  E. **Treatment**: Associated infections usually respond well to antibiotics and plasma, although treatment is not recommended since the disease is hereditary.

V. TRANSIENT HYPOGAMMAGLOBULINEMIA[4,5]

A. Normal fetus starts to produce IgM at 190 days gestational age. Delayed onset of immunoglobulin synthesis (up to 3 months of age). Has been reported in Arabians and Thoroughbreds.
B. Genetic basis is suspected, but unproven yet.
C. Clinical signs start when maternal antibodies begin to wane.
D. Diagnosis is made with Gamma-globulin quantification. B- and T-cell numbers are normal.
E. Essential to differentiate form agammaglobulinemia, since the prognosis is excellent if they receive appropriate supportive care.

VI. FELL PONY SYNDROME (anemia, immunodeficiency and peripherial ganglionopathy) [3,4,6]

A. **Recently described** in Fell-ponies. No sex predilection. Affected foals are normal at birth. This is a congenital fatal disease. Inheritance is suspected but has not been proven yet. Exact etiology is unknown.
B. **Clinical signs** at occur at 2-4 weeks of age. Foals become weak and lethargic, and start losing weight. Diarrhea, coughing, hypersalivation and chewing motions are common.
C. **Presumptive diagnosis** can be made on the presence of clinical signs and on significant reduction of immunoglobulin levels. Affected foals are anemic that is unrelated to hemolysis or blood loss. Opportunistic infections include bronchopneumonia and cryptosporidial enteritis.
D. **Other immunodeficiencies** should be considered and ruled out. Anemia has not been reported in any other primary immunodeficiencies. Secondary immunodeficiencies manifest earlier in life.
E. **Foals fail** to respond to therapy with recurrence of clinical signs. Progressive anemia always present. Affected foals die before 3 months of age.
F. **Postmortem lesions** show bone marrow hypoplasia, thymus hypoplasia, and lymphoid depletion of the

lymphoid tissues, bronchopneumonia, enteritis and glossal hyperkeratosis. Peripherial ganglionopathy has been reported in some cases.

VIII. SECONDARY IMMUNODEFICIENCIES

A. **FAILURE OF PASSIVE TRANSFER** (See Chapter 10)
B. **CONGENITAL EQUINE HERPES VIRUS INFECTION**
It causes lymphoid depletion in the thymus and spleen. Foals that are born alive may be premature and have severe lymphopenia (< 1000/ul) and neutropenia.

References:
1. Morris, D. Deem: Immunological diseases of foals. Compend Cont Educ for Pract Vet 8(3):S139-S150, March 1986.
2. Lunn, DP, McClure, JT.: Clinico-pathological diagnosis of immunodeficiency. Equine Vet Educ 5:30, 1993.
3. Galvin, N.: The immune system in McAuliffe, SB.,Slovis NM.: Color Atlas of Diseases and Disorders of the Foal. 293-296. Saunders, Philadelphia. 2008.
4. Finno, C.: Inherited Disorders in foals. Teaching Material. UC Davis. 2007
5. Crisman MV, Scarratt WK Immunodeficiency disorders in horses. Vet Clin North Am Equine Pract. 24(2):299-310, 2008.
6. Scholes SF, Holliman A, May PD, Holmes MA A syndrome of anaemia, immunodeficiency and peripheral ganglionopathy in Fell pony foals. Vet Rec. 142(6):128-34, 1998.

CHAPTER 33
DIARRHEA

I. FOAL HEAT DIARRHEA

   A. Most frequently occurs at a time that would correspond with dam's first postpartum estrus; foal is 6-10 days old.
   B. Foals are bright and alert.
   C. Duration is usually 2-5 days.
   D. Usually no therapy required other than perineum cleaning.

II. NUTRITIONAL

   A. Consumption of excessive amount of milk after a foal is separated from its dam for a period of time, or in overfeeding ill or orphaned foals.
   B. Sudden changes in diet of the mare or foal.
   C. Foreign material (sand, dirt).
      1. Examine feces for sand, digital exam of rectal mucosa for grit.
   D. Carbohydrate intolerance. While primary carbohydrate intolerances are uncommon, they are often transient and associated with viral diarrhea.

III. PARASITES

   A. *Strongyloides westeri*[1]
      1. May cause diarrhea in foals at 1-4 weeks of age.
      2. Larvae in mare's milk beginning at 4 days post partum and peak at 10-12 days.
      3. Prepatent period in foal 6-14 days; - use fresh feces and sugar flotation.
      4. Treatment with thiabendazole, cambendazole, ivermectin.
      5. Administering ivermectin to mares on day of parturition prevents transmission to foals.
   B. *Parascaris equorum*. Heaviest infections of *P. equorum* occur in late suckling or weanling foals. Diarrhea is unlikely manifestation.

Chapter 33 Diarrhea

- **C. Crytosporidium sp** [2,3]
  1. Associated with diarrhea in both immunocompetent and immunosuppressed foals.
  2. Incubation 9-28 days.
  3. Oocysts found in feces by sugar float or direct FA test (FA is the best test).[3]
  4. Found in 15-31% of normal foals beginning at 4 weeks; very rare in yearlings and adults.[3]
  5. Duration of excretion of oocysts can be up to 14 weeks.
  6. Infected foals considered the source of infection for other foals.
- **D. Giardia**[3]
  1. Found in 17-35% of foals in one study; all age groups including nursing mares.
  2. Foals shed cysts between 2 and 22 weeks of age.
  3. May be concurrently infected with cryptosporidium.
  4. Infected mares considered the source for foals.
  5. Relationship to diarrhea in most cases is not observed.

IV. BACTERIA

In a retrospective study at University of Florida, at least 1 infectious agent was detected in 122/223 (55%) foals. Rotavirus was most frequently isolated (20%), followed by *C. perfringens* (18%), *Salmonella spp.* (12%), and *C. difficile* (5%). The survival rate was 87% (191/223)[4].

- **A. *E. coli*** is a frequent cause of septicemia in which diarrhea may be a component; however, *E. coli* has not been frequently documented as a primary cause of foal diarrhea.
  1. Effacing *E. coli* can cause bloody diarrhea.
- **B. *Salmonella spp***. endotoxemia/diarrhea. (See Chapter 30)
- **C. *Clostridium perfringens*** type C, has been responsible for high mortality in neonatal foals during the first two days of life. These organisms have been isolated from the gut in large numbers from foals with a necrotizing hemorrhagic enteritis characterized by colic, depression, hemorrhagic diarrhea, shock and death; however,

peracute cases may manifest as sudden death without diarrhea.
1. Produces hemorrhagic necrotizing enteritis characterized by colic, depression, shock and death in 12 hr - 4 day old foals. It may manifest as **sudden death** without diarrhea.
2. May affect more than 1 foal on a farm, causes illness in newborn foals within 72 hours of birth.
    a. Changing foaling environment and hygiene usually not successful.
3. Clinical pathology - leukopenia, neutropenia, ± azotemia, metabolic acidosis.
4. Therapy of ill foals consists of supportive care (IV fluids, acid-base) IV antibiotics because gut is often eroded and may have concurrent gram-negative bacteremia, IV Clostridium perfringens type C & D antiserum, no milk for 24 hours, IV and oral plasma, oral metronidazole.
5. Diagnosis via pathology - hemorrhagic necrotizing enteritis, large number of gram-positive rods, *Clostridium perfringens* α and β toxin in fresh gut contents.
6. **EC** In outbreaks on a farm try this: wash mares udder and remove smegma and dirt between sides of mammary gland, disinfect, lessen caloric intake of mare to reduce milk, milk out 1 side of mammary gland to lessen foals milk intake, oral metronidazole at 10 mg/kg BID beginning at 8-12 hours of age (**EC**: no sooner because of open gut) for 5 days may prevent disease. Use *C. perfringens* antitoxin orally during first 6 hrs of life.

D. *Clostridium difficile*
1. In foals < 3 days of age; two presentations:
    a. Fatal hemorrhagic necrotizing enterocolitis[5]
    b. Severe watery diarrhea[6]
2. Diagnosis by fecal culture (direct plating of fecal specimen in selective media) or cytotoxin via assay
    a. Submit 25-50 ml of liquid feces
    b. Must evaluate within 24 hours - keep refrigerated or freeze

3. Therapy with metronidazole may be beneficial if administered early
E. Necrotizing enterocolitis[7]
1. Associated with high risk and premature foals.
2. Clinical signs seen at 3-24 hours of age are abdominal distension and ileus, colic and signs of septicemia.
   a. Foals are acidotic, hypotensive.
3. Diagnosis via abdominal radiographs for pneumatosis intestinalis.
4. Therapy is ICU support, parenteral nutrition, ± surgical removal of affected bowel.

F. *Rhodococcus equi*.
Occasionally causes diarrhea in foals between 1 and 4 months of age, but has not been a neonatal problem.

G. *Actinobacillus equuli*.
Diarrhea attributed to the organism is frequently a secondary manifestation of septicemia in the neonate from birth to 2 weeks of age.

V. VIRUSES

A. Rotavirus
1. Epidemiology[8]
   a. Affects ages 2 days to 4-5 months.
   b. Younger foals more severely affected.
   c. Outbreaks of rapid spreading diarrhea reported.
   d. Low mortality, high morbidity.
   e. 1/3 of foals positive for rotavirus are asymptomatic.
   f. Phenolic disinfectants required to disinfect. (Bleach not effective).
   g. Recovered foals shed virus for 4-10 days following recovery and can perpetuate spread of infection during that time.
   h. Virus persists in environment for up to 9 months.
      i. Control is sanitation, isolation and quarantine of affected premises, protective clothing, team effort.
2. Diagnosis[8]
   a. Virogen Rotatest ® (Wampole Laboratories) rapid detection of rotavirus antigen in feces.

i. Elisa test is sensitive and specific.
ii. Clinical signs should be compatible.
3. Clinical Signs[8]
   a. Fever, depression, watery diarrhea, ± anorexia.
   b. Younger foals more severely affected.
   c. Dehydration, electrolyte and acid-base problems.
   d. Synergistic infection with other agents may potentiate severity of clinical signs[9]
   e. CBC usually normal except for evidence of dehydration.
4. Prevention
   a. Immunity is based on local gut immunity.
      Vaccine for horses - administer to pregnant mares. Fort Dodge Laboratories, PO Box 518, Fort Dodge, Iowa 50501, www.fortdodge.com[10]
   c. Minimize stress and crowding, isolate diarrhea cases.

B. Other viruses[8]
1. Corona virus isolated from foals with and without diarrhea; significance is unknown.
2. Adenovirus isolated from diarrheic foal, significance unknown.

C. Immunodeficiency
1. Regardless of the type of deficiency (i.e., failure of passive transfer, combined immunodeficiency, humoral immune system abnormalities, cellular immune system abnormalities, etc.) such immunocompromised foals are more susceptible to all infections and diarrhea is a common manifestation.

VI. SOME ORALLY AND SYSTEMICALLY-ADMINISTERED ANTIBIOTICS (e.g., oxytetracycline, erythromycin, rifampin, trimethoprim-sulfa, ampicillin) have been incriminated as causal agents of diarrhea due to toxic effects, alterations in normal intestinal flora, superinfections by pathogens (*Clostridium difficile*), and the emergence of resistant strains of bacteria.

VII. EVALUATION

A. **History**. Particular attention must be paid to the age of the affected foal because of the age of occurrence of some etiologic types of diarrhea, i.e., foal heat diarrhea, enterotoxemia, etc.
B. **Physical examination.**
C. **Overeating confirmed by:**
   1. History
   2. Acid fecal pH
   3. Presence of reducing sugars in feces (Clinitest®, Ames Co., Division Miles Laboratories, Elkharter, IN.)
D. **Carbohydrate intolerance**
   1. Lactose tolerance test. (See absorption tests)
   2. Response to treatment with lactase preparation (Lact-Aid ®Lactaid Inc., Pleasantville, NJ).
E. **Blood**
   1. Blood cultures in suspect neonatal septicemia. Most bacteremias are gram-negative and yield more than one isolate.
   2. Complete blood count.
      a. Leukopenia associated with Salmonellosis, *E. coli* septicemia, *Clostridia sp*, endotoxemia.
      b. May be unremarkable in viral diarrheas.
   3. Electrolytes
      a. Diarrhea causes losses of sodium, bicarbonate, chloride, potassium and calcium.
   4. BUN, creatinine, may be elevated due to hemodynamic (pre-renal) nephritis from infectious agents, or tubular damage from concurrent use of aminoglycoside antibiotics.
   5. IgG - often is low (< 400 mg/dl)
   6. Acid/base status.
      a. Can be determined by measuring total CO_2 with Harleco® CO_2 Apparatus.
      b. Milliequivalent of bicarbonate needed = base excess X body weight (Kg) X 0.4.
F. **Hydration**
   1. Indicators of dehydration include poor jugular distensibility; enophthalmos, increased skin turgor, prolonged CRT, and elevated HCT & TPP.

G. Absorption studies
1. <u>Oral lactose tolerance</u> test to determine diarrhea attributed to maldigestion.
   a. 1 gram lactose/kg body weight as a 20% solution via nasogastric tube.
   b. Curve normally peaks at 90 minutes following lactose administration.
   c. Normal: should see ≥ 35 mg/dl 92 mmol/l) increase in blood glucose

VIII. THERAPY

A. Foal Heat diarrhea
1. Uncomplicated cases require no specific therapy other than cleansing of the foal's perineum and subsequent application of a water repellent ointment to prevent scalding and hair loss.

B. **Lactose-intolerant foals** should have limited access to mare's milk.
1. Mare's milk can be "stripped" or foal can be muzzled. Foal may be given commercial milk replacer with yeast-derived lactase enzyme (Lactaid ®, SugarLo Co., Pleasantville, NJ).

C. Parasites
1. *Strongyloides westeri*. Benzimidazoles are effective against adults in small intestine. Thiabendazole (44 mg/kg); cambendazole (20 mg/kg); oxibendazole (10 mg/kg).

D. **Fluids** in light of the consequences of dehydration and electrolyte imbalances (Chapter 22). Fluid and electrolyte replacement and maintenance should be of utmost concern. Fluids with sodium chloride, bicarbonate and potassium replacement can be accomplished by oral or intravenous therapy.
1. Commercially available glucose-electrolyte supplements can be administered free-choice to diarrheic foals that are able to drink from a bucket; otherwise, they can be administered via nasogastric tube.
   a. Withhold milk from foal while administering oral fluids.

  b. Monitor plasma glucose closely and supplement as needed. These preparations will predispose to hypoglycemia if no other source of energy is available and should be used on a short term basis.
 2. I.V. fluid and electrolyte solutions should be isotonic as fluid loss is isotonic. (See Chapter 22).

E. Plasma Transfusion (Chapter 10)
 1. Indications
  a. Failure of passive transfer in presence of diarrhea + septicemia.
  b. Protein loss through inflamed bowel wall may lead to hypoproteinemia.

F. Antimicrobial Therapy (Chapter 70)
 1. Indicated in the neonate with diarrhea **and** signs of depression and anorexia because they frequently become septicemic. Selection of appropriate antimicrobials should be based on blood culture and susceptibility results.
  a. Rotavirus infected foals will not need antimicrobials if CBC is normal.
 2. Be aware of enhanced nephrotoxic potential of aminoglycosides due to decreased renal perfusion in diarrheic, hypovolemic and dehydrated foals.

G. Internal Protectants
 1. Bismuth subsalicylate. It also acts to neutralize bacterial toxins; 3-4 ounces/45 kg PO, every 6-8 hours.
 2. Kaolin and pectin; 3-4 ounces/45 kg PO, every 2-3 hours.
 3. Activated charcoal. It may act to neutralize toxins of some organisms, i.e., *Salmonella spp., Clostridium spp.*, and *E. coli*. 0.5-1.0 oz (15-30 g) /45 kg, every 12 hours, via nasogastric tube.
 4. Di-tri-octahedral smectite (Biosponge, Platinum Performance, Buellton, CA) can bind endotoxin and has been shown to neutralize toxins of C. difficile and C perfringens. 15-30 ml every 6 hours

H. Intestinal lubricant/cathartic
 1. Mineral oil. It may be used in managing overeating-induced enteritis.

2. Mucilloid via stomach tube beneficial in managing sand-induced enteritis. 1-2 ounces mucilloid (Metamucil ®, Searle and Co., San Juan, PR; Mucilose ®, Winthrop-Breon Laboratories, New York, NY).
- **I. Nonsteroidal anti-inflammatory drugs (NSAID)**
    1. Caution must be exercised because of their potential nephrotoxicity and role in gastroduodenal ulceration.
        a. Minimum effective dosage should be used.
        b. Flunixin meglumine appears to be safer than phenylbutazone.
- **J. Total Parenteral Nutrition (TPN)** should be considered along with making the severely diarrheic foal NPO if it is not so already (Chapter 23, 24).
- **K. Gastrointestinal ulcer prevention** (Chapter 34)

IX. EPIDEMIOLOGY OF FOAL DIARRHEA

- **A.** Risk factors associated with **increased** incidence of foal diarrhea.[11]
    1. Shavings for stall bedding.
    2. Prophylactic treatment of foals with antibiotics.
    3. Treatment of foals with vitamins.
    4. Foals born to non-farm resident mares.
- **B.** Risk factors associated with **decreased** incidence of foal diarrhea.[11]
    1. Stall disinfection between foaling mares.
    2. Tail wrapping and udder washing mares.
    3. Use of straw for stall bedding.
- **C.** *Salmonella spp* infections.
    1. In foals <12 weeks of age *Salmonella spp* tend to be primary cause of death whereas in older animals *Salmonella* not correlated with lesions.
    2. Serotypes include (from most common to least): *S. typhimurium, S. typhimurium var copenhagen, S. saint-paul, S. kentucky, S. muenchen, S. montevideo*, and many other serotypes.

References:

1. Pietro, J.A.: A review of *Strongyloides westeri* infection in foals. Equine Pract 11:35-39, 1989.
2. Coleman, S.V., Klei, T.R., French, D.D., et al.: Prevalence of *Cryptosporidium sp* in equids in Louisiana. Am J Vet Res 50:575-577, 1989.
3. Xiao, L, Herd, RP.: Epidemiology of equine Cryptosporidium and Giardia infections. Equine Vet J 26:14-17, 1994.
4. Frederick J, Giguère S, Sanchez LC. Infectious agents detected in the feces of diarrheic foals: a retrospective study of 233 cases (2003-2008). J Vet Intern Med. 23(6):1254-60, 2009.
5. Jones, R.L., Adney, W.S., Alexander, A.F., et al.: Hemorrhagic necrotizing enterocolitis associated with *Clostridium difficile* infection in four foals. JAVMA 193:76-79, 1988.
6. Jones, R.L., Adney, W.S., Shiderler, R.K.: Isolation of *Clostridium difficile* and detection of cytotoxin in the feces of diarrheic foals in the absence of antimicrobial treatment. J Clin Microb 25:1225-1227, 1987.
7. Cudd, T.A., Parly, T.H.: Necrotizing enterocolitis in two equine neonates. Compend Cont Educ Pract 9:88-96, 1987.
8. Dwyer, R.M.: The third report of Lloyd's foal disease project. University of Kentucky, 1989.
9. Tzipori, S., Makin, T., Smith, M., et al: Enteritis in foals induced by rotavirus and enterotoxigenic *E. coli*. Aust Vet J 58:20-23, 1982.
10. Dreyer, RM, Powell, DG, Fulker, RH, et al.: Safety and initial results of an equine rotavirus vaccine. Proceed. Amer Assoc Equine Pract. 42:316-317, 1996.
11. Traub-Dargatz, J.L., Gay, C.C., Evermann, J.F., et al: Epidemiologic survey of diarrhea in foals. JAVMA 192:1553-1556, 1988.

CHAPTER 34
GASTRODUODENAL ULCERS

The occurrence of gastric ulcer disease is not limited to foals treated with non-steroidal anti-inflammatory drugs (NSAIDS). Many foals that have not been treated with NSAIDs have gastric ulcer disease. Endoscopic studies reveal erosions and ulcers in a high percentage of foals without signs of gastric disease.

I. CLINICAL SYNDROMES[1]

A. **Asymptomatic ulcers** are subclinical ulcers usually located in the non-glandular stomach along the margo plicatus.
B. **Symptomatic ulcers** are usually non-perforating ulcers, unless there is progression to perforation, in the glandular or non-glandular stomach.
C. **Perforative ulcers** in the gastric wall or duodenum. Clinical signs are associated with acute severe peritonitis and cardiovascular collapse.
D. **Pyloric or duodenal stricture** secondary to healing and scarring of non-perforating ulcers.

II. GASTROENDOSCOPIC FINDINGS

A. **Healthy foals**.[2,3]
   1. Most lesions prevalent in foals < 10 days of age are found in the squamous mucosa immediately adjacent the margo plicatus along greater curvature.
   2. Squamous mucosa of fundus lesions less common.
   3. Squamous epithelial desquamation observed in 80% of foals < 40 days of age.
   4. Glandular mucosal lesions uncommon unless foal has symptoms.
   5. Presence of concurrent or recent **diarrhea** increases prevalence of lesions.
B. **Ill foals**.[2,3]
   1. Severe ulceration of stratified squamous mucosal epithelium adjacent to margo plicatus in young foals.
   2. Ulceration of glandular mucosa.

Chapter 34 Gastroduodenal Ulcers

3. Ulceration of stratified squamous mucosal epithelium along the lesser curvature and around cardia in older foals.
4. Diarrhea is most frequent clinical sign in foals with gastric ulcers.

III. CLINICAL SIGNS

Some of the signs of gastroduodenal ulcers in foals vary with the clinical syndrome.

A. **Diarrhea**[2,3] is the most common sign according to some studies.
B. **Teeth grinding**, salivation, gastric reflux (may be hemorrhagic), colic, dorsal recumbency, anorexia, fever, weight loss, diarrhea, "stretching-like" episodes.[1]
C. **Fever**
D. **Development of clinical signs** may follow a stressful situation such as shipping, surgery, or concurrent illness (respiratory tract disease, diarrhea, or may occur in outbreaks involving a number of foals).
E. **Because gastric ulcers** frequently develop with other problems, early accurate diagnosis is difficult.

IV. DIAGNOSIS

A. **History** of foals having diarrhea, an induced stressful situation, i.e., shipping, surgery or other illnesses; history of having been administered NSAIDs; history of farm outbreak of gastroduodenal ulcer disease. Rotavirus thought to have a role in the development of duodenal ulcers.
B. **Clinical signs**. The observation of diarrhea alone, colic, excessive salivation and teeth grinding (bruxism) is very suggestive of gastroduodenal ulcers. Other signs, as listed above, are nonspecific for gastroduodenal ulcers.
   1. Abdominal pain can sometimes be localized to xiphoid region by abdominal palpation.
C. **Gastric reflux** of foul smelling, hemorrhagic fluid.
   1. **Fecal occult blood** (Hematest™, Ames Co.), while not specific for ulcerative disease, may be positive in

diarrheas associated with gastroduodenal ulceration, parasites or mucosal ulceration associated with infectious agents.
- D. **Gastroscopy** may afford direct observation of ulcers but can be hampered by:
  1. Ingesta and gastric secretions obscuring visualization.
  2. Acute angle between cardia and pylorus.
  3. Solid food and milk should be withheld for 12 and 4 hours respectively, before gastroscopy if possible in foals over 20 days of age.
- E. **Contrast radiographic findings** consistent with duodenal stricture include a flaccid esophagus with fluid that refluxes into the esophagus from stomach, large gastric silhouette, and delayed gastric emptying (> 2 hours).
- F. **Sucrose test:** this disaccharide has been used experimentally to diagnose gastric ulceration in horses. Sucrose gets hydrolyzed to glucose and fructose in the small intestine although in gastric ulceration the sucrose gets absorbed through the injured gastric mucosa. Detection of sucrose in the blood or urine indicates gastric ulcers. The test has not been validated yet.
- G. **Abdominal ultrasound** may reveal thickened, edematous (>5mm) stomach wall. Duodenal wall may also be thickened (>3 mm) and its lumen is dilated (>3 cm). Small intestinal loops are often dilated (>3cm) with sluggish motility, all suggestive of ileus.

V. TREATMENT

- A. **Agents to decrease gastric acid via H_2 receptor antagonism**
  1. Cimetidine (Tagamet™ Glaxo, North Carolina) 4.4-6.6 mg/kg 4-6 times daily IV or 20-25mg/kg orally QID for minimum of 2 weeks. Not frequently used anymore, because of side effects and short half life.
  2. Ranitidine (Zantac™ Glaxo, North Carolina) 6.6 mg/kg BID or TID PO or 1.5 mg/kg IV TID for minimum of 2 weeks. Should be the drug of choice as an H_2-blocker.

EC - With higher dose watch for increase in liver enzymes.
3. Famotidine (Pepcid) 0.25-0.5mg/kg IV TID or 2-4mg/kg orally TID. Minimal pharmacokinetic data is available.

B. Agents to decrease gastric acid via proton pump inhibition[4-6]
1. Omeprazole (Gastrogard® Merial) is a very potent proton pump blocker. 1-4 mg/kg orally SID for 2-4 weeks or 0.5 mg/kg IV SID.
   a. Omeprazole may disrupt normal GI flora, by increasing gastric pH, and allow the proliferation of pathogens (Salmonella).
   b. Some studies suggest that sick neonates actually do not have acidic gastric environment.
2. Pantoprazole has been shown to effectively increase gastric pH, when given iv. at a dose of 1.5mg/kg SID.

C. Antacids
1. Can be used at end of other therapies to prevent reoccurrence.
2. Mylanta II™, Maalox™.

D. Mucosal protectant
1. Carafate™ (Sucralfate) 22 mg/kg 2 to 4 times daily orally.[7]
2. Can administer at same time as H_2 blockers;[8] others suggest giving 1 hour before H_2 blockers.
3. Did not heal asymptomatic ulcers.[9]

E. Therapeutic agents for reflux esophagitis or delayed gastric emptying.
1. Use agents described above.
2. Bethanecol (Urecholine®) 0.025 - 0.03 mg/kg. subcutaneously q 4 hours to aid gastric emptying.
   a. Follow by oral dosages of 0.3-0.75 mg/kg 3 to 4 times daily.
   b. Side effects: diarrhea, colic, salivation; decrease dosage.
   c. Make sure no GI obstruction is present prior to use.
3. Metoclopramide (Reglan®)
   a. 0.10-0.25 mg/kg 3 to 4 times daily orally or 0.04 mg/kg as a CRI

       b. May see adverse CNS effects, facial sweating, tachycardia.
    4. Cisapride: dose is 0.8 mg/kg orally TID.

F. Prostaglandin E synthetic agents
    1. Misoprostol (Cytotec®) (5 ug/kg TID orally) has been used to prevent ulcers in foals receiving NSAIDs and in treatment of ulcers.
       a. If colic develops may need to lower dosage.
       b. Only drug approved in humans to prevent NSAID associated gastric ulcers.
       c. Expense and concern about side effects have limited use.

    EC - May be under utilized therapy.

VI. DRUGS THAT MAY CAUSE GASTRIC ULCERS

A. Phenylbutazone
    1. 10 mg/kg/day for 10 to 42 days produces severe oral, gastrointestinal ulcers and diarrhea as early as day 3 of treatment.[10]

B. Flunixin meglumine
    1. 1.1 mg/kg/day for 30 days produces oral and gastric ulcers.
       a. Less ulcerogenic than phenylbutazone.[11]
    2. Intramuscular route produces less oral ulceration.
    3. Dosages of 0.5-1.1 mg/kg/day intravenously in 2 day old foals for 5 days did not produce gastric ulceration.[12]

B. Prevention of ulcers when using NSAIDS in foals.
    1. Study with ranitidine during phenylbutazone administration - failed to protect against ulcers[10].
    2. Misoprostol only drug that has been shown to be effective.

References:
1. Becht, J.L., Byars, T.D.: Gastroduodenal ulceration in foals. Equine Vet J 18:307, 1986.
2. Murray, M.J., Murray, C.M.: Prevalence of gastric lesions in foals without signs of gastric diseases: an endoscopic survey. Equine Vet J 22:6-8, 1990.

3. Murray, M.J.: Endoscopic appearance of gastric lesions in foals: 94 cases (1987-1988). JAVMA 195:1135-1141, 1989.
4. Sanchez, LC et. al Effect of omeperazole paste on intragastric pH in clinical normal neonatal foals. Am J Vet Res 2004.
5. Ryan CA, Sanchez LC, Giguère S, VickroyT.: Pharmacokinetics and pharmacodynamics of pantoprazole in clinically normal neonatal foals. Equine Vet J. 37(4):336-41, 2005.
6. Javsicas LH, Sanchez LC.: The effect of omeprazole paste on intragastric pH in clinically ill neonatal foals. Equine Vet J. 40(1):41-44, 2008.
7. Murray, M.J.: Gastric ulceration. In: Smith, B.P. (ed) Large Animal Internal Medicine, 4th Edition. Saunders, Philadelphia. pp 695-700, 2008.
8. Panesh, J.Z., et al: Is an acid pH medium required for the protective effect of sucralfate against mucosal injury? Amer J Med 83(Suppl 3B):11-15, 1987.
9. Borne, AT, MacAllister, CG.: Effect of sucralfate on healing of subclinical gastric ulcers in foals. J Am Vet Med Assoc 202:1465-1468, 1993.
10. Traub, J.L., Gallina, A.M., Grand, B.D., Reed, S.M., Gavin, P.R., Paulsen, L.M.: Phenylbutazone toxicosis in the foal. Am J Vet Res 44:1410, 1983.
11. Traub-Dargatz, J.L., Bertone, J.J., Gould, D.H.: Chronic flunixin meglumine therapy in foals. Am J Vet Res 49:7-12, 1988.
12. Carrick, J.B., Papich, M., Middleton, D.: The effect of the administration of flunixin meglumine on the gastrointestinal tract of foals. Abstract. Proceed ACVIM, 5th forum, p 902, 1987.

CHAPTER 35
NEONATAL ISOERYTHROLYSIS

Neonatal isoerythrolysis (N.I.) is an immune-mediated hemolytic disorder of newborn foals due to absorption of colostral immunoglobulins which contain antibodies against red cell antigens inherited from the stallion. The problem is seen most commonly in multiparous Aa or Qa negative mares due to sensitization to blood group factors during pregnancy or blood transfusion. Other antigens may cause NI occasionally (Ua, Pa, Qc, Db). Recent reports indicate some donkey-mare matings have produced NI in mule foals. Ca antibodies may prevent NI through antibody-mediated immunosuppresion[1].

I. CLINICAL FEATURES

A. **Foal from high risk mare** - foals are normal at birth and only develop clinical signs after ingestion of colostrum.
B. **Signs vary** with rate and severity of erythrocyte destruction.
C. **Progressively developing anemia**, icterus or rarely hemoglobinuria leading to depression, anorexia, collapse, death.
D. **Symptoms more severe** and prognosis poorer in foals with obvious signs at 12 to 24 hours of age due to rapid loss of red cells. Significant signs may not be apparent until 3 to 4 days of age in foals with milder forms.
E. **Neonatal isoerythrolysis in mule foals**[2,3]
A RBC antigen of some donkeys is not found in mares. Donkeys with this antigen mated to mares may sensitize mares to produce antibody to this antigen which may be inherited by the mule foal offspring of the mating. Typical NI reported in several mule foals. Test by screening serum of mares bred to donkeys when mares are in last trimester. If positive for antibody to donkey antigen, withhold colostrum from newborn and provide alternate source of colostrum to newborn mule.

II. LABORATORY FEATURES AND DIAGNOSIS[4]

A. **Progressive hemolytic anemia.**
B. **Hyperbilirubinemia** - elevation of both direct and indirect bilirubin.
C. **Blood typing** (Serology Laboratory).
D. **Hypoglycemia** and acidosis may be present concurrently.
E. **Coombs test**
F. **Flow cytometry**
G. **Serial tube agglutination test**[5] (Jaundice Foal Agglutination Test- JFA-test)
   1. **Collect EDTA** tube blood sample from the foal before it nurses.
   2. **Collect colostrum** from the mare and filter though gauze.
   3. **Set out** 6 clean test tubes in a rack. Add 1 ml of normal saline at room temperature to each tube and label each tube.
   4. **In the first tube**, add 1 ml of colostrum and mix well. This will be a 1:1 ratio.
   5. **In the second tube**, a 1:2 ratio is established. This is done by pipetting 1 ml of the mixture of the first tube and mixing it in the second tube.
   6. **Pipet out** 1 ml of the mixture of the second tube and put in the third tube to obtain a 1:4 ratio.
   7. **Continue** this procedure down to the sixth tube until a 1:32 ratio is obtained. Pipet 1 ml from this mixture and save for further dilution if necessary.
   8. **Place one drop** of whole blood from the foal into each of the test tubes, mix gently and centrifuge at 1500 rpm for 3 minutes. The ratios should be:
      Tube #1 1:1   Tube #4 1:8
      Tube #2 1:2   Tube #5 1:16
      Tube #3 1:4   Tube #6 1:32

Interpretation of the Results:
Negative test: hold the test tube at a 30 degree tilt. A precipitate will form a streak which will stretch one inch and more.
Positive test: If the precipitate (plug) doesn't streak (or very little).
If the test shows a strong positive at a 1:4 dilution but a weak positive at 1:8, let the foal nurse but watch very carefully!

If the result shows a strong positive at a 1:8 dilution, or greater, don't let the foal nurse!

If there is a positive reaction with foal's cells repeat with mare's RBC to validate procedure.

III. TREATMENT BLOOD TRANSFUSION

A. **Best results** when administered prior to the onset of severe signs.
B. **Indications**
1. RBC <3 X 10^6/ul, PCV <14%, Hgb <5 g/dl.
2. Evidence of progressive decline in these parameters and hypovolemia.
C. **Erythrocyte donor**
1. Washed erythrocytes (0.5-2L) from the dam. (Washed 1-3 times by centrifugation in isotonic (0.9%) saline under sterile conditions).
   a. Administer shortly after washing because cells do not store well and risk of bacterial contamination is high.
   b. Resuspend cells to make a 50% solution of red cells and isotonic saline (0.9% NaCl).
   c. Administer 1 L/hour of this 50% suspension I.V.
      i. Blood from an unrelated donor whose blood is compatible with the dam and the foal (may be difficult to find).
      ii. Do not use sire of foal as donor.
D. **Monitor** clinical and hematologic response. Repeat transfusion may be necessary.
E. **Multiple transfusions** associated with histologic evidence of iron-toxicity, development of liver failure and decreased survival rates[6].
F. **Synthetic Hemoglobin products** (Oxyglobin®, Biopure, Cambridge, MA) can be used if blood is not readily available (5-7.5ml/kg).
G. **Exchange Transfusion**- to avoid kernicterus, practitioners in New Zealand often do an exchange transfusion on severe acute NI cases. Better success and long RBC life occurs when done with washed RBCs from the mare: 4-5 liters of washed maternal RBC is

administered in one jugular vein and an equal amount of blood is taken from other jugular at the same rate into a collection vial that allows matching of volumes in and out. This removes bilirubin and anti-RBC antibody that would be active against remaining foal RBC inherited from sire.

IV. SUPPORTIVE CARE

A. **Minimize stress**, and exercise- stall rest is imperative.
B. **Provide monitoring** and supportive care depending on degree of clinical signs. N.I. foals need a warm, dry environment, adequate IV fluids, correction of hypoglycemia, or acidosis and monitoring for concurrent infection. **EC** - be careful with volumes of IV fluids - can drop PCV even lower.
C. **Hyperbilirubinemia** is a very serious complication and can produce permanent damage to basal ganglia region of brain (kernicterus). Mild cases have clinical signs of dysphagia and inability to suck and prehend food. Moderate and severe cases will develop coma and eventually die (usually if total bilirubin>20-30 mg/dl). (See Exchange Transfusion)
D. **Sepsis** due to partial failure of passive transfer of adequate antibodies, due to compromised hepatobiliary function, or due to tissue hypoxia and enhanced translocation. Administer antimicrobials to minimize the risk.
E. **Liver failure** can occur in severe cases. Several contributing factors have been proposed including hypoxia, immune complex deposition, cholangiopathy due to bile stasis and iron toxicity. Recent study has shown histologic evidence of centrolobular necrosis and increased number of siderophages within the liver supporting the theory of iron toxicity[6].

V. MANAGEMENT OF THE N.I. MARE

A. **Observe** foaling and do not allow foal to nurse mare.
B. **Milk mare by hand.**
C. **Provide alternative** colostrum from colostrum bank tested negative for alloantibodies.

D. Allow visual access to mare or muzzle foal until colostrum milked from mare. Allow a minimum of 18 hours to pass before foal nurses. Make sure that the foal has received adequate colostrum or plasma transfusion from another source and serum IgG indicates adequate passive transfer. Check milk via colostrometer and it may be possible to return the foal to the mare earlier.

VI. PREVENTION[5]

A. **Screen mares** to be bred by blood typing. Blood for typing and detection of the presence of antierythrocyte antibodies is collected and mailed to Serology Lab.[a] One clotted or serum tube and one whole blood tube with acid-citrate-dextrose (ACD) anticoagulant are required. Mares that are Aa or Qa negative are at higher risk delivering a possible NI foal.
B. **Mares at risk:**
   1. Known to have had a previous foal with N.I.
   2. Known to be Aa or Qa negative.
C. **Evaluate antierythrocyte antibody titer** in the last 2-3 weeks of pregnancy. Earlier blood tests may be negative because the antierythrocyte antibodies rise during pregnancy.
   1. If hemolysin titer >1:4, withhold colostrum.
   2. Anti Ca antibody not known to produce NI.
   3. Provide antibodies to foal via alternate source of colostrum or plasma tested free of alloantibodies.
D. **Breed to a stallion without A or Q antigens.**
E. **Anti-C antibody** is found in mares with C negative blood type.
   1. No documented cases of an anti C mediated N.I. disease.
   2. If extremely high titers of anti C are found in a pregnant mare, should run the colostrum Serial Tube Agglutination Test (JFA test).
F. **Serial tube agglutination test (Laboratory Features, Section G).**
   1. This field test has been used for many years by veterinary practitioners and appears to be an aid in

determining if the foal should be prevented from nursing.
2. It is based on presence of agglutinins and not hemolysins. Agglutinins are believed present with hemolysins in all but Q system with R or S factors. The serial tube agglutination test will fail to indicate the presence of antibodies to these factors in the colostrum and regular serum screening for iso-antibodies must be used.

References:
1. Horohov, D., Lunn, P.: The equine immune system in Reed, S. M., Bayly, W. M., Sellon, D. C. (eds.): Equine Internal Medicine, 2nd Edition 1-59. WB. Saunders, St. Louis, 2004.
2. Boyle AG, Magdesian KG, Ruby RE: Neonatal isoerythrolysis in horse foals and a mule foal: 18 cases (1988-2003). J Am Vet Med Assoc. 15;227(8):1276-83, 2005.
3. Traub-Dargatz, JL, McClure, JJ, Kosh, C. et al.: Neonatal isoerythrolysis in mule foals. JAVMA. 206:67-70, 1995.
4. Haggett, E.: Icterus in foals. Teaching Material. UC Davis. 2008.
5. Bailey, E., Conboy, H.S., McCarthy, P.F.: Neonatal isoerythrolysis of foals; an update on testing. Proced Amer Assoc Equine Pract 1987, pp 123-132.
6. Polkes AC, Giguère S, Lester GD, Bain FT.: Factors associated with outcome in foals with neonatal isoerythrolysis (72 cases, 1988-2003). J Vet Intern Med. 2008 Sep-Oct;22(5):1216-22
    [a] Veterinary Genetics Laboratory
    University of California
    School of Veterinary Medicine
    One Shields Ave, Davis CA-95616, USA
    +1 530-752-2211. www.vgl.ucdavis.edu

CHAPTER 36
RENAL DISORDERS OF EQUINE NEONATES

The equine neonatal kidney is reasonably mature in its ability to excrete electrolytes (except Na), and excrete drugs via glomerular filtration[1]. **EC-** This means that neonatal foals are NOT more sensitive to aminoglycosides like gentamicin and amikacin than adults provided they are not dehydrated.

I. ETIOLOGY OF RENAL DISEASE IN EQUINE NEONATE

A. **Pre-renal** cause due to inadequate perfusion of functional kidneys is the most common condition.
  1. Dehydration - sunken eyes, poor pulse.
  2. Asphyxia damage occurring during cesarean section, dystocia, induction of parturition.
  3. Diarrhea, inadequate fluid intake.
B. **Renal causes are primarily due to gram negative sepsis** causing inflammatory foci, bacterial colonization of the kidney, and tubular necrosis from prolonged reduced renal blood flow and ischemia associated with shock, enteritis or surgical and gastrointestinal problems. Fibrin may also deposited in the renal capillaries and glomeruli due to DIC.
  1. Neonatal isoerthyrolysis can produce hemoglobin nephrosis.
  2. NSAID drugs accompanied by hypovolemia may significantly reduce renal blood flow.
  3. Aminoglycoside toxicity is uncommon if hydration is maintained in ill foals.
      a. Ill foals treated with aminoglycosides and undergoing anesthesia may be most susceptible to aminoglycosides.
  4. Tetracycline overdose associated with attempts to treat contracted tendons has been observed.
C. **Post-renal causes include**, urachal tearing, urethral obstruction, ruptured bladder, ureter rents.
  1. Ureter defect in foals aged 5-6 days - off feed, urinalysis normal, peritoneal tap normal, post renal azotemia, vaginal edema, perineal edema, swollen

sheath. Urine accumulates in retroperitoneal space; bilateral defect adjacent to kidney. May be repairable.

II. CLINICAL SIGNS AND DIAGNOSIS

A. **Oliguria** is uncommon with acute renal failure in neonates.
   1. Foals produce approximately 6-10 ml/kg/hr of urine
   2. Catheterize bladder to confirm after IV fluid treatment
   3. Lasix to induce urine formation.
   4. Dobutamine drip at 2-10 ug/kg/min IV.
   5. Norepinephrine at 0.1-1.5 µg/kg/min IV.
B. **Specific clinical signs** may not be seen but suspect renal involvement with sepsis, dehydration, prematurity and other disorders.
C. **Creatinine levels**[2]
   1. Some <24 hour old foals **without** severe renal disease can have elevated serum creatinine concentrations (4-23 mg/dl). Cause is usually placentitis and creatinine is lower on day two and drops over 3-5 days to normal (<2 mg/dl).
   2. A single elevated serum creatinine determination is not diagnostic. However, serial determination over several days with fluid support and rising creatinine is indicative of renal disease or post renal problems.
D. **BUN levels rise with renal disease**. Values on day 1 and 2 reflect maternal levels.
E. **Urinalysis**[2]
   1. Caution must be used because the normal foal values are distinctly different than adults. Normal equine neonate has proteinuria for first 36 hours of life, urine pH 6-7, and specific gravity 1.001-1.012.
   2. Mild hematuria can be seen nonspecifically in sick foals.
   3. Abnormalities are > 2 + occult blood, casts, bacteria and leukocytes.
   4. Fractional excretion of electrolytes has been estimated in a limited number of foals < 7 days of age, on a milk diet FxNa 0.31% ± 0.18, Fx K 13.26% ± 4.49, Fx PO_4 3.11% ± 3.81[3]

5. Urine Gamma GT/creatinine ratio 12.5 - 46.15 in normal foals < 14 days of age.[2]
6. Urine volume produced is ≈148 l/kg/day.[3]

III. MANAGEMENT OF RENAL DISEASE

A. **Provide** adequate fluids by oral or intravenous route. Weigh foal twice daily and observe for overhydration.
B. **Determine** if post-renal problems exist.
C. **Avoid** NSAID if possible.
D. **Limit** sodium and potassium containing fluids because foal has limited ability to excrete - monitor serum levels.
E. **Modify** dose of aminoglycosides.
F. **Hyperkalemia (life threatening) may be treated with:**
   1. Sodium bicarbonate 1-2 mEq/kg IV over 30 minutes.
      a. Check pH and be sure foal is ventilating adequately.
   2. Calcium gluconate 10% 0.5-1.0 ml/kg IV over 15 minutes.
   3. Glucose infusion 5% IV 100 ml over 15 minutes.
   4. Glucose IV plus 0.1 units of insulin/kg (regular insulin).
      a. Closely monitor for hypoglycemia.
   5. Sodium polystyrene sulfonate exchange resin 15 gms/100 ml of 10% dextrose via enema. Monitor serum K^+ and Na^+ closely.

IV. CONGENITAL PROBLEMS

A. Bilateral renal dysplasia with nephron hypoplasia.[4]
   1. Depression and lethargy at < 48 hours of age.
   2. Hyponatremia, hypochloremia, azotemia, hypoproteinemia.
   3. Urinalysis - 1+ blood, 3+ proteinuria, increased FE Na, increased GGT/Cr ratio.
   4. Renal biopsy - tubular hypoplasia with secondary necrosis.
   5. Ultrasound - cystic appearing lesions.
B. Renal hypoplasia and dysplasia.
   1. Disease may manifest in neonatal period.

References:
1. Brewer, B.D., Clement, S.F., Lotz, W.S., et al.: A comparison of Inulin, para-aminohippuric acid, and endogenous creatinine clearances as measures of renal functions in neonatal foals. J Vet Int Med 4:301-305, 1990.
2. Koterba A.M., Adams R., McClure J.R., et al.: Renal and urinary tract function and dysfunction in the neonatal foal. Proc of Amer Assoc Equine Pract 659-671, 1985.
3. Brewer, B.D., et al: Renal clearance, urinary excretion of exogenous substances and urinary diagnostic indices in healthy neonatal foals. J Vet Int Med 5: 28-33, 1991.
4. Zicker, S.C., Marty, G.D., Carlson, G.P., et al.: Bilateral renal hypoplasia with nephron hypoplasia in a foal. JAVMA 196:2001-2005, 1990.

CHAPTER 37
RUPTURED BLADDER & UROPERITONEUM

There are several causes of uroperitoneum in the neonatal foal. Ruptured bladder is the most common. Urachal rents (tears) can also produce uroperitoneum. Congenital or traumatic lesions of the ureter may produce uroperitoneum or retroperitoneal urine accumulation.[1]

I. RUPTURED BLADDER

A. History
1. **Male & female foals**.
2. **Clinical** signs develop by less than 7 days of age, usually after day 2.
3. **Foal** appears normal at birth.
    a. Exception is megavesica secondary to umbilical cord torsion and obstruction of urachus.[2]
        i. Signs seen at birth.
4. In some hypoxic ischemic encephalopathy (HIE) foals occurs because for a period of time foals don't perceive bladder as full.
   EC- always check the bladder with ultrasound on HIE foals

B. Clinical Signs[3-5]
1. **Depression**, gradual anorexia (milk may accumulate on foal's head from mammary gland dripping).
2. **± abdominal pain**, usually mild.
3. **Abdominal distension** (uroperitoneum) - may feel percussion waves across abdomen; rapid shallow breathing.
4. **Intestinal ileus.**
5. **Dysuria and/or stranguria** (dorsal-ventral flexion of the back and legs extended caudally), decreased frequency and volume of urine.
6. **Dribbling urine.**
7. **Some septicemic** foals develop ruptured bladder associated with cystitis.

C. Diagnosis
1. **History** and clinic signs.

2. **Abdominal ultrasonography**
   a. Free peritoneal fluid.
   b. Inability to identify intact bladder.
3. **Abdominal paracentesis** - large volume of fluid. May occasionally smell like ammonia.
4. **Compare serum creatinine** vs. that in peritoneal fluid.
   a. If abdominal fluid is urine, creatinine measured in peritoneal fluid should be higher (1.75 - 2X) than that of serum.
   b. BUN is not as reliable due to equilibration with plasma.
   c. K^+ in serum compared to peritoneal fluid is not reliable.
   d. Foals may or may not be azotemic.
5. **Retrograde injection** of new methylene-blue into bladder and look for dye in peritoneal fluid via paracentesis.[5]
   EC - Make sure new methylene-blue is sterile.
6. **Contrast bladder radiography** - use aqueous based organic iodine solutions.
7. **Blood gas and electrolyte imbalances** (hyponatremia, hypochloremia, hyperkalemia and acidosis).
   a. These may be seen with conditions other than ruptured bladder.
   b. Electrolytes may be normal if foal has been on IV fluids.

D. **Differential**
   1. **Most often** confused with septic foal or neurologic case when presented in semi coma.
   2. **Hyponatremia** may produce neurologic symptoms.

E. **Subcutaneous rupture of the urachus.**[6]
   1. Fluctuant non painful swelling in umbilical region noted at 5-30 hours of age.
   2. Differentiate from hernia because cannot reduce this swelling with palpation.
   3. Aspirated fluid has increased creatinine or BUN.
   4. Urine may be confined to subcutaneous tissue or dissect to peritoneum and cause uroperitoneum.
   5. Prompt surgical correction indicated.

II. URACHAL RENT AND UROPERITONEUM

- **A. History and clinical signs** are similar to ruptured bladder.
- **B. Concurrent infection of the urachus**.
    1. Associated with septicemia, prematurity, or ICU foal.
    2. Associated with patent urachus.
    3. Associated with urachal infection and cystitis.
- **C. Peritoneal fluid**
    1. Inflammatory cells and increased protein.
    2. Creatinine - is 2X that of serum creatinine.
- **D. Treatment is** immediate surgical correction and aggressive antibiotic therapy and nursing care; plasma transfusion, etc.
- **E.** Ureter stenosis and ureter defect has been described as a cause of uroperitoneum in a foal[7].

III. RUPTURED BLADDER TREATMENT - MEDICAL

- **A. Nonsurgical**
    1. Small leaks have been managed with an indwelling urinary catheter[8] (Levine naso-gastric tube) especially if foal has other problems and is a surgical risk (respiratory problems-pneumonia).
    2. Hyperkalemia can cause death; Do not administer K^+ containing antibiotics or I.V. fluids (use 0.9% saline).

IV. SURGICAL CONSIDERATIONS [9]

- **A. Necessary** for all large defects in the bladder or urachus.
- **B. Detailed surgical** description can be found in Reference 9
- **C. Replace and correct** fluid, electrolyte and blood gas abnormalities before anesthetic induction[10, 11]
- **D. Slowly draining** urine from abdomen before surgery is controversial. Foals have developed peritonitis from this effort; conversely rapid loss of fluid from abdomen during surgery may potentiate shock.
- **E. Incision** is made 2-3 cm paramedian to prepuce or prepuce can be reflected and incisions made on midline.

- F. If urachus is the site of the tear, remove along with umbilicus and use Parker-Kerr over sew with Vicryl®.
- G. **Tears** are usually located dorsally on the bladder.
- H. **If tear** is not easily visible, bladder can be distended with a pre-placed urinary catheter (Levine tube). Leave tube in place 2-3 days post-surgically.
- I. **Drain urine** off slowly, if not accomplished before surgery.
- J. Use Vicryl ® Ethicon Sutures (absorbable) in bladder.
  1. Non-absorbable sutures serve as nidus for stones and infection.
- K. **Post operative care** -Leave catheter in bladder if not voiding urine post-surgically. <u>Some foals may need 2-5 days of catheterization because they do not perceive bladder distension</u>. That is how it ruptured in the first place in some foals.

V. PROGNOSIS

- A. In non-infected foals outcome is good.
- B. In those with concurrent infection or other gastrointestinal problems - 50% survival.[5]
- C. Repeat rupture in some foals- need catheterization – some for 7 days.

References:
1. Robertson, J.T., Spurlock, G.H., Bramlage, and L.L., et al.: Repair of a ureteral defect in a foal. <u>J Am Vet Med Assoc</u> 183:799-800, 1983.
2. Rossdale, P.D., Greet, T.R.C.: Mega Vesica in a newborn foal. <u>ISVP Newsletter</u> 2:10-13, 1989.
3. <u>The Practice of Large Animal Surgery.</u> Jennings P.B. (ed). W.B. Saunders, Philadelphia, 1984.
4. Vaughn J.T., Walker D.F.: <u>Bovine and Equine Urogenital Surgery</u>. Lea and Febiger, Philadelphia, 1980.
5. Adams, R., Koterba, and A.M.: Exploratory celiotomy for suspected urinary tract disruption in neonatal foals: A review of 18 cases. <u>Equine Vet J</u> 20:13-17, 1988.
6. Lees, M.J., Easley, K.J., Sutherland, R.J., et al. Subcutaneous rupture of the urachus, its diagnosis and surgical management in three foals. <u>Equine Vet J</u> 21:462-464, 1989.

7. Morisset S, Hawkins JF, Frank N, Sojka JE, Berg D, Blevins WE Surgical management of a ureteral defect with ureterorrhaphy and of ureteritis with ureteroneocystostomy in a foal. J Am Vet Med Assoc. 220(3):354-358, 323, 2002.
8. Lavoie J.P., Harnagel, S.H.: Nonsurgical management of ruptured urinary bladder in a critically ill foal. JAVMA 192:1577-80, 1988.
9. Auer, J. A. Equine Surgery: Stick, J. A. (Ed). *3rd. ed.*, WB Saunders, Philadelphia, pp. 202-218, 616-623., 623-629, 2006.
10. Kablack KA, Embertson RM, Bernard WV, et al. Uroperitoneum in the hospitalized equine neonate: Retrospective study of 31 cases, 1988–1997. Equine Vet J. 32:505–508, 2000.
11. Dunkel B, Palmer JE, Olson KN, Boston RC, Wilkins PA. Uroperitoneum in 32 foals: influence of intravenous fluid therapy, infection, and sepsis. J Vet Intern Med. 19:889–893, 2005.

CHAPTER 38
SEPTIC ARTHRITIS AND OSTEOMEYLITIS

Joint and bone infection are a sequel to bacteremia in neonatal foals. Common names for this condition are: joint-ill, navel ill, infectious arthritis, septic polyarthritis, septic epiphysitis, and septic physitis.[1] Rapid diagnosis and aggressive therapy are important in preventing irreversible cartilage or bone damage. It is most common in foals less than 30 days. Most commonly isolated organisms are gram-negative enteric organisms including *E. coli*, *Actinobacillus suis* like spp., *Klebsiella pneumoniae,* and less commonly *Salmonella* spp.[2] Several bacterial species may be recovered from the same foal or joint.

I. **SOURCES OF INFECTION**
   Previous or concurrent bacteremia ± failure of passive transfer

   A. **Gastrointestinal tract**
      1. Probably most common portal of entry
      2. May or may not be associated with obvious signs of diarrhea or enteritis
      3. Diarrhea may have occurred 20 to 30 days previously - signs of a single joint infection then develop in a bright, alert foal
   B. **Umbilical infection**
      1. Often exterior of navel appears normal, but can also be enlarged or swollen.
      2. Infection may be associated with umbilical arteries, vein or urachus
      3. Ultrasound may assist with diagnosis
   C. **Concurrent pneumonia**
      1. Concurrent pneumonia in approximately 35% cases
      2. Pneumonic lesion often focal
   D. **Penetrating wounds** - rare in young foals (<60 day). More common in older foals
   E. Extension into joint from adjacent osteomyelitis
   F. Intra-muscular abscess - uncommon

Chapter 38 Septic Arthritis and Osteomeylitis

II. CLINICAL SIGNS

- A. Sudden onset of lameness with or without joint distension, pain and edema.
- B. Swollen joints with or without periarticular edema in a recumbent foal
- C. Sudden onset of lameness with systemic signs of illness - i.e. fever, depression, diarrhea or anorexia
- D. Sudden onset of lameness without systemic signs of illness - i.e. bright, alert foal
- E. Onset of stiffness, with back or neck pain and a low grade fever - consider vertebral osteomeylitis
- F. Sudden onset of lameness with owner history of trauma to foal (mare stepped on foal). In foal less than 45 days, any lameness should be <u>proven NOT to be related to an infectious</u> etiology.
- G. More than one joint may be involved in approximately 50% of cases

III. DIAGNOSIS

- A. Evidence of septicemia and above clinical signs. Older foals can be bright and alert.
- B. Fever, lameness (joint swelling in recumbent foal), inflammation, hemogram, leukocytosis ± joint swelling and periarticular edema
- C. **Ultrasound of joint** (See Chapter 52 section V. MUSCULOSKELETAL IMAGING)
- D. **Joint aspiration**
    1. Aseptic technique; shave or clip, prep, gloves, etc
    2. If concerned about passing needle through periarticular edema, may instill 0.5 ml gentomicin following aspiration of synovial fluid
    3. Synovial fluid examination[2]
        - a. May be normal with bone infection prior to invasion into synovia or with an open draining wound
        - b. Color - cloudy, turbid, flocculent fluid and low viscosity
        - c. Normal 800 WBC/µl - greater than 1000 WBC/µl with 70% neutrophils suspect infection

d. Normal total protein <1g/dl - greater than 2.5 g/dl may be infection or trauma
 e. Fibrin clots may clump and lower WBC count - may cause difficulty in aspirating fluid
 f. Gram stain may reveal intracellular and extracellular bacteria

D. Culture synovial fluid[2]
 1. Aseptic technique
 2. Aerobic and anaerobic cultures
 3. Media - thioglycolate broth or brain, heart broth w/agar slant and SPS to prevent clotting
 4. Attempt culture even if foal is receiving antimicrobials - recovery of bacteria only slightly less than foals not receiving antimicrobials

E. Culture of blood
 1. Culture any foal with systemic signs or those foals <14 days
 2. Greater probability of obtaining causative organism than joint culture - do both joint and blood culture
 3. Excellent correlation between joint and culture of blood - if joint culture negative assume infected with organism(s) cultured from blood[2]
 4. Significant number of foals have more than one bacterial species

F. Ultrasonography (Chapter 52 Section V Musculoskeletal Ultrasound)
 1. Very sensitive at determining synovial effusion, proliferative synovial membrane and presence of intra-articular fibrin
 2. Useful in determining location for needle placement to obtain synovial fluid
 3. Assess cartilage damage
 4. Appearance: Normal - small amount anechoic fluid; Synovial effusion without infection - large quantity anechoic fluid; Synovial effusion with infection - large quantity echoic fluid (note: echoic may be blood - require synovial aspirate)
 5. Very sensitive to detect osteomeylitis - echoic fluid >2mm between periosteum and bone cortex

G. Radiography
1. May be normal on initial examination - repeat in 5-7 days
2. Examine metaphysis, physis or epiphysis for osteolysis, sclerosis, or reactive cortical bone
3. Soft tissue swelling

IV. TREATMENT

A. **Treat early** - within hours. Consider as a medical emergency. If suspect infection due to clinical signs and synovial fluid appearance - treat aggressively before obtaining results of synovial aspirate[3]
B. Broad spectrum bacteriocidal antimicrobials given systemically with activity against gram negative and gram positive bacteria. Commence immediately - prior to results of culture and sensitivity. Ideal choice amikacin and ampicillin or first generation cephalosporin - effective against 93% isolates.[2] Other less broad spectrum: gentocin with ampicillin/penicillin; chloramphicol, 3rd generation cephalosporins. Procaine penicillin is least appropriate. Cases of resistant Salmonella strains may be treated with Enrofloxacin or Imipenem. (Chapter 70)
C. **Intra-articular antimicrobials**[4]
   1. Can combine with systemic antimicrobial therapy
   2. Inject 0.5 mls of 50mg/ml gentocin (25mg) or 0.5 mls 250 mg/ml amikacin (125 mg) into joint
   3. Do not buffer solution
   4. Use along with drainage and lavage and systemic antimicrobials and anti-inflammatory drugs
   5. Injecting multiple joints could potentially raise gentocin or amikacin levels to toxic levels
D. **Regional Limb Perfusion**[5-7]
   1. **Advantages**
      a. High and persistent concentrations in joints (up to 100 x concentration after IV administration)
      b. MIC of many bacteria exceeded for 24 hours
      c. Infusate reaches peri-articular tissues, bone, synovium
      d. Infusate reaches normal, inflamed, necrotic tissue

    e. Outcome of treatment of orthopedic infection better than with conventional IV administration
  2. **Method**
     a. Anesthesia or deep sedation
     b. Catheter - 20 gauge x 2.5 inch
     c. Tourniquet placed proximal to the joint involved - 30 minute duration
     d. Dosages used in foals
        - Amikacin - 50 mg in 10 to 12 ml of saline
        - Gentamicin - 50 mg in 10 to 12 ml of saline
        - Imipenem may be used in very valuable animals with resistant infections, 200 mg in 10 ml of saline
E. **Assure adequate serum immunoglobulin concentration**
F. **Drainage** - mechanical lavage and removal of debris.
  1. Removal of degenerative neutrophils, fibrin, high WBC, proteolytic enzymes, will benefit from aspiration and flush.
  2. Flush
     a. Distension - irrigation with one puncture and 3-way stopcock and 2 syringes with saline or preferably lactated Ringer's. Use 500 ml to 1 liter total volume.
     b. Through and through - two needles in joint and continuous lavage of 1 - 2 liters sterile fluid.
  3. Dilute Betadine® **no** advantage over saline
  4. **Arthroscopy** - allows look at cartilage, removal of fibrin and synovectomy (removal of bacteria sequestered in synovial membrane) in addition to flushing joint. Submit synovial biopsy for culture
  5. **Flushing** generally repeated until WBC <30,000 cell/µl (clinical impression)
  6. **Arthrotomy**
     a. Previously indicated for advanced cases which were refractory to flushing, but is effective in acute cases.
     b. Arthrotomy in distal portion of joint ± penrose drain (I do not use due to risk of ascending infection) and sterile wraps (changable stent bandage over more proximal joints) - healing by

second intention or delayed primary healing if joint infection resolved.
G. **Curettage** of physeal lesions
H. **Use of antimicrobial impregnated beads** placed adjacent to bone - under sterile conditions mix antimicrobial with poly methyl methacrolate, string together beads and place surgically adjacent to lesion. Gives increased concentrations locally.
I. **Interosseous antimicrobial perfusion**.[6] Useful to increase concentration of antimicrobial agent to infected joint and bone in distal limb. Place tourniquet proximal to lesion - place canulated screw distal to tourniquet into medullary cavity - infuse systemic dose of antimicrobial into medullary cavity. Care to avoid toxicity if systemic antimicrobials are being administered.
J. **Immobilization of joint** - splints and support wraps
K. **Pain control**
   1. Low dose NSAID over short time - weigh foal to prevent overdose and measure dose carefully.
   2. Banamine™ (flunixin meglumine) IM or IV for five days did not produce ulcers in foals. Phenylbutazone more ulcerogenic[9]
L. **Post infection treatment**
   1. Synovial fluid transfer or intra-articular hyaluronic acid to decrease pain and persistent inflammation. **EC** –Consider avoiding intra-articular Adequan™ following therapy-some joints have re-inflamed-unknown if potentiates infection if organisms remain in joint?
   2. Systemic hyalauronic acid or Adequan™ may improve joint environment
M. **Correction or treatment of underlying nidus** of infection or systemic disorders

V. **PROGNOSIS- General comments**

Good with early treatment (1st day), broad spectrum systemically administered antimicrobials, aggressive flushing/drainage of joint, regional limb perfusion where indicated and better prognosis with the absence of bone involvement.

Poor with a delay in treatment, use of procaine penicillin only and radiographic evidence of bone involvement, and failure to treat underlying septicemia.

References:
1. Martins R.J., Ayer J.A., Carter G.K.: Equine pediatrics: Septic arthritis and osteomeylitis. JAVMA 188:582, 1986.
2. Vatistas N.J., Wilson W.D., JR Pascoe J.R. et al.: Septic arthritis in foals: Bacterial isolates and antimicrobial susceptibility. Proc. 7th Int Conference Equine Infectious Disease, Tokyo, Japan Nakajima, H.Plowright, W. (eds.). R and W Publications Ltd. p. 359-360 1994,
3. Vatistas N.J., Wilson W.D., JR Pascoe J.R. et al. Septic arthritis in 140 neonatal foals (1978-1992): factors affecting prognosis, and long term outlook. (In press)
4. Lloyd K.C., Stover S.M., Pascoe J.R. Et al.: Synovial fluid pH, cytologic characteristics, and gentamicin concentration after intra-articular administration of the drug in an experimental model of infectious arthritis in horses. Am J Vet Res 51:1363-1369, 1990.
5. Scheuch BC et. al. Comparison of intraosseous or intravenous infusion for delivery of amikacin sulfate to the tibiotarsal joint of horses. Am J Vet Res 63-374-380, 2002.
6. Rubio-Martínez LM, Cruz AM.: Antimicrobial regional limb perfusion in horses. J Am Vet Med Assoc. 228(5):706-12, 655, 2006,
7. Rubio-Martínez LM, López-Sanromán J, Cruz AM, Santos M, Andrés MS, Román FS.: Evaluation of safety and pharmacokinetics of vancomycin after intravenous regional limb perfusion in horses. Am J Vet Res. 66(12):2107-13, 2005.
8. Whitehair K.J., Bowersock T.L., Blevins W.E., et al: Regional limb perfusion for antibiotic treatment of experimentally induced septic arthritis. Veterinary Surgery. 21:367-373, 1992.
9. Carreck J.B., et al.: The effect of the administration of flunixin meglumine on the gastrointestinal tract of foals. Abstract Proceed ACVIM 5th forum. P 702, 1987.

CHAPTER 39
UMBILICAL PROBLEMS

The umbilicus consists of 3 structures and undergoes functional and anatomic changes at birth. **Two umbilical arteries** connect internal iliac arteries; these regress to become the round ligaments of the bladder. One **umbilical vein** connecting the placenta to the liver and portal cava, regresses to become the round ligament of the liver within the falciform ligament. The **urachus** connects the fetal bladder to the allantoic cavity.

I. DIAGNOSIS OF UMBILICAL DISORDERS

   A. **Palpation**
      1. Allows detection of gross enlargement, hernias, etc.
   B. **Ultrasonography**[1,2] - (See chapter 52).
      1. Use 7.5-10 MHz with standoff transducer and sector scanner.
      2. Valuable in detecting enlargements of the umbilical arteries, vein and urachus.

II. UMBILICAL ABSCESSATION – Extra-abdominal

   A. **Clinical signs** are enlarged navel, which may be hot, swollen and painful, in a foal usually >1 week of age that often is showing no signs of systemic infection because abscess is extra-abdominal.
   B. **Diagnosis**
      1. History and clinical signs with or without ultrasound examination of area.
      2. Differentiate from a hernia by palpation and needle aspiration.
      3. Include a good physical exam and hematology to evaluate systemic component.
   C. **Treatment**
      1. **Medical** - if the foal is clinically normal and laboratory values and physical exam reveal no abnormalities, manage by hot packs, and drainage ± systemic antibiotics.
         a. Foals showing signs of systemic infection should be evaluated as a septicemic case and

consider abdominal paracentesis away from umbilicus if fluid is present.
2. **Surgical** - indicated if nonresponsive to topical and systemic management or if foal begins to show signs of septicemia.
   a. Combine with ultrasound to make decision to operate.

III. SEPTIC OMPHALOPHLEBITIS

A. **Foal may have a completely normal,** dry appearing external navel and be severely ill from an infected urachus, umbilical arteries or vein.
B. **May extend to peritonitis**, and produce a bacteremia and subsequent septic arthritis, also liver abscesses, pneumonia, or osteomyelitis.
C. **When involving the urachus** can produce
   1. Uroperitoneum by abscessing the tip of the bladder.
   2. Cystitis and white blood cells on urinalysis.
D. **Diagnosis**
   1. External umbilical stump may appear normal.
   2. Ultrasound of umbilical artery, vein or urachus for abnormalities[1,2].
   3. Leukogram may or may not be inflammatory.
   4. In cases of septic arthritis examine umbilicus for evidence of infection.
E. **Treatment** has traditionally consisted of surgical removal of the suspected infected tissue under general anesthesia and administration of systemic antimicrobials. However, many cases are managed by medical means and long term antibiotics.

IV. ACUTE, DIFFUSE, EDEMATOUS UMBILICUS SYNDROME

A. **Foals develop a painful**, swollen umbilicus with surrounding tissue edema along with fever and anorexia.
B. **Consider as an emergency situation.**
   1. Involvement of abdominal wall fascia.
   2. Cellulitis appears to be differentiating feature.
   3. Foal may die in 12-24 hours in spite of aggressive therapy.

4. Decision to operate on these foals is not clear cut.

V. PATENT URACHUS is seen as a dribble of urine from the umbilicus during normal urination or as moisture around umbilicus. Foals usually behave as clinically normal unless infection develops.

A. **May remain open** immediately after birth or close and re-open several days later.
B. **May leak urine** into the abdominal cavity or subcutaneous tissue from a rent between the umbilicus and bladder.
C. **Foals <14 days of age and sick from other problems** may develop a patent urachus secondarily. An increased incidence may occur when umbilical cords are ligated at birth.
D. **Restraint and lifting** of foals can force urine from bladder into urachus and create condition.
   Therapy is medical or surgical.
   1. Conservative therapy consists of daily dipping of the navel. Daily cauterization of the first 1-2 cm of the urachus with silver nitrate sticks or phenol solution flushed into the urachus have been suggested.
      EC: be very careful or avoid performing this procedure - frequent complications. Determine IgG status and provide systemic antimicrobials if indicated by hemogram; should respond in 7 days.
   2. Surgery is indicated in refractory cases or those that develop systemic signs of infection. General anesthesia and removal of the entire urachus to the tip of the bladder is performed. Merely ligating the exterior stump can trap organisms and cause infection. Associated arteries and veins should be ligated and removed if infected or necrotic.
F. **Potential complications** are cystitis, bladder wall necrosis, septicemia, and uroperitoneum.

VI. UMBILICAL HERNIAS[3,4]

A. **Rupture at birth** (Chapter 48).
B. **Most umbilical hernias** occur or are noticed weeks after foaling.

- **C. Decision on whether to repair** depends on the size of the opening.
    1. Very small opening with large amount of bowel or omentum - repair soon.
    2. Repair is either with clamps or surgical reduction[4].
- **D. Strangulating hernias** in neonates are presented as acute abdominal pain cases.
    1. Uncommon occurrence.
    2. Often associated with a small hernia.
    3. Umbilical area is swollen and hernia may be irreducible.
    4. Aspiration reveals bowel contents.
    5. May require surgery and enlargement of umbilical defect, inspection of bowel and resection of any damaged intestine.
- **E.** Enlarging umbilical mass due to evagination of urinary bladder can occur.[5]
    1. Clinical signs in <12 hr old foal with enlarging umbilical mass and stranguria.

References:
1. Reef, V.B., Collatos, C.: Ultrasonography of umbilical structures in clinically normal foals. Am J Vet Res 49:2143-2146, 1988.
2. Reef, V.B., Collatos, C., Spencer, P.A., et al.: Clinical, ultrasonographic, and surgical findings in foals with umbilical remnant infections. JAVMA 195:69-72, 1989.
3. C B Riley, A M Cruz, J V Bailey, S M Barber, and P B Fretz Comparison of herniorrhaphy versus clamping of umbilical hernias in horses: a retrospective study of 93 cases (1982-1994). Can Vet J. 1996 May; 37(5): 295–298.
4. Enzerink E, van Weeren PR, van der Velden MA.: Closure of the abdominal wall at the umbilicus and the development of umbilical hernias in a group of foals from birth to 11 months of age. Vet Rec. 147(2):37-39, 2000.
5. Textor JA, Goodrich L, Wion L. Umbilical evagination of the urinary bladder in a neonatal filly. J Am Vet Med Assoc. 219(7):953-6, 939, 2001.

CHAPTER 40
EYE PROBLEMS

There are numerous ocular diseases and congenital problems (See Chapter 42) seen in ill neonatal foals.[1,2] Only the common ocular problems seen with critical care management of the premature and ill foal are mentioned here. A recent study indicated frequent eye problems in referral foal units: abnormalities found in 70 foals included conjunctival hyperemia or episcleral injection 42.9%, uveitis 25.7%, ulcerative keratitis 18.6%, nonulcerative keratitis 14.3%, entropion 11.4%, retinal hemorrhage 11.4%, and cataract 8.6%. Foals with sepsis were significantly more likely to have uveitis than were those without sepsis. Foals with sepsis and uveitis were also significantly less likely to survive to discharge than were foals that had sepsis without uveitis.[2] **EC** we better start calling the ophthalmologists in at 3 am more often.

I. **CORNEAL ULCERS**

   A. **Most commonly** develop secondary to trauma while recumbent due to weakness and incoordination, seizures, flailing during transport, ocular drying and entropion.
   B. **Preventive measures** are head protectors, sedation and supervised restraint, lubricating drops or ointments 4 times daily and frequent examination for ulcers by staining with fluorescence strips.
   C. **May be responsible** for considerable prolongation of hospitalization.
   D. **Treatment is broad spectrum** antibiotic ointments applied every 4-6 hours. Severe or persistent ulcers and keratitis require culture and sensitivity. Small amounts of atropine drops for blepharospasm is helpful. **EC** Use with caution due to systemic absorption and GI motility problems.

II. **ENTROPION**

   A. **Seen frequently** in premature and severely ill foals.
   B. **Infolding of the eyelid** may cause corneal conjunctival irritation, and ulceration.
   C. **Correction** is via temporary sutures to evert the lid.

D. **Eye lid injections** of various substances included procaine penicillin, Vitamin E-Se, have been used to evert lid.

III. **IRIDOCYCLITIS, UVEITIS** -- seen accompanying systemic bacterial infection (septicemia), viral infections or rarely after blood/plasma product administration.

 A. **Eye may appear cloudy** due to corneal edema with hemorrhage seen in the anterior chamber. Flare, miosis, and corneal vascularization may be present.
 B. **Treatment** - correction of primary inciting problem. Atropine drops are used and **without** evidence of corneal ulcer, documented by frequent staining, an antibiotic-steroid ointment too.
  1. Systemic NSAIDs may be helpful but side effects in foals may preclude frequent use.

IV. **CONJUNCTIVITIS**

 A. **Secondary to entropion.**
 B. **Secondary to trauma**, stall bedding contamination and shavings or sawdust.
 C. **Associated with bacterial** and viral infection.
 D. **Subconjunctival** and episcleral hemorrhages are seen with compression from parturition.

V. **STROMAL ABSCESS**[3,4]

 A. **Often** present as a medical emergency.
 B. **Primary** due to micropunctures or **secondary** to steroid use on an ulcerated corneal surface.
 C. **Focal, yellow** stromal infiltrate with corneal edema.
 D. **Blepharospasm, epiphora** secondary to iridocyclitis.
 E. **Corneal vascularization, hypopyon, and fibrin accumulation** may be present.
 F. **Treatment** consists of topical antifungal and antimicrobial therapy with DMSO. Highly lipophilic antibiotics (fluoroquinolones, chloramphenicol) are recommended. Atropine is indicated in patients with concurrent iridocyclitis.

- **G. Systemic antibiotics and anti-inflammatories** may be useful especially if stroma is vascularized.
- **H. Severe cases** require surgical interventions (keratoplasty).
- **I. Long term treatment** is essential for success (4-8 weeks)

VI. EYE TRAUMA

- **A.** Both **primary** and **secondary traumas** are fairly common in foals. They require surgical or medical treatment depending on the type of injury.

References:
1. Latimer, C.A., Wyman, M.: Neonatal ophthalmology. Neonatal Equine Disease. Vet. Clinic. North America. W.B. Saunders Co. 235-260, 1985.
2. Labelle,A.I.; Hamor, RE; Townsend, W. et. al. Ophthalmic lesions in neonatal foals evaluated for nonophthalmic disease at referral hospitals. Journal of the American Veterinary Medical Association. Vol. 239, (4): 486-492, 2011.
3. Slovis, NM.:The eye and related structures in McAuliffe, SB., Slovis, NM.: Color Atlas of Diseases and Disorders of the Foal. 326-346. Saunders, Philadelphia. 2008.
4. Gilger, B.: Equine ophthalmology. Saunders, Philadelphia, 2005.

CHAPTER 41
CONGENITAL CARDIAC ANOMALIES

Recognition of congenital heart defects in foals is important both in determining the cause of clinical signs such as fatigue, tachypnea, weakness or cyanosis, and in evaluating the potential future utility of a young horse.

I. **CONGENITAL CARDIAC DEFECTS** reported in the horse include[1-4]:

   A. **Simple defects**, including ventricular septal defect[5], patent ductus arteriosus[6,7], patent foramen ovale or atrial septal defect, and pulmonic stenosis.
   B. **Complex defects**[8], including tetralogy of Fallot, tricuspid atresia, truncus arteriosus, pentalogy of Fallot (tetralogy + PDA), double outlet right ventricle, Eisenmenger VSD or PDA, single ventricle and others.
   C. **Vascular anomalies**, including persistent right aortic arch and anomalous coronary arteries.

II. **DIAGNOSTIC STUDIES** - accurate diagnosis almost always requires the combination of findings from more than one examination.

   A. **Physical examination** - jugular pulse, arterial pulse, percussion, timing and location of heart murmur(s).
   B. **Electrocardiograms** - evidence of atrial or ventricular enlargement.
   C. **Thoracic radiographs** - degree of cardiomegaly, left atrial enlargement, pulmonary vascularity, and pulmonary/pleural signs of left or right heart failure.
   D. **Echocardiography** - atrial/ventricular dilation, ventricular hypertrophy, atrial and ventricular septa, heart valves, position of great vessels.
   E. **Cardiac catheterization**/angiography - systolic and diastolic pressures, blood oximetry, and abnormal blood flow patterns including valvular regurgitation and shunts.

III. CLINICAL FEATURES OF COMMON CONGENITAL CARDIAC DEFECTS

A. **Ventricular septal defect (VSD)[5].**
1. Physical exam - a loud, harsh holosystolic murmur is usually heard best on the right cranial precordium and equally well or softer over the left heart base.
2. ECG - often normal with small defects. Larger defects may cause increased QRS voltages.
3. Radiographs - depending on defect size, heart size may be normal to moderately increased. Left atrium and pulmonary vasculature may be enlarged with large left-to-right shunts.
4. Echo - may be near normal with small defects. Larger defects produce increased diastolic dimension/volume of the left atrium and both left and right ventricles, and increased LV SF% due to volume overload. Large defect may be recognized by M-mode, but 2D is superior, often showing aortic-septal discontinuity even with small defects. LV saline injection can prove L-R shunt.
5. Cath/angiography - pressures may be normal until heart failure increases atrial and ventricular diastolic pressures. Increased oxygen saturation/content occurs between the RA/RV apex and RV outflow/pulmonary artery. Confirmation of anatomy usually requires LV contrast injection to demonstrate L-R shunt.

B. **Patent ductus arteriosus (PDA)**
1. Physical exam
   a. Continuous murmur localized or loudest over the left heart base. Diastolic portion of the murmur is often heard poorly elsewhere.
   b. With large L-R shunt the arterial pulse is hyperkinetic (bounding).
   c. If pulmonary hypertension develops, the murmur shortens into a transystolic or purely systolic murmur with a normal arterial pulse.
   d. The continuous or transystolic murmur of a slightly patent ductus arteriosus may be present

in normal foals for at least 3-4 days, and occasionally up to 7-8 days of age[6,7].
2. ECG - normal unless shunt is large, causing increasing QRS amplitudes due to LV enlargement.
3. Radiographs - mild to moderate cardiomegaly, enlarged LA and increased pulmonary vascularity.
4. Echo - increased LA and LV diastolic dimension/volume and hyperdynamic septal and LV wall systolic motion (increased SF%) commensurate with size of the L-R shunt. If pulmonary hypertension develops, the RV becomes dilated and the RV wall thickens. The ductus **may** be visible by 2D imaging from the left caudal transducer location in some foals.
5. Cath/angiography - wide arterial pulse pressure, slightly to moderately increased LV diastolic pressure, increased PA oxygen saturation/content, L-R shunt visible following LV or aortic root injection. With pulmonary hypertension the RV and PA systolic pressures are increased, sometime equivalent to arterial pressure, R-L (PA -->Aorta) shunt following IV, RV or PA injection.

C. Tetralogy of Fallot
1. Physical exam - systolic ejection murmur of pulmonic stenosis is heard at the left heart base. Normal arterial pulse, normal to slight jugular venous pulse. Symmetrical cyanosis may be present at rest or following mild exercise.
2. ECG - RV hypertrophy may be indicated by negative QRS complexes in leads I, II, and aVF.
3. Radiographs - mild to moderate cardiomegaly, rounding of the silhouette, and decreased pulmonary vascularity may be seen.
4. Echo - thickened RV wall, septal echo dropout in the area of the VSD, rightward displacement of the aortic root, and abnormal pulmonary outflow region (2D). Injection of saline IV demonstrates R-L flow from RV to LV or aorta.
5. Cath/angiography - systolic pressure gradient across pulmonary outflow region (pulmonic stenosis), increased RV systolic pressure equivalent to LV or aortic pressure. Decreased oxygen

saturation/content between LV apex and ascending aorta. RV contrast injection shows pulmonic stenosis and R-L shunt from RV to LV/aorta.

D. Tricuspid atresia
1. Physical exam - symmetrical cyanosis at rest or following very mild exertion (due to obligatory presence of atrial septal defect), holosystolic murmur loudest at the left heart base, normal to weak arterial pulse, increased jugular venous pulse.
2. ECG - increased P wave amplitude and duration are common, increased QRS amplitudes due to LV enlargement may occur.
3. Radiographs - may be deceptively normal or show mild cardiomegaly and decreased pulmonary vascularity.
4. Echo - enlarged LV, very small RV, enlarged atria, atretic tricuspid valve, atrial and/or ventricular septal defects are best seen by 2D echo examination. The R-L interatrial shunt can be easily demonstrated by IV saline injection.
5. Cath/angiography - decreased oxygen saturation/content in the left heart, equal LV and RV systolic and diastolic pressures, RA contrast injection shows small RV and R-L shunt.

E. Other types of complex malformations may occur.
1. Accurate diagnosis requires echocardiography and/or cardiac catheterization/angiography.
2. Total anomalous pulmonary venous connection in a foal[9] seen in an Arabian-Morgan cross foal at 8 days with weakness and murmur.
3. Parachute left atrioventricular valve causing stenosis and regurgitation in a Thoroughbred foal.[10]
4. Giant right atrial diverticulum in a foal.[11]

References:
1. Huston, R., Saperstein, G., Leipold, H.W.: Congenital defects in foals J Equine Med Surg 1:146-161, 1977.
2. Rooney, J.R., Franks, W.C.: Congenital cardiac anomalies in horses. Pathol Vet 1:454-464, 1964.

3. Fregin, G.F.: The cardiovascular system. In: Mansmann R.A., McAllister E.S., Pratt P.W. (eds): <u>Equine Medicine and Surgery</u> 3rd ed., American Veterinary Publications, Inc., Santa Barbara, 645-704, 1982.
4. Reef, V.B.: Cardiovascular disease in the equine neonate. <u>Vet Clin North Am: Equine Pract</u> 1:117-129, 1985.
5. Lombard, C.W., Scarratt, W.K., Buergeit, C.D.: Ventricular septal defects in the horse. <u>J Am Vet Med Assoc</u> 183:562-565, 1983.
6. Amorosao, E.C., Dawes, G.S., Mott, J.C.: Patency of the ductus arteriosus in the newborn foal. <u>Brit Heart J</u> 20:92-96, 1958.
7. Scott, E.A., Kneller, S.K., Witherspoon, D.M.: Closure of ductus arteriosus determined by cardiac catheterization and angiography in newborn foals. <u>Am J Vet Res</u> 36:1021-1023, 1975.
8. Bayly, W.M., Reed, S.M., Leathers, C.W., et al.: Multiple congenital heart anomalies in five Arabian foals. <u>J Am Vet Med Assoc</u> 181:684-689, 1982.
9. Seco Diaz O, Desrochers A, Hoffmann V, Reef VB. Total anomalous pulmonary venous connection in a foal. <u>Vet Radiol Ultrasound</u>. Jan-Feb;46:83-5, 2005
10. McGurrin MK, Physick-Sheard PW, Southorn E. Parachute left atrioventricular valve causing stenosis and regurgitation in a Thoroughbred foal. <u>J Vet Intern Med</u>. Jul-Aug;17:579-82. 2003
11. Patterson-Kane JC, Harrison LR**.** Giant right atrial diverticulum in a foal. <u>J Vet Diagn Invest</u>. 14(4):335-7. 2002.

CHAPTER 42
CONGENITAL ANOMALIES AND GENETIC DISORDERS

With congenital (existing at birth) abnormalities genetic influences are often suspected, but difficult to substantiate. Effects of nutrition, toxins, infections (i.e. environment) can have profound effects on genetic expression. The following list is not intended to cover every case report or every treatment associated with congenital/genetic diseases. An attempt was made to include the most common.

I. **OPHTHALMOLOGY**

   A. **Microphthalmia**[1] (unilateral or bilateral small globes)
      1. Eye may occasionally be functional, but more commonly are nonfunctional.
      2. Sporadic - believed non-heritable.
   B. **Ectropion** - eversion of eyelid - correct surgically.
   C. **Entropion**
      1. Infolded eyelid causes corneal and conjunctival irritation, tearing, conjunctivitis, corneal ulceration.
      2. Treatment: vertical mattress sutures to temporarily evert the lid plus appropriate medical therapy of the eye.
   D. **Nasolacrimal Duct Obstruction**[1]
      1. Usually via atresia of the nasolacrimal meatus.
      2. Clinical signs: epiphora (clear to mucopurulent), no nasolacrimal meatus upon exam of nostril.
      3. Treatment is normograde passage of 3.5 or 5 French catheter with incision over end to create patency. Suture catheter in place for 10 days and treat associated dacryocystitis.
   E. **Corneal dermoid**[1]
      1. Focal skin-like tissue that involves temporal limbus and adjacent cornea and conjunctiva.
      2. Unilateral or bilateral.
      3. Treatment - nothing or superficial keratectomy.
   F. **Cataracts**[1]
      1. Most commonly reported ocular anomaly of foals.
      2. May be unilateral or bilateral, focal or diffuse and most common cause of blindness in young horses. Most often present as only ocular defect, but it may

be associated with persistent pupillary membranes, persistent hyaloid structures, or multiple ocular anomalies.
3. Treatment - depends on severity (focal or diffuse) - surgical extraction of lens, phaecoemulsification or euthanasia.

G. Persistent Pupillary Membrane
1. Pigmented strands that arise from iris stroma.
2. May traverse pupillary opening (iris to iris) or anterior chamber (iris to cornea).
3. Also may contact anterior lens capsule leading to anterior capsular and cortical cataracts.

H. Persistent Hyaloid Vasculation[1]
1. Remnant of vessel from optic disc to posterior lens. It may persist normally until approximately 3 weeks of age.
2. Remnants on posterior lens may be associated with posterior capsular and cortical cataracts.

I. Retinal Detachment
1. Usually bilateral and complete with dilated pupil and hyper-reflective tapetum. Pupils are non-responsive to light. Retina is folded and gray.
2. Have not been treated with success.

J. Congenital Corneal Vascularization[2] has been reported in a Thoroughbred foal.
Bulbar and palpebral conjunctivae were inflamed with superficial corneal vascularization which resolved spontaneously within 7 days. It is believed to be related to alterations in amniotic fluid and eye irritation.

K. Others[1]
1. Microcornea, megalocornea
2. Lenticonus/lentiglobus - defect in lens shape
3. Microphakia - small lens
4. Luxated lens
5. Aniridia - complete absence of iris. Autosomal dominant trait in Belgians with secondary cataracts.

II. GASTROINTESTINAL

A. Cleft Palate[3]
1. Failure of the hard or soft palate to close along its midline prior to birth.
2. Diagnosis - palpation or visualization during physical exam for clefts in hard palate or visualization via endoscopy for soft palate. Foal will expel milk through nostrils during and after nursing. Secondary aspiration pneumonia frequently develops.
   a. Differentiate from temporary pharyngeal paresis; no lesion and improves after 1-7 days of tube feeding.
3. Treatment - euthanasia or surgical correction of smaller clefts of the soft palate or hard palate, or some foals without significant aspiration pneumonia become riding horses.

B. Atresia ani and Atresia recti[3]
1. Diagnosis - physical exam, unable to defecate.
2. Potential surgical correction.

C. Ileocolonic aganglionosis ("Lethal White Foal")[4]
1. Seen in overo - overo Paint horse crosses.
2. Congenital absence of myenteric ganglia in terminal portion of ileum, cecum and entire colon.
3. Associated with colonic atresia, but there are actually contracted areas of small colon often with meconium impaction.
4. Diagnosis - white foal from overo spotted x overo spotted breeding - foals normal at birth but cannot defecate leading to colic and death.
5. Condition is fatal.
4. Genetics: Overo lethal white gene is an allele to the recessive overo spotting gene which is lethal in the homozygote.[5]
5. For information on genetic testing go to: www.vgl.ucdavis.edu/services/coatcolorhorse.php

D. Atresia Coli[6]
1. Any breed.
2. Signs similar to meconium impactions; pain, straining, abdominal distension, lack of meconium.

3. May have membranous atresia, cord atresia with gut remnant connecting blind ends or blind end with no connection.[6]
4. Surgical correction is difficult.

E. Parrot Mouth (Prognathism)[3]
1. Malformation of the "bite" via maxilla overgrowth or a short mandible.
2. Genetically transmitted.
3. Diagnosis - physical exam.
4. Many severe cases manage quite well.

F. Esophageal stricture[3]
1. Found in association with persistent right aortic arch.
2. Found in mid esophagus - cause unknown - may be congenital or traumatic.

G. Esophageal stenosis[7]
1. Reported in Thoroughbred colt; onset at 3 days.
2. Milk discharge from both nostrils when head lowered after nursing.
3. Endoscope or contrast studies reveal narrowed area near base of heart.
4. Tube feeding for several weeks lead to recovery.

H. Diaphragmatic Hernia
1. May be due to failure of fusion of embryonic development or rupture from birth trauma.
2. Signs may be colic - especially after nursing.
3. Diagnosis auscultation, ultrasound and chest radiograph.
4. Surgical repair possible.

III. CARDIOVASCULAR DISEASE (See Chapter 41)

IV. URINARY SYSTEM

A. Rupture of Urinary Bladder (See Chapter 37).
B. Bilateral Ureter Defect (Chapter 37).
C. Persistent Membrane Over Glans Penis
1. Foals cannot extend penis and consequently urinate within the sheath.
2. Most resolve spontaneously or require minor surgery to correct; wait for several weeks.

D. Posterior Urethral Valves

1. Uncommon but has been recognized in colt foals.
2. Characterized by stranguria, pollakuria, azotemia.
3. May be present as a ruptured bladder or as a hydronephrosis.
4. Failure or difficulty to perform urinary catheterization.
5. Successful treatment has not been documented in the veterinary literature.

V. MUSCULOSKELETAL SYSTEM

A. Rupture of Common Digital Extensor Tendon[8]
1. Usually present at birth or shortly after.
2. Characteristic swelling over dorsal lateral surface of carpus via tendon rupture within carpal synovial sheath.
3. Diagnosis - clinical signs, palpation - can develop associated with flexor tendon contracture.
4. Treatment - stall rest for 4-8 weeks with or without splints.

B. Angular Limb Deformities - congenital or acquired (See Chapter 78-80)

C. Wry Mouth or Campylognathy or Deviated Premaxilla[3]
1. If severe may not allow foal to nurse.
2. Less severe cases may improve somewhat with time if foal can nurse.

D. Contracted Foal Syndrome[9]
1. Bilateral contraction of the joints of the fore or hind limbs, or both.
2. Usually involves 3rd metacarpal or 3rd metatarsal articulation of first phalanx.
3. Scoliosis or torticollis seen in conjunction.
4. Frequently associated with cranial asymmetry or curvature.

VI. NERVOUS SYSTEM

A. Cerebellar abiotrophy (hypoplasia)[10]
1. Seen at birth to 6 months of age in Arabian foals.
2. Ataxia, intention tremors, dysmetria, and no menace response.

3. Familiar in the Arabian and Gotland pony breeds only.
4. Genetic test available: www.vgl.ucdavis.edu/services/CA

B. Hydrocephalus
1. May have domed head appearance.
2. Signs usually present at birth and may improve temporally with treatment.
3. May present with signs suggesting Neonatal Maladjustment Syndrome.
4. Uniformly fatal.

C. Congenital Myoclonus of Peruvian Pasos[11]
1. Foals cannot rise without assistance.
2. When assisted to standing, foals can move but have stilted, rabbit hopping type gait.
3. With auditory and tactile stimulation have myoclonic contractions.
4. Bright alert responsive and good suckle.
5. No treatment is successful. Valium and muscle relaxants help symptomatically.
6. May erode hip joint due to myoclonic contractions.
7. Have deficiency of glycine receptor in spinal cord for synaptic inhibition.

VII. SKIN

A. Junctional Epidermiolysis Bullosa[12,13]
1. Moderate to severe blistering of the skin and sloughing of the hooves at birth.
2. Lesions often develop after mild trauma
3. Ulcers on mucosal surfaces.
4. Biopsy - epidermis separating from dermis by subepidermal clefts.[14]
5. A loss of cohesion of basal epithelial cells along lamina lucida of basement membrane.
5. Seen in Belgian foals, autosomal recessive heritable condition (laminin 5 formation defect).
6. Genetic testing is available: www.vgl.ucdavis.edu/services/jeb.php

B. Hereditary equine regional dermal asthenia (HERDA)[15]

1. Predominantly in American Quarter horse lines.
2. Hyperextensible skin, scarring, and severe lesions along the back of affected horses
3. Affected foals rarely show symptoms at birth. The condition typically occurs by the age of two, most notably when the horse is first being broken to saddle
4. Treatment is not available, and the majority of diagnosed horses are euthanized because they are unable to be ridden and are inappropriate for future breeding
5. HERDA has an autosomal recessive mode of inheritance and affects stallions and mares in equal proportions. Research carried out in Dr. Danika Bannasch's laboratory at the University of California, Davis, has identified the gene and mutation associated with HERDA.
6. For genetic testing go to: www.vgl.ucdavis.edu/services/herda.php

VIII. MUSCULAR SYSTEM

A. Glycogen branching enzyme deficiency[16-19]

This is a recently recognized disease mainly of quarter horses.

1. **Clinical Signs**
   a. Abortion or still birth of foals
   b. Sudden death on pasture from the heart stopping or from seizures (associated with hypoglycemia)
   c. Weakness, low body temperature at birth.
   d. High respiratory rate leading to fatigue.
   e. Contracted tendons in all four legs.
   f. Weakness and inability to rise.

2. **Diagnosis**
   a. Compatible hematology and chemistry; low WBC count, elevated CK, AST and liver GGT
   b. Hypoglycemia even with normal feeding
   c. A muscle biopsy can be performed to screen for muscle diseases at the University of Minnesota. To determine if the foal has GBED hair samples can be submitted to the Veterinary Genetics Laboratory at the University of California, Davis

to test for the GBED genetic mutation. Submission forms and information are available on their website www.vgl.ucdavis.edu/services/gbed.php
   d. Dr. Valberg's web site has more information: www.academicserver.cvm.umn.edu/neuromuscularlab/GBED.htm#symptoms
   e. Genetic testing - University of California, Davis, Veterinary Genetics Laboratory performs GBED testing. www.vgl.ucdavis.edu/services/gbed.php

3. Treatment
All foals with GBED have died. No treatment is effective.

B. Hyperkalaemic periodic paralysis[20]

1. Etiology
   a. Quarter horses and Quarter horse crosses
   a. Autosomal dominant
   b. Defect in the voltage dependent skeletal muscle Na^+ channel alpha subunit

2. Clinical signs
   a. Sweating, muscle fasciculations, 3rd eyelid prolapse.
   b. Severe muscle cramping.
   c. Episodes last 15-60 minutes.
   d. Respiratory distress (paralysis of upper respiratory muscles).
   e. Homozygous: respiratory stridor and upper respiratory tract obstruction.

3. Diagnosis
   a. Hyperkalemia (6-9 mEq/l) or normokalemia during mild episodes.
   b. Hyponatremia
   c. Hemoconcentration
   d. Mane or hair tail with the follicle for DNA testing, for more information go to: www.vgl.ucdavis.edu/services/hypp.php

4. Treatment
   a. Mild episodes - mild exercise, grain or corn syrup.
   b. Severe episodes - calcium gluconate, IV dextrose, insulin.

5. Prevention
   a. Decrease dietary potassium intake; feed timothy hay or bermuda grass and grain.
   b. Do not feed alfalfa or supplemental oils!
   c. Multiple feedings.
   d. Regular exercise and turn-out
   e. Acetazolamide(2-4mg/kg) or hydrochlorthiazide (0.5-1mg/kg)

C. Polysaccharide storage myopathy (EPSM, PSSM, EPSSM)[21-24]
1. Etiology
   a. Equine polysaccharide storage myopathy Type I and Type II are characterized by a defect in glycogen storage in skeletal muscle.
   b. This disease is seen in many different breeds including Quarter horses, draft horses, Warmbloods and crosses of these breeds.
   c. Skeletal muscles in affected horses have higher amounts of stored glycogen than in normal horses.
   d. Affected horses also have higher levels of a complex polysaccharide which is resistant to amylase digestion, aiding identification of the disease by histopathology
   e. **Clinical signs – not reported in foals- see references for adult information**

D. Myotonia congenita
   1. Quarter horses and Quarter horse crosses.
   2. Periods of involuntary muscle contractions following stimulation or activity.
   3. Animals show signs usually < 1 year of age.
   4. Well developed musculature, pelvic limb stiffness or lameness.
   5. Only skeletal muscles are affected, no progression seen beyond 1 year.
   6. **Myotonic dystrophy** is a separate condition and it progresses to severe muscle atrophy and involves other organs.

E. Malignant hyperthermia[24-27]
   1. Has been recognized in Quarter horses and Thoroughbreds.

2. The condition is inherited, autosomal dominant.
3. A defect of the ryanodine receptor leads to the condition and causes increased intracellular calcium accumulation.
4. The process of reabsorbing this excess Ca^{2+} consumes large amounts of ATP, and generates hyperthermia. The muscle cell is damaged by the depletion of ATP and possibly the high temperatures, and cellular constituents "leak" into the circulation.
5. The process is triggered by certain drugs used for general anesthesia (inhalational anesthetics: halothane, isoflurane).
6. Treatment is available. Dantrolene can be given 4-5mg/kg iv although it is very expensive.

IX. OTHER

A. **Inguinal (scrotal) hernias**
   1. Usually seen within first few days of life. Manage by reduction into abdomen on a daily basis can often result in correction.
   2. If extensive, treatment is surgery with removal of testicle on side of hernia.
B. **Cryptorchidism**[2]
   1. Unilateral or bilateral - believed genetic.
C. **Umbilical hernia (See Chapter 39 & 48)**
D. **Severe Combined Immunodeficiency (SCID See Chapter 32)**[28,29]
   1. Lethal genetic disease inherited as an autosomal recessive trait; identified only in Arabians.
   2. Lack of functional B and T lymphocytes.
   3. Death usually is due to infectious causes.
   4. Genetic test is available:
      www.vgl.ucdavis.edu/services/scid.php
E. **Agenesis of a lung lobe**
F. **Autosomal trisomy**[30].
   1. Standardbreds.
   2. Developmental defects - facial asymmetry (one eye higher than other), dorsomedial strabismus, dysmetric gait, small testes, poor condition.

G. Lavender Foal Syndrome
1. Seen in Egyptian and ½ Egyptian Arabians.
2. Foals are born of normal gestation length and cannot rise from lateral recumbency, struggle severely to rise, are bright and alert mentally but cannot stand and walk. If propped up, foal will temporarily assume abnormal position and collapse and resume struggling.
3. Physical exam normal - bright, alert, responsive.
4. Foals are born a lavender color or best described as a diluted color appearance.
5. Have not improved with nursing care for 1 week.
6. CNS lesions consisting of vacuolization in some neurons at post mortem.

References:
1. Munroe, G.A., Barnett, K.C.: Congenital ocular disease in the foal. Vet Clin North Am (Large Anim Pract) 6(3):519-540, 1984.
2. Munroe, GA.: Congenital corneal vascularisation in a neonatal Thoroughbred foal. Equine Vet J 27:156-157, 1995.
3. Huston, R., Saperstein, G., Leipold, H.W.: Congenital defects in foals. J Equine Med Surg 1:146-161, 1977.
4. Hultgren, B.D.: Ileocolonic aganglionosis in white progeny of overo spotted horses. JAVMA 289-292, 1982.
5. McCabe, L., Griffin, L.D., Kinzer, A., et al.: Overo lethal white foal syndrome: Equine model of aganglionic megacolon (Hirschsprung Disease). Amer J of Med Genetics 36:336-340, 1990.
6. Shires, G.M.: Congenital and familial diseases. In: Equine Medicine and Surgery, 4th Edition, American Veterinary Publications, 1991, p 34.
7. Clabough, DL, Roberts, MC, Robertson, I. Probable congenital esophageal stenosis in a Thoroughbred foal. JAVMA 199:483-485, 1991.
8. Yovich, J.V.: Rupture of common digital extensor tendon in foals. Compend Cont Educ 6(7):S373-S378, 1984.
9. Leitch, M.: Musculoskeletal disorders in neonatal foals. Vet Clin North Am (Equine Practice) 1(1):189-207, 1985.
10. Beatty, M.T., Leipold, H.W., Cash, et al.: Cerebellar disease in

Arabian horses. Proceed of Amer Assoc Equine Pract, 31st Meeting 1985, p 241-245.Caron, J.P., Angular limb deformities in foals. Equine Vet J 20:255-258, 1988.
11. Gundlach, A.L., Kortz, G., Burazin, T.C.D., Madigan, J.E., et al.: Deficit of inhibitory glycine receptors in spinal cord from Peruvian pasos: Evidence for an equine form of inherited myoclonus. Brain Res 628:263-270, 1993.
12. Spirito F, Charlesworth A, Linder K, et al: Animal models for skin blistering conditions: absence of laminin 5 causes hereditary junctional mechanobullous disease in the Belgian horse, J Invest Dermatol 119(3):684, 2002.
13. Milenkovic D, Chaffaux S, Taourit S, Guerin G: A mutation in the LAMC2 gene causes the Herlitz junctional epidermolysis bullosa (H-JEB) in two French draft horse breeds, Genet Sel Evol 35(2):249, 2003.
14. Frame, S.R., Harrington, D.D., Fessler, J., et al: Hereditary junctional mechanobullous disease in a foal. JAVMA 193:1420-1424, 1988.
15. Tryon RC, White SD, Famula TR, Schultheiss PC, Hamar DW, Bannasch DL.: Inheritance of hereditary equine regional dermal asthenia in Quarter Horses. Am J Vet Res. 2005 Mar; 66(3):437-42.
16. Valberg SJ, Mickelson JR, Ward TL, Rush B, Kinde H, Hiraragi H, Nahey D, and Fyfe J. Glycogen branching enzyme activity in Quarter Horse foals. JVIM. 2001; 15:572-580.
17. Render JA, Common RS, Kennedy FA, Jones MZ, Fyfe JC: Amylopectinosis in fetal and neonatal Quarter Horses. Veterinary Pathology 1999: 36(2):157-60.
18. Sponseller BT, Valberg SJ, Ward T, Williams AJ. And Mickelson JR. Muscular weakness and recumbency in a quarter horse colt due to glycogen branching enzyme deficiency. Equine Vet Educ 2003;14:182-188.
19. Ward TL, Valberg SJ, Adelson DL, Abby CA3, and James R Mickelson JR Glycogen Branching Enzyme (GBE1) Mutation Causing Fatal Glycogen Storage Disease IV in American Quarter Horse Foals Mammalian Genome 2004;15:570-577.
20. Rudolph JA, Spier SJ, Byrns G, et al: Periodic paralysis in quarter horses: a sodium channel mutation disseminated by selective breeding. Nat Genet 2(2):144, 1992.

21. Hunt LM, Valberg SJ, Steffenhagen K and McCue ME. An Epidemiologic Study of Myopathies in Warmblood Horses. Equine Vet J. 2008 Mar;40(2):171-7
22. McCue ME, Valberg SJ. Estimated prevalence of polysaccharide storage myopathy among overtly healthy Quarter Horses in the United States. J Am Vet Med Assoc. 2007; 231(5):746-50.
23. McCue, M, Ribiero W, Lewis S and Valberg SJ. Prevalence of polysaccharide storage myopathy in horses with neuromuscular disorders. Equine Veterinary Journal Suppl.36 2006:340-344.
24. Perkins G, Valberg SJ, Madigan JE, Carlson GP, and Jones SL. Fluid, electrolyte and renal abnormalities associated with acute rhabdomyolysis in four neonatal foals. J Vet Int Med 1998; 12:173-177.
25. Aleman M, Brosnan RJ, Williams DC, LeCouteur RA, Imai A, Tharp BR, Steffey EP.: Malignant hyperthermia in a horse anesthetized with halothane. J Vet Intern Med. 2005 May-Jun;19(3):363-6.
26. Aleman M. A review of equine muscle disorders. Neuromuscul Disord. 2008 Apr;18(4):277-87.
27. Wiler R, Leber R, Moore BB, et al: Equine severe combined immunodeficiency: a defect in V(D)J recombination and DNA-dependent protein kinase activity. Proc Natl Acad Sci USA 92(25):11485, 1995.
28. Aleman M, Riehl J, Aldridge BM, Lecouteur RA, Stott JL, Pessah IN.: Association of a mutation in the ryanodine receptor 1 gene with equine malignant hyperthermia. Muscle Nerve. 2004 Sep;30(3):356-65
29. Genetzky, R.M., et al.: Combined immunodeficiency in an Arabian filly. Compend Cont Educ 7(5):S319-S324, 1985.
30. Klunder, L.R., McFeely, R.A., Beech, J.: Autosomal trisomy in a standardbred colt. Equine Vet J 21:67-70, 1989.

CHAPTER 43
WHITE MUSCLE DISEASE

Nutritional myodegeneration (NMD) associated with inadequate selenium and perhaps Vitamin E in diet. Seen in Pacific Northwest and Eastern states in equine neonates.[1] May also be precipitated by birth asphyxia and oxidative stress. There are two types of the disease based on the organs affected: the peracute or cardiac form and the skeletal or sub acute form.

I. **CLINICAL SIGNS**
   Peracute or cardiac form

   A. **Fulminant onset.**
   B. Animals **found dead** or exhibit cardiac failure, or cardiogenic shock.
   C. Intercostal muscles and diaphragm may also be affected.

   Subacute or skeletal form
   A. **Signs from birth to 11 months of age.**
   B. **Weakness** - unable to rise without assistance, falls on attempting to rise, often resembles colic.
   C. **Dysphagia** - seen as oral and nasal regurgitation of milk.
   D. **Stiff painful gait or neck.**
   E. **Tense or painful muscles.**
   F. **Temperature** may be elevated due to thrashing and straining and secondary infections.
   G. **Elevated respiratory rate.**
   H. **Dark urine**

II. **CLINICAL PATHOLOGY**[2]

   A. **Elevated serum CK** (subtypes for myocardium or skeletal muscle can be differentiated)
   B. **Elevated serum AST**
   C. **Elevated LDH**
   D. **Occult blood or myoglobin in urine.**
      1. Dip stick orthotoluidine reagent reacts with both blood and myoglobin.
   E. **Low serum glutathione peroxidase activity**
      1. Submit whole blood in EDTA tube.

2. Normal level is 20-50 U/mg of hemoglobin/min
- **F. Low blood selenium**<0.07 ppm suggests deficiency.
- **G. Vitamin E level** should be >1-2 ppm.
- **H. Hyperkalemia and hyponatremia can be severe.**

III. DIFFERENTIAL DIAGNOSIS

- **A. Botulism**
    1. Lack tone to muscles.
    2. Shaking of muscles.
    3. Dilated pupils
    4. Weak eye lids
- **B. Hemolytic Anemia**
- **C. Polyarthritis**
- **D. Tetanus**
- **E. Asphyxia**
- **F. Polysaccharide storage myopathy**
- **G. Glycogen branching enzyme deficiency**
- **H. Malignant Hyperthermia**[3]
    1. Recently described and gene identified by Dr. Monica Aleman- horses have similar signs of 'white muscle disease'. Test all suspect cases for MH (**Chapter 42**).

IV. TREATMENT

- **A. Vitamin E** - Selenium injection - 1 ml E-Se/45 kg IM. It may need to be repeated daily or q 2 - 6 weeks. Also use oral vitamin E 1000 unit/day during acute phase.- **EC** use natural form of alpha tocopherol and not synthetic - better absorption.
- **B. Supplementation** of pregnant mares at risk.
    1. 1 mg/day Selenium to ration.
    2. 10 ml Vitamin E-Se ® intramuscularly.
- **C. Metabolic support** - I.V. fluids, correction of hyperkalemia (Chapter 22, 24) and hyponatremia, diuresis for myoglobinuria, limit movement.

V. PROGNOSIS is poor to guarded, treatment must be started early to be beneficial.

References:
1. Dill, S.G., Rebhun, W.C.: White muscle disease in foals. <u>Compend Cont Educ Pract Vet</u> 7:S627-S635, 1985.
2. Maas, J., Valberg, SJ.: Nutritional and toxic rhabdomyolysis in Smith, BP.:<u>Large Animal Internal Medicine.</u> 4th Edition, 1405-1411. WB Saunders, Philadelphia. 2008.
3. Aleman M, Riehl J, Aldridge BM, Lecouteur RA, Stott JL, Pessah IN.: Association of a mutation in the ryanodine receptor 1 gene with equine malignant hyperthermia. <u>Muscle Nerve.</u> 2004 Sep;30(3):356.

CHAPTER 44
HYPOGLYCEMIA

I. FOALS AT RISK

A. **Cesarean section or dystocia with anesthesia**
B. **Premature or small for gestational age**
C. **Neonatal Isoerythrolysis foals**
D. **Hypothermia**
E. **Asphyxia and hypoxia**
F. **Septicemia**
G. **Maladjustment syndrome**
H. **Inherited metabolic defects**
 1. Lysosomal storage disease
 2. Glycogen Branching Enzyme deficiency (Chapter 42)
I. **Previous bolus injections** of glucose or rapid rate of glucose infusion and sudden cessation.
 1. "Rebound" hypoglycemia following bolus.
 2. When parenteral nutrition discontinued.
J. **Orphan foals.**
K. **Liver failure - Tyzzer's disease.**
L. **Hyperlipidemia.**

II. SYMPTOMS

A. **Many foals** merely look weak, or are floppy and falling when attempting to rise. It may manifest as decreased nursing, apathy or lethargic appearance.
B. **Seizures** are not a consistent clinical sign even with prolonged hypoglycemia.

III. DIAGNOSIS

A. **Asymptomatic hypoglycemia.**
 1. Suspect when dextrose stick is less than 60 mg/dl (3.3 mmol/l).
 2. Order Stat quantitative blood glucose.
 3. Diagnosis is glucose less than 40 mg/dl (2.2 mmol/l) in a presuckle foal and less than 80 mg/dl (4.4 mmol/l) in a foal > 2 hours which has suckled.

B. **Symptomatic hypoglycemia** is defined as symptoms that disappear with glucose infusion regardless of blood glucose level.

IV. THERAPY

A. **Draw pretreatment blood** for quantitative glucose.
B. **Symptomatic foal:** foal that has not nursed with no measurement - 8 mg/kg/min glucose (high end of the dose range) which translates to 200 ml/h of 10% dextrose in an isotonic crystalloid like LRS or Plasmalyte 148A for an average sized foal (which is a dose rate of 4 ml/kg/h of a 10 % dextrose solution) for the first hour, then decrease to 4 mg/kg/min after that (200 ml/h of 5% dextrose). Recheck glucose in 1 hour. (See section on Fluid therapy).
C. **Attempt** to maintain blood sugar at 100-160 (80-180) mg/dl (4.4-10 mmol/l). Check serum Na to avoid hyponatremia.
D. **Begin oral feedings** of milk or 10% dextrose or karo (corn) syrup in a syringe or by nasogastric tube.
E. **Correct predisposing causes** and provide nursing care.
F. **Monitor glucose** every 4 to 6 hours via dextrose sticks.
G. **Correct** any concurrent acid base imbalance or hypoxemia.

V. PROGNOSIS

A. **Prolonged hypoglycemia** can result in permanent neurologic defects.
B. **We have found a reasonable response** to severe (10-15 mg/dl [0.6-0.8 mmol/l] blood glucose) hypoglycemias if correction of the concurrent initiating factors can be accomplished.
C. A recent multicenter study evaluated the association between blood glucose and survival rates of critically ill neonatal foals. 29.1% of the study population had blood glucose concentrations within the reference range of 4-7 mmol/l (76-131 mg/dL) at admission, 36.5% were hyperglycemic, and 34.4% were hypoglycaemic. Foals with blood glucose concentrations <2.8 mmol/L (50 mg/dL) or >10 mmol/L (180 mg/dL) at admission were less likely to survive[1].

References:
1. Hollis AR, Furr MO, Magdesian KG, Axon JE, Ludlow V, Boston RC, Corley KT.: Blood glucose concentrations in critically ill neonatal foals. J Vet Intern Med. 2008 Sep-Oct; 22(5):1223-7.

CHAPTER 45
HEMOSTATIC DISORDERS

Primary bleeding disorders of the neonatal foal are relatively uncommon but may occasionally require investigation.

I. **NORMAL VALUES**

   A. **Platelet numbers similar to adults**.
      1. Significantly decreased function of platelets in foals in first 12 hours of life may predispose to platelet related bleeding[1].
   B. **Prothrombin time - (PT) & activated partial thromboplastin time (APPT)** are slightly longer than adult.
      1. PT 13.1 ± 0.3 sec (mean ± SD).
      2. APTT 44.4 ± 2.4 sec (mean ± SD).

II. **INHERITED DEFECTS**

   A. **Hemophilia**[2]
      1. Documented in male Thoroughbreds, Standardbred, Arabian and Quarter horses.
      2. Factor VIII deficiency.
      3. Signs develop from 2 months to 3 years of age.
      4. Diagnosis
         a. Normal PT
         b. Prolonged APTT
         c. Low factor VIII activity.
      5. Inherited as X-chromosome homozygous recessive.
   B. **von Willebrand Disease**[3]
      1. Prolonged breeding noted at injections or wounds.
      2. Prolonged activated partial thromboplastin time (APTT); normal PT. APTT findings are variable.
      3. von Willebrand factor required for platelet adhesions and plug formation.
      4. Need specific assay.
      5. Is heritable - test sire and dam.
   C. **Prekallikrein deficiency**[4]
      1. Prolonged bleeding with wounds.
      2. Marked prolonged APTT, normal PT.

a. APTT becomes normal with plasma added.
3. Belgian horses, is familial.

III. DISSEMINATED INTRAVASCULAR COAGULATION[5]

A. **A thrombotic and hemorrhagic** disorder secondary to shock, septicemia, endotoxemia, viremia, renal disease, liver disease, peritonitis, pneumonia or post operative hemorrhage.
B. **May present clinically** as a thrombotic crisis or hemorrhagic diathesis.
   1. Petechiation and ecchymoses on mucous membranes, nictating membrane, inner pinna of ear and retina.
C. **Diagnosis** - Presence of three of these four clinical pathologic findings.
   1. Thrombocytopenia.
   2. Elevated fibrin degradation products.
   3. PT increased.
   4. APTT increased.
D. **Therapy**
   1. Correct primary disorder.
   2. Use of systemic anticoagulants to inhibit consumptive process has not been evaluated in foals.
   3. NSAID - antiprostaglandin drugs to decrease platelet aggregation may be helpful but must be evaluated relative to their potential side effects in severely ill foals.

IV. IMMUNE-MEDIATED THROMBOCYTOPENIC BULLOUS PEMPHIGOID[3,4]

This is a recently described disorder which is most likely an immune-mediated due to absorption of colostral immunoglobulins which contain antibodies against thrombocytes and possibly dermal components. Foals often have oral ulcers, crusty miliary skin, and on blood work leucopenia and thrombocytopenia, which can be very severe. It has been described in several different breeds including Quarter horse and Friesian.

Prevention

A. **If a mare** has previously produced one of these foals: if a similar repeat mating is done, withhold mare colostrum, provide alternative colostrum and treat as NI foal.
B. **Mares at risk:**
Unknown.

Clinical Features

A. **Foals** born healthy, nurse, and then seen at 12-36 hrs for not nursing, lethargy, and inflammation of mouth, lips, nasal mucosa with ulceration and sometimes bleeding.
B. **Biopsy** of ulcers compatible with bullous pemphigus.[1]

Laboratory Features

A. Thrombocytopenia- very low (often <50000/µl)
B. May have leucopenia
C. PCV normal

Treatment

A. Dexamethasone, antimicrobials, nursing and supportive care.
B. Most foals will recover.

References:
1. Clemmons, R.M., Dorsey-Lee, M.R., Gorman, N.T., Sturtevant, F.L.: Hemostatic mechanisms of the newborn foal: Reduced plated responsiveness. Eq Vet J 16:354, 1984.
2. Byars, T.D.: Hemophilia. Current Ther Equine Pract. W.B. Saunders Co., Philadelphia, pp 309-310, 1986.
3. Ginn, PE, Hillier, A, Lester, GD. Self Limiting subepidermal bullous disease in a neonatal foal. Veterinary Dermatology, 9, 249-256, 1998.
4. Perkins GA, Miller WH, Divers TJ, et. al. Ulcerative dermatitis, thrombocytopenia, and neutropenia in neonatal foals. J Vet Intern Med. 19(2):211-6, 2005

5. Brooks, M., Leith, G.S., Allen, K.H., et al. Bleeding disorder: von Willebrand disease in a Quarter Horse. <u>JAVMA</u> 198:114-116, 1991.
6. Geor, R.J., Jackson, M.L., Lewis, K.D., et al. Prekallikrein deficiency in a family of Belgian horses. <u>JAVMA</u> 197:741-745, 1990.
7. Byars, T.D.: Disseminated intravascular coagulation. <u>Current Ther Eq Pract</u> W.B. Saunders Co., Philadelphia, pp 306-309, 1986.

CHAPTER 46
ENDOCRINE PROBLEMS

I. GOITER

A. Hyperplastic goiter is the most common thyroid disorder in the foal.

B. Cause is ingestion of excess iodine by the dam in the form of kelp containing feed supplements or plant goitrogens (*Brassica spp.*).

C. Idiopathic hyperplastic goiter is reported in western Canada.

D. High levels of iodine inhibit thyroid function and foals with goiter may be hypothyroid or may have normal T_3 and T_4 levels.

II. THYROID ACTIVITY OF NORMAL NEONATAL FOAL

A. The newborn foal has the highest levels of thyroid hormones (T_3 and T_4) of domestic animal species[1] (Table I).

B. Thyroid stimulating hormone administered to 1 day old foals increases T_3 in 3 hours by 50% and 16% increase in T_4 at 6 hours.[2]

III. HYPOTHYROIDISM occurs in three forms.

A. Hypometabolic[3]
1. Thyroid may be of normal size.
2. Incoordination, poor sucking and righting reflexes, hypothermia, depression, poor growth, rough hair coat, angular limb deformities, anemia, lipemia, and abnormal bone ossification.
3. Be aware that severe illness may non-specifically lower T_3 and T_4 but thyroid "function" remains normal ('euthyroid sick').
4. Thyroid hormone levels may be low.
5. Poor response to TSH stimulation.

B. Developmental Lesions[4,5]
1. Thyroid levels may be normal at the time the abnormalities are noted, and foals may be bright, alert and growing.

2. Ruptured common digital extensor tendons, forelimb contracture, mandibular prognathism and immature carpal or tarsal bones are seen.
C. **Hypothyroid and Respiratory Insufficiency**[6]
   1. Weak, persistent hypothermia, poor suckle, hypoxemia, respiratory acidosis.
   2. Large thyroid glands with large follicles containing eosinophilic colloid.
   3. Diffuse atelectasis - incomplete surfactant development.
D. **Treatment** - after signs have developed, if thyroid levels are normal, no treatment is indicated. If T_3 and T_4 are low, replacement by Cytobin ®(Norden) at 1 µg/kg PO daily or 20-50 µg/kg Synthroid® PO daily is indicated. Measure values at 1 week to avoid over-dosing. Irvine suggests dose calculation of T_4 in µg/day = fractional turnover (0.22) X (Kg body wt. X 0.08) X plasma T_4 in µg/L X 10 for oral administration.[3]

IV. **HYPOADRENOCORTICISM** is seen in foals which are premature or normal gestation but dysmature.

A. **Clinical signs** of a premature foal is described in detail previously (See Chapter 12)
B. **Hematology and clinical pathology**: Abnormally low neutrophil to lymphocyte ratio (<0.5-1.0 without bands or immature neutrophils) is common. Hypoglycemia or hypoinsulinemia may also be present.
C. **Plasma cortisol** < 30 ng/ml 2 hours after birth -normal values 120-140 ng/ml.[7]
D. **In healthy neonates** significant elevation in cortisol concentration should be observed after the administration of low dose (10µg) or high dose of ACTH (100µg)[8].
E. **Aqueous ACTH** (Synachten® Cosyntropin®) 0.125 mg (0.003 - 0.006 mg/kg) IM produces only 28% increase in plasma cortisol and no change in neutrophil - lymphocyte ratio in foals with hypoadrenocorticism. Normal foals should have an increase of about 200% in plasma cortisol.
F. In one study, a small percentage of ill neonatal foals exhibited HPA insufficiency after the administration of aqueous ACTH (Cosyntropin®).[9]

G. A different study showed an increased ACTH/cortisol ratio in non-surviving septic foals in comparison to surviving septic foals which could indicate hypothalamic-pituitary-adrenal axis dysfunction at the level of the adrenal gland in these animals.[10]

H. Vasopressin and ACTH levels of septic neonatal foals showed increased plasma AVP (Vasopressin) and ACTH concentrations in septic foals that did not survive. Several septic foals had increased AVP: ACTH and ACTH: cortisol ratios, which indicate relative adenohypophyseal and adrenal insufficiency[11]. See also treatment of relative adrenal insufficiency, Chapter 12, Prematurity.

References:

1. Irvine, C.H.G., Evans, M.J.: Postnatal changes in total and free thyroxine and triiodothyronine in foal serum. J Reprod Fert Suppl 23:709-715, 1975.
2. Shaftoe, S., Schick, M.F., Chen, C.L.: Thyroid-stimulation hormone response tests in one day old foals. Equine Vet Sci 8:310-312, 1988.
3. Irvine, C.H.G.: Hypothyroidism in the foal. Equine Vet J 16:302-305, 1984.
4. McLaughlin, B.G.: Thyroid hormone levels in foals with congenital musculoskeletal lesions. Can Vet J 27:264-267, 1986.
5. Vivrette, S.L., Reimers T.J. and Knook L.: Skeletal disease in a hypothyroid foal. Cornell Vet 74:373-386, 1984.
6. Murray, M.J.: Hypothyroidism and respiratory insufficiency in a neonatal foal. JAVMA 197:1635-1638, 1990.
7. Vaala, W.E.: Diagnosis and treatment of prematurity and neonatal maladjustment syndrome in newborn foals. Compend Cont Educ for Pract Vet 8:S211-S222, 1986.
8. Hart KA, Heusner GL, Norton NA, Barton, MH. Hypothalamic-Pituitary-Adrenal Axis Assessment in Healthy Term Neonatal Foals Utilizing a Paired Low Dose/High Dose ACTH Stimulation Test. J Vet Intern Med. 2009 Feb 3.
9. Wong DM, Vo DT, Alcott CJ, Peterson AD, Sponseller BA, Hsu WH.: Baseline plasma cortisol and ACTH concentrations and response to low-dose ACTH stimulation testing in ill foals. J Am Vet Med Assoc. 2009 Jan 1;234(1):126-32.

10. Gold JR, Divers TJ, Barton MH, Lamb SV, Place NJ, Mohammed HO, Bain FT.: Plasma adrenocorticotropin, cortisol, and adrenocorticotropin/cortisol ratios in septic and normal-term foals. J Vet Intern Med. 2007 Jul-Aug;21(4):791-6.

11. Hurcombe SD, Toribio RE, Slovis N, Kohn CW, Refsal K, Saville W, Mudge MC.: Blood arginine vasopressin, adrenocorticotropin hormone, and cortisol concentrations at admission in septic and critically ill foals and their association with survival. J Vet Intern Med. 2008 May-Jun;22(3):639-47.

12. Chen, C., Riley, A.: Serum thyroxin and triiodothyronine concentrations in neonatal foals and mature horses. Am J Vet Res 42:1415, 1981.

Table I. Normal Equine Neonatal Thyroid Levels

Age	Total T_4 (µg/dl) ± S.D. [*]	Total T_3 (ng/dl) ± S.D. [*]
Birth	43.3 ± 8.4	527.7 ± 136
1 day	13.6 ± 5.1	366.5 ± 222.5 [2]
4-6 days	11.1 ± 5.1	935.1 ± 441
7-10 days	7.4 ± 1.9	629.0 ± 15
21-90 days	2.62 ± 72	194.8 ± 45
1.5-4 months	4.02 ± 0.19 [**]	192.86 ± 8.54 [**]

[*] Tri-Tab Radioimmunoassay [1,4]

[**] Gamma coat Radioimmunoassay [12]

[2] Clinical Assays, Division of Travenol, Laboratories, Cambridge, MA

CHAPTER 47
RESPIRATORY DISTRESS

Respiratory distress is a clinical feature. The signs of labored or rapid breathing, flared nostrils and increased breathing efforts are not specific for a single cause. Remember that non pulmonary causes can be fever, neurological disease, pain, anxiety, excitement, severe anemia or drug induced hyperthermia.

I. ACUTE RESPIRATORY DISTRESS SYNDROME (ARDS)

ARDS is a poorly understood condition with the common feature of impairment of the lung to adequately exchange gas at the alveolar level, which produces hypoxemia and carbon dioxide retention. Diffuse atelectasis and reduced lung compliance are features of the syndrome. Foals that experience asphyxia, deprivation of placental blood, or are premature or small for gestational age are at increased risk.[1] Surfactant deficiency has not been documented in term foals as a component of the syndrome.

II. DIAGNOSIS

A   Clinical Findings
  1. Flared nostrils and rapid breathing with chest wall collapsing inward during inspiration.
  2. Poor entry of air into lungs on auscultation. Bronchovesicular sounds are diminished compared to the degree of effort, crackles may be audible.
  3. Expiratory grunting and cyanosis may be present.
B. **Blood gas abnormalities:** PaO_2 <50 mmHg and $PaCO_2$ >60 mmHg without metabolic alkalosis[1].
C. **Chest radiographs** in foals with respiratory distress do not resemble the ground glass or reticulated pattern seen in human infants with ARDS. Air bronchogram indicating diffuse atelectasis can occasionally be seen but a generalized increase in interstitial density is the more common finding.
D. **Ultrasonography** reveals diffuse wide comet tails in most cases of ARDS (See Chapter 52).

III. CONCURRENT OR PREDISPOSING FACTORS

A. **Any factor** that leads to a decrease in efficiency of respiration or an increased demand can produce fatigue and progressive atelectasis.[1]
   1. Pneumonia; viral, bacterial.
   2. Pneumocystis carinii[2]
   3. Increased vascular permeability.
   4. Pulmonary hypertension.
   5. Fractured ribs.

B. **Prematurity**
   1. Prematurity may lead to ARDS.
   2. Whether or not ARDS develops in a premature foal, is not necessarily predictable based on gestational age alone.
      a. Foals that are born at 300-320 day gestation or that have experienced in-utero stress (twins or other conditions) may have hastened pulmonary maturation and have mature lungs.
   3. Amniotic fluid analysis for surfactant (Lecithin/sphingomyelin (L/S) ratio and phosphatidylglycerol (PG)) has not been able to predict lung maturity in foals.[3]
      a. **Preliminary** evidence does suggest L/S ratio of 2.2 and 2+ PG indicative of some degree of lung maturity in foals.
   4. Corticosteroids to mare may hasten lung maturity.
   5. **Preventive measures** are limited to avoiding elective early induction of labor. Avoid induction entirely unless absolutely essential.

C. **Premature placental separation**, dystocia or cesarean section, maternal medication, placentitis, in utero infection.

D. **Sepsis** or other conditions which cause a foal to be in prolonged recumbency can produce atelectasis.

E. **Reversion to fetal circulation** with high pulmonary arterial pressure and a shunting of blood through the ductus arteriosus away from the lung has been documented by the author by cardiac catheterization in a premature foal with ARDS and diagnosed via ultrasonography in a foal.[4]

F. **Meconium Aspiration** - foals may have meconium staining on eyes, face and skin.
  1. Occurs due to defecation associated with pre or intrapartum asphyxia.
  2. Causes surfactant inactivation and inflammation.
  3. Treatment is suctioning of airways, oxygen insufflation, mechanical ventilation, surfactant administration.

III. **MANAGEMENT - GENERAL PRINCIPLES**

The object is to support the respiratory system and entire patient while correcting undesirable conditions or allowing spontaneous resolution to occur. Sternal position to improve oxygenation efficiency is extremely important.

A. **Airway Management**
  1. Coupage, airway suction as needed and early ambulation (Chapter 66).
B. **Oxygen Therapy**
  1. **Warm, humidified**, O_2 at sufficient rates to maintain PaO_2 in lateral recumbency of 80-100 mmHg (Chapter 13).
  2. **Useful in** foals with low O_2 and normal or low $PaCO_2$ (<60 mmHg).
  3. **Hypoventilation** as evidenced by elevated $PaCO_2$ may require ventilation therapy.
C. **Vascular Catheters**
  1. **An indwelling** arterial catheter for monitoring of blood gases is helpful.
  2. **Sites used** have all been somewhat difficult to maintain but have included facial, brachial, femoral, and dorsal metatarsal artery.
  3. **Swan-Ganz thermodilution catheters** to determine cardiac output, mixed venous blood gases, and pressures within pulmonary artery, atrium and right ventricle have been used by the author in management in conjunction with a cardiac output computer.[5]
D. **Acidosis**
  1. **Metabolic acidosis** with a base deficit of ≥ 6 mEq/L requires evaluation of causes including shock,

hypovolemia, hypoglycemia, hypothermia, infection, renal disease and sequelae of asphyxia.
2. **If the arterial pH** is less than 7.25 with a base deficiency of 6, correction is via volume expansion, glucose infusion if hypoglycemic, or plasma or whole blood. If refractory to volume expansion, use I.V. administration of diluted sodium bicarbonate if ventilation is adequate. Bicarbonate is converted to CO_2 which must be capable of being eliminated by the lung.
3. **Bicarbonate** amounts are calculated by base deficit x body weight in kg x 0.4, due to the larger extracellular fluid of newborn foals.
4. **Administer bicarbonate** slowly – use an isotonic solution (See Fluid therapy, Chapter 22). Monitor arterial blood gas for evidence of CO_2 increases.
5. **A pure respiratory acidosis** in the range of 7.2 - 7.3 may be tolerable. When the pH falls below 7.2 due to respiratory acidosis, assisted ventilation is indicated.
   a. If assisted ventilation not possible, consider CRI of Doxapram.

E. **Sudden Deterioration in Condition**
   1. **Check mechanical portions of oxygen delivery system.**
      a. O_2 amounts and pressure in tanks.
      b. Obstruction of endotracheal tube by secretions.
      c. Inadvertent positioning of the endotracheal tube into the esophagus or too far distal in an airway into a bronchus.
   2. **Check metabolic causes** such as hypoglycemia and acidosis.

F. **Respiratory Failure Management**[1]
   1. **Reasons to intervene** with pulmonary support techniques other than supplemental oxygen are inability to maintain a PaO_2 >52 mmHg in lateral recumbency and/or steadily rising $PaCO_2$ above 60 mmHg (See Chapter 13).
   2. **See Section** on nasotracheal intubation and positive pressure ventilation (Chapter 67).
   3. **Be prepared** and make a commitment for the significant degree of effort to manage these patients.

4. Bronchopulmonary dysplasia has developed following treatment for ARDS in foals.[6]

G. **Differential Diagnosis** - Transient Tachypnea Syndrome
1. Resembles respiratory distress
2. Has been seen in foals with significantly elevated respiratory rates of 60-120/min.
3. **May have elevated body temperature** but foals are alert, nurse, and not cyanotic or pale.
4. **Differentiate by normal CBC**, clinical chemistry, blood gases and acid base and chest x-ray.
   a. Even though foals are hyperventilating, $PaCO_2$ is normal which means foals are "panting".
5. **Condition is self limited** over 1-2 weeks. Clipping body hair in warm climates and keep in a neutral thermal environment. Avoiding higher environmental temperatures is helpful.
6. **Cause is unknown** but believed associated with immature or delayed development of central brain regulation of ventilation and thermoregulation.

References:
1. Sonea, J.: Respiratory Distress Syndrome in neonatal foals. Compend Cont Educ for Pract Vet 7(8):S412-S419, 1985.
2. Wilson WD: Foal Pneumonia in Robinson NE (ed). Current Therapy in Equine Medicine. 5th Edition. WB Saunders. Philadelphia. 2003. 666-677.
3. Paradis, M.R.: Lecithin/sphingomyelin ratios and phosphatidyl - glycerol in term and premature equine amniotic fluid. Proceed ACVIM p. 789-792, 1987.
4. Cottrill, C.M., O'Conner, W.N., Cudd, T, et al.: Persistence of fetal circulation pathways in a newborn foal. Equine Vet J 19:252-254, 1987.
5. Thomas, W.P., Madigan, J.E., Backus, K.Q., Powell, W.E.: Systemic and pulmonary hemodynamics in normal neonatal foals. J Reprod Fert Suppl 35:623-628, 1987.
6. Freeman, K.P., et al: Recognition of bronchopulmonary dysplasia in a newborn foal. Equine Vet J 21:272-274, 1989.

CHAPTER 48
HERNIA

I. **SCROTAL HERNIA**

   A. **Clinical signs**
      1. Enlarged scrotal sac.
      2. Usually non-strangulating and easily reduced.
      3. Noticed between birth and the first week of age.
      4. Unilateral (most common) or bilateral.
      5. Foal is normal acting with uncomplicated hernias.
      6. **Complicated** hernias
         a. Associated with rent in the common vaginal tunic.[1]
         b. Persistent colic, edema of prepuce and scrotum, mechanical trauma to skin over hernia.[2]
         c. Difficult to manually reduce.[2]
         d. Loops of small intestine palpable in subcutaneous tissue of scrotum or thigh.[2]
   B. **Diagnosis** clinical signs and palpation.
   C. **Differential diagnosis**
      1. Strangulation of intestine.
      2. Excessive uroperitoneum or peritoneal fluid.
      3. Testicular torsion or hematoma - testicle is painful to palpation and firm.
   D. **Treatment**
      1. **Nonsurgical**
         a. Most regress or improve within 7-10 days with repeated manual reduction.
      2. **Surgical**[2,3]
         a. Strangulated hernias are best handled by a combination of scrotal and midline incisions. This allows for exteriorization of affected bowel and easier resection and anastomosis.
         b. Hernia is usually inside tunica vaginalis, but may be subcutaneous.
         c. Best (least complications) to remove testicle of affected side, although not absolutely necessary.

d. Manual reduction of bowel, transfixation ligature of spermatic cord, distal emasculation or amputation is performed.
e. The external inguinal ring is closed with interrupted ligatures incorporating distal stump.
f. Wound may be closed 1° or allowed to heal by second intention.
g.

II. PERSISTENT PREPUTIAL RING OR MEMBRANE

A. Clinical Signs
1. Foal cannot "drop penis" during urination.
2. Urine scald around prepuce and hind limbs.

Diagnosis
1. History, clinical signs.
2. Manual examination of prepuce.

Treatment
1. Requires short general anesthesia.
2. Resect membrane to expose glans penis. May require partial resection of preputial folds.

III. UMBILICAL HERNIAS

A. Standard care (See Chapter 39)
B. Rupture during parturition has occasionally occurred.
   1. Congenital umbilical hernias may rupture out of hernia at umbilicus at foaling or soon after.
   2. Often follows a dystocia.
   3. If bowel is not damaged, clean with saline or Lactated Ringers, replace and ligate cord. Stabilize the foal medically and consider if surgical repair of defect is indicated.

IV. DIAPHRAGMATIC HERNIAS

A. Congenital (abnormal closure of the crura).
B. Acquired (most commonly associated with fractured ribs, dystocia, blunt trauma).

C. Characterized by violent intermittent colic and respiratory distress.
   D. Diagnosis with x-ray, ultrasound.
   E. Surgical repair possible (primary or mesh technique).

References:
1. Spurlock, G.H., Robertson, J.T.: Congenital acquired hernias associated with a rent in the common vaginal tunic in five foals. JAVMA 193:1087-1088, 1987.
2. Auer, J. A. – Stick, J. A.: Equine Surgery. 3rd. Ed., WB Saunders, Philadelphia, 2006.
3. Vaughan, J.T., Walker, D.F.: Bovine and Equine Urogenital Surgery. Lea and Febiger, Philadelphia, 1980.

CHAPTER 49
FRACTURED RIBS

This is a condition that occurs in larger foals or from dystocia foals. Foals of primiparous mares should be considered at a higher risk for thoracic trauma. May be subclinical and be overlooked by the practitioner.[1]

A. **Clinical Signs**[1]
 1. Lethargic, spend time down, may get up stiffly with groaning.
 2. Pericardial and lung lacerations may lead to hemopericardium, hemothorax, pulmonary tamponade, pneumothorax and respiratory difficulty.
 3. May produce diaphragmatic lesions and hemoperitoneum.
B. **Diagnosis**[1]
 1. While foal is standing palpate ribs with both hands feeling for asymmetry and crepitus.
 2. Series of ribs may be indented on one side; rarely are fractures bilateral.
 3. Ultrasound for rib displacement.
 4. Sudden death due to laceration of large vessels.
C. **Treatment**[1, 2]
 1. Early detection and stall rest for 2-4 weeks.
 2. More severe cases require chest drainage and taping or padding chest for flail chest problems.
 3. Surgical repair is possible[2], ribs repaired by internal fixation.
    a. surgical stabilization utilizing reconstruction plates, self-tapping cortical screws and cerclage wire for selected cases.
 4. Analgesics and respiratory support if indicated.
 5. Antibiotics if delayed nursing from mare.
 6. Foals may develop pneumothorax during surgical repair.

References:
1. Byars, TD. Fractured Ribs in Neonatal Foals. AAEP Report 1997, Pediatric Perusals. P 13.
2. Bellezzo F, Hunt RJ, Provost R, Bain FT, Kirker-Head C. Surgical repair of rib fractures in 14 neonatal foals: case selection, surgical technique and results. Equine Vet J. 36(7):557-62, 2004

CHAPTER 50
COLIC IN THE NEONATAL FOAL

Abdominal pain is a common problem in neonates. It is may be difficult to distinguish cases that require surgery from those that can be treated medically, therefore a thorough history and physical exam utilizing ultrasound of the abdomen must be performed, along with laboratory evaluation.

I. CLINICAL SIGNS

- **A.** Restlessness, attempts to defecate, swishing of the tail, walking around the stall, tail elevation and straining.
- **B.** Advanced signs of abdominal pain are lying down and getting up repeatedly, dorsal recumbency, rolling.
- **C.** May appear to be attempting to urinate frequently.
- **D.** Abdominal distention may or may not be present.
- **E.** Fever in cases of infectious enteritis.
- **F.** Bruxism, salivation, dorsal recumbency, diarrhea, interrupted nursing in cases of gastrointestinal ulceration.

II. DIFFERENTIAL DIAGNOSIS

Common causes	Less common causes
1. Meconium impaction	1. Congenital defects (atresia coli, ani)
2. Enteritis (viral, bacterial)	2. Pyloric stenosis
3. Overfeeding (iatrogenic)	3. Torsion, volvulus, intussusception
4. Ruptured bladder	4. Ileal impaction
5. Gastroduodenal ulceration	5. Hernias: umbilical, scrotal, diaphragmatic

6. Ascarid impaction
   post deworming
   older foals/ weanlings
	6. Fecalith impaction

	7. Peritonitis/adhesions[1]
	8. Intra-abdominal masses
	9. Agangliosis (overo-overo)
	10. Incarceration in mesodiverticulum band
	11. Hemoperitoneum[2]
	12. Thromoembolism (previous surgery)
	13. Post enema – "fire butt"

III. DIAGNOSTIC APPROACH[3]

A. **Complete history**, considerations:
1. Breed (overo-overo: agangliosis) and sex (colts more predisposed to meconium retention than fillies).
2. Age of the foal at presentation and at the onset of clinical signs.
3. Urination and defecation (frequency and characteristics).
4. Diet: mare's milk or milk replacers, amount and frequency of feedings if supplementing.
5. Peripartum events and farm history of current or past enteritis.

B. **Physical exam**, including:
1. Observation of the patient. Gastric distention can cause dilation of the caudal rib cage. Severe distention may indicate a colonic disorder.
2. Auscultation and percussion of the abdomen. Absence of borborygmi sounds indicates ileus; the presence of high pitched resonant sounds (ping) indicates gas distention.
3. External palpation of the abdomen. Urinary bladder and occasionally colonic impactions and masses can be felt.
4. Ballottement of the abdomen may help differentiating gas from fluid abdominal distention.
5. Rectal digital palpation can reveal rectal impaction with meconium.
6. Measurement of abdominal circumference. Serial determinations are helpful to monitor progression or regression of abdominal distention.
7. Nasogastric intubation to determine the presence of reflux and/or gas. Reflux suggests intestinal obstruction or ileus, although its absence does not rule it out. In every case of abdominal pain, NGT must be passed for diagnostic and/or therapeutic purposes.

C. **Clinicopathologic data**
1. Acute bacterial enteritis (leukopenia with left shift, toxic neutrophils, hyperfibrinogemia). (See Chapter 33 diarrhea).

2. **Chemistry panel and blood gases** - ruptured bladder (marked hyperkalemia), or metabolic acidosis with electrolyte imbalances in diarrhea cases.
3. Lactate levels elevated in severely compromised cases.

D. **Abdominal Radiography and Ultrasound (See Chapter 52&53) may assist with a specific diagnosis**
   1. Volvulus of small intestine
   2. Large colon torsion
   3. Meconium impaction (high)
   4. Diaphragmatic hernia
   5. Gastroduodenal ulcers and subsequent pyloric stenosis and delayed gastric emptying.
   6. Enteritis

E. **Abdominal ultrasonography** is considered valuable (See Chapter 52).

F. **Abdominocentesis** should be performed carefully in the recumbent or standing foal. Perform a sterile prep and block the skin. Some prefer using a needle (20 ga) while others have used bitch catheter or teat cannula. Sedation may be required. Nucleated cell counts are lower in foals than in adults (greater than 1500/µl are considered elevated).[4] Normal peritoneal fluid protein concentration ranges from 0.3 to 1.8g/dl[4]. Cytologic examination may reveal bacteria, ingesta, or degenerated cells. If peritonitis suspected, culture of the fluid is indicated. Peritoneal tap is often normal in cases of **enteritis**. In foals with suspected uroperitoneum, the creatinine concentration of peritoneal fluid and serum must be obtained (see Chapter 37).

G. **Fecal analysis (flotation, culture, microscopic evaluation)** is indicated in cases of diarrhea, especially if stools are bloody. Pathogens associated with diarrhea and colic are *Salmonella spp.* and *Clostridium spp.* (See Chapter 33, Diarrhea)

H. **Gastroscopy** should be used to detect gastric ulceration, pyloric stenosis, **colonoscopy** to detect malformations of rectum and small colon.

I. **Exploratory celiotomy** indicated if surgical condition is identified or in unidentified cause of persistent or severe pain/distention. Surgical considerations (see references for detailed descriptions).

1. Correct fluid, electrolytes and blood gas abnormalities before surgery if possible.
2. Avoid damaging umbilicus and associated vessels. [If suspect umbilical infections or involvement (patent urachus) then remove at time of surgery].
3. Use wound protectors whenever possible
4. Use copious abdominal lavage (warm Lactated or buffered Ringers solution ± antibiotics as foals are more prone to get adhesions.
5. Minimize tissue handling - intestine is easily irritated and damaged.
6. Recent reports suggests prevention of ischemia-induced small intestinal adhesions in foals using flunixin meglumine and Penicillin and gentamicin treatment[5]; others have suggested treat with IV DMSO at 20 mg/kg diluted in 500 ml saline.

IV. SPECIFIC CONDITIONS WITH SEVERE PAIN MANIFESTATIONS

D. Enteritis
1. Auxiliary lab tests: CBC, fibrinogen, electrolytes, blood gases and paracentesis are indicated.
2. Blood may have low white blood cell count (degenerative left shift) and peritoneal fluid analysis is usually normal.
3. Clostridium enteritis requires **immediate therapy** (see Chapter 33 Diarrhea).
4. Ultrasound reveals fluid-filled hypermotile small and large intestine.

B. Duodenal-pyloric stenosis
Clinical signs (See Section 34 gastroduodenal ulcers).
1. Advanced stages of gastric ulcers.
2. Persistent bruxism, salivation and/or regurgitation, endoscopic and radiographic evidence of gastric outflow obstruction.
3. Progressive debilitation and unresponsive to medical therapy.

Diagnosis
1. History and clinical signs

2. Upper G.I. barium study - delayed gastric emptying.
    a. Normal 2 hour gastric emptying time after 12 hour fast using 5 ml/kg of a 30% weight/volume barium suspension.[6]
    b. Gastric endoscopy.

Surgery
1. Improved outcome if done before severe debilitation and peritonitis develop. May develop into racing and performance horses based on a report[7]
2. Gastrojejunostomy - most common procedure.
3. Gastroduodenostomy - ideal, but more difficult.
4. Must continue ulcer therapy after surgery.
5. Often have secondary hepatitis problem (retrograde infection) or blind loop syndrome.
6. Recent report showed 50% survival rate long term on 16 foals with gastrojejunostomy[7].

C. **SMALL OR LARGE INTESTINAL STRANGULATION**
   Clinical signs
   1. Depression, anorexia, milk stained face.
   2. Elevated respiratory and heart rates ± increased temperature.
   3. ± Abdominal distension and tympany.
   4. Progressive systemic deterioration.
   5. May occasionally see milk regurgitation.
   6. Persistent pain, even with most analgesics.

   Diagnosis - large bowel problems often have slower onset.
   1. Clinical signs.
   2. Abdominal US, thoracic radiographs can be very useful.
   3. Differential diagnosis
      a. Intussusception (jejunal-jejunal, ileo-cecal, etc).
      b. Diaphragmatic hernia - thoracic radiographs show distended loop of intestine (usually small).
      c. Intra-abdominal hernias (mesenteric rents, etc).
      d. Strangulated scrotal hernia - see below.
      e. Thromboembolism (large or small bowel) - usually seen after a previous surgery.
      f. Volvulus of large intestine.

V. THERAPY

- **E.** Treat cause if determined.
- **B.** Stabilize with fluids and pain relief.
- **C.** Prevent/treat sepsis
  1. Plasma (failure of passive transfer or high risk foal) (See Chapter 10).
  2. Antimicrobial therapy (high risk foal) (See Chapter 70):
     - a. Broad spectrum
     - b. Anaerobe coverage (if suspected)
- **D. Analgesia**[8,9]
  1. **NSAIDs**, <u>important to maintain adequate hydration</u>. Use low doses due to potential side effects — GI ulceration and nephrotoxicity.
     - a. Dipyrone (10-20 mg/kg IV or IM), off the market in the US.
     - b. Ketoprofen (less ulcerogenic) 2.2 mg/kg IV.
     - c. Flunixin-meglumine (0.25-1.5 mg/kg IV or IM), lower dose used to prevent deleterious effects of endotoxemia.
     - d. Phenylbutazone (2.2 mg/kg PO or IV) more ulcerogenic.
     - e. COX-2 specific blockers have not been extensively studied in neonates.
     - f. **Opiate agonists**
       - i. Butorphanol tartrate (0.02-0.1 mg/kg IV or IM). It has been shown to decrease intestinal motility in adults although still the most convenient opioid currently available.
       - ii. Morphine can be used in foals at a dose of 0.1-0.2 mg/kg IM.
       - iii. Fentanyl is a highly potent opioid and is most commonly used for musculoskeletal conditions (available as a patch 100 μg/hr release)
  2. **Tramadol** has not been extensively studied in neonatal foals. It has been used to eliminate moderate to severe pain in adult horses at a dose of 1-2 mg/kg IV, IM[9].

3. **Anticholinergics: Buscopan (N-butylscopolamine bromide)** can be used as a spasmolytic in cases of inflamed bowel or meconium impaction. It has minimal side-effects (mild tachycardia) and can be given at a dose of 0.2-0.3 mg/kg IV q12 hrs.
4. **Alpha 2 adrenergic agonists:** Xylazine hydrochloride (0.2-0.5 mg/kg IV). More potent in neonates than in adults which will decrease GI motility, can cause marked depression, bradycardia. Whenever possible avoid its use in compromised foals ≤2 weeks old.
5. **Prevent/treat gastrointestinal ulceration**[10] (See Chapter 34)
    a. Proton pump inhibitors
    b   Mucosal protectants
    c. Histamine type 2 receptor antagonists
    d. Antacids

References:
1. Lundin C.S., Sullins K.E., White N.A., Pfeiffer C.J., Clem M.F. and Debowes R.M. The pathogenesis of peritoneal adhesions in the foal. Vet Surgery 18:66, 1989.
2. Green S.L., Specht T.E., Dowling S.C., Nixon A.J., Wilson J.H. and Carrick J.B. Hemoperitoneum caused by rupture of a juvenile granulosa cell tumor in an equine neonate. JAVMA 193:11, 1417-1419, 1988.
3. Cohen N.D. and Chaffin K.: Assessment and initial management of colic in foals. Compend Contin Educ Pract Vet 17:1, 93-103, 1995.
4. Grinden C.B., Fairley N.M., Uhlinger C.A. and Crane S.A. Peritoneal fluid values from healthy foals. Equine Vet J 22:359-361, 1990.
5. Sullins KE, White NA, Lundin CS, Dabareiner R, Gaulin G. Prevention of ischaemia-induced small intestinal adhesions in foals. Equine Vet J. 36(5):370-5, 2004
6. Fischer A.T., Kerr L.Y. and O'Brien T.R. Radiographic diagnosis of gastrointestinal disorders in the foal. Vet Radiology 28:2, 42-48, 1987.
7. Coleman, MC, Slovis, NM, Hunt RJ: Long-term prognosis of Gastrojejunostomy in foals with gastic outflow obstruction: 16

cases. (2001-2006). <u>Equine Vet J</u>. 41: 653-657. 2009
8. Mair TS, Divers T, Ducharme N: Manual of Equine Gastroenterology. WB. Saunders. Philadelphia 2002.
9. Doherty, T., Valverde, A.: Manual of Equine Anesthesia and Analgesia. Blackwell. UK. 2006
10. Murray M.J. Gastric ulceration, in Smith B.P. (ed): <u>Large animal Internal Medicine</u>, 4th ed. Mosby, 710-716, 2008.

CHAPTER 51
SEDATION AND ANESTHESIA

Sedation and anesthesia may be required in neonatal foals to allow diagnostic and therapeutic procedures to be carried out in a safe fashion. There are several differences in foals compared to adult horses that require consideration.[1]

I   **NEONATAL CHARACTERISTICS**

   A.   The newborn foal (especially during the first 72 hrs of life) and the premature foal are in circulatory transition from in utero right ventricular dominance to left ventricular dominance and can revert to fetal circulation following birth (See Chapter 47 section IIIE).
   1.   The ductus arteriosus and the foramen ovale may re-open under conditions of hypoxia, hypotension and bradycardia. Therefore caution needs to be used with the use of agents affecting circulatory status to prevent hypoxia and hypotension.
   2.   Neonates rely on heart rate to maintain cardiac output compared to adults.[7]
   3.   Foals may have altered responses to hypoxemia and hypercapnia leading to alveolar hypoventilation, ventilation perfusion mismatch and R-L shunts.
   B.   Immature drug metabolism may also cause different outcomes compared to adult horses using the same agents. (See Chapter 71).
   C.   Susceptibility to hypothermia requires efforts to prevent heat loss and maintain body temperature during some procedures with sedation and anesthesia.
   D.   Low energy stores will cause hypoglycemia and thus foals should have dextrose containing solutions infused during anesthesia.
   E.   Because of limitations in stroke volume in neonates cardiac output depends more on heart rate.
   1.   Drugs that lower the heart rate (xylazine and detomidine) and those that decrease preload (acepromazine) may produce diminished cardiac output and tissue perfusion.

II SEDATION

A. α2-agonists

1. **Xylazine** is not recommended as a preanesthetic agent in **ill** foals - significant effects on decreasing heart rate and can compromise circulatory status.

    a. In sick neonatal foals doses of 0.44 mg/kg IV (about 22 mg in a 50 kg foal) produced blanching of mucous membranes, marked depression and prolonged recovery and 2 sick foals died that received 0.55 mg/kg IV (about 28 mg in a 50 kg foal) [5]

    EC - Use diazepam in sick foals for sedation.

    b. Healthy foals 10 days to 28 days of age received a dose of 1.1 mg/kg IV which produced sedation and ataxia and recumbency in 4 of 6 foals with no adverse effects.[3]

    c. Xylazine at lower doses 0.25 to 0.5 mg/kg IV (12-25 mg in 50 kg foal) combined with butorphanol 0.02 - 0.04 mg/kg (1-2 mg in a 50 kg foal) produces good sedation and analgesia[4]

    d. Xylazine (0.5-1.0 mg/kg) mixed with pentazocine 0.03-0.08mg/kg (Talwin®).

2. **Detomidine** widely used with safety in healthy foals at 10-20 µg/kg (0.5 to 1 mg in a 50 kg foal).[6]

    a. Combination with butorphanol 20-40 µg/kg (2-4 mg in 50 kg foal) produces good analgesia and sedation.

3. **Medetomidine** has been used by infusion in experimental settings in ponies. It is used as a component of TIVA or PIVA in adult horses although it has not been evaluated in neonatal foals yet. It is very potent and should be carefully dosed (0.001-0.01 mg/kg).

4. **Romifidine** is not used commonly in foals. The dose is 0.04-0.12 mg/kg. It has a shorter duration compared to detomidine.

B. Benzodiazepines

1. **Diazepam** (Valium) 0.1 - 0.2 mg/kg (5-10 mg in a 50 kg foal) is a safe and effective tranquilizer in neonatal foals but has no analgesia. Good for sick foals

because it has minimal cardiovascular effects. Catheter placement is consequently easier in foals sedated with diazepam as jugular distensibility is less affected.

EC - I use this when I get a sick foal that is flopping around, can't stand and won't lie quietly.

2. **Midazolam** (0.05-0.1 mg/kg iv) is a shorter acting agent. Doses can be repeated frequently or used as a CRI if needed.

C. **Phenothiazine tranquillizers**
1. **Acepromazine** has its major drawback as it causes dose dependent cardiovascular effects and vasodilatation that produces hypothermia.
   EC - We don't use this in neonatal foals

III. ANESTHESIA

A. **Premedication**
1. Premedication of neonatal foals with a sedative or tranquilizer is not usually performed when using inhalation anesthetics.
2. A report of 2 cases of cardiac dysrhythmias with xylazine premedication and halothane anesthesia.
3. If needed, use diazepam 0.1 - 0.2 mg/kg
4. In foals >1 month and that are less tractable can use alpha-2 agent and butorphanol followed by mask or tube induction. [6]

B. **Induction agents** (See references for more details and consult[10])
EC-with inhalational anesthesia, withhold milk from neonates 30- 60 minutes prior.

C. **Inhalational agents**
1. *Isoflurane* produce a smooth induction and rapid recovery[8].
2. *Sevoflurane* has become the most popular and the safest inhalational anesthetic in young foals. MAC is slightly higher for sevoflurane than for isoflurane (2.31% vs. 1.31%)
3. *Halothane* is not recommended for equine neonates.
4. *Inhalational methods*

- a. Face mask - can be used to deliver oxygen and inhalant
- b. Naso-tracheal intubation with cuffed silicone tubes (Bivona) 55 cm or longer with internal diameters of 8-14 mm.
- c. Large clear plastic canine mask or 1liter plastic bottles if nothing else is available.
- d. Single carbon dioxide absorber canisters suitable for foals up to 60 kg and double canisters for foals up to 150 kg.[4]
5. Keep mare next to foal during induction to prevent stress. May wish to tranquilize mare in preparation for separation
6. Small animal anesthesia machines will work on most neonatal foals.
7. Keep body temperature stable with warm water blankets, warm IV fluids, etc.[4]

D. Induction with intravenous anesthetics (following sedation)
1. Ketamine (2-3mg/kg)
    a. Ketamine (2-3 mg/kg)+diazepam (0.05-0.2 mg/kg)
    b. Ketamine (2-3mg/kg)+ midazolam (0.05-0.1mg/kg)
    c. Propofol (2 mg/kg) can be used in foals alone or in combination with ketamine or a benzodiazepine for induction[9, 10]

E. Maintenance of anesthesia[8,10]
1. Inhalational anesthesia
    a. Isoflurane (1-3%)
    b. Sevoflurane (1-5%)
2. TIVA (Total Intravenous Anesthesia)
    a. Ketamine + benzodiazepine
    b. Ketamine + α_2 -agonists + guaiphenesin (older, healthy foals only)
    c. Propofol
    d. Propofol + Ketamine
3. PIVA (Partial Intravenous Anesthesia)
    This technique is widely used nowadays because of the safety and lower mortality rate. It will result in a

significant decrease of the inhalational anesthetic use (25-90% reduction in MAC).
   a. Ketamine
   b. α_2–agonists (older, healthy foals only)
   c. Ketamine + α_2 –agonists (older healthy foals only)
   d. Lidocaine
   e. Lidocaine + Ketamine
   f. Lidocaine + Ketamine + α_2 –agonists (older healthy foals only)

IV. SUPPORTIVE THERAPY

A. **Intravenous fluids and electrolytes (Chapter 22)** should be administered based on laboratory and blood gas values. Monitor for glucose levels during prolonged anesthesia and give isotonic fluids with 1-2.5% dextrose depending on the blood glucose.
B. **Heart rate problems**
   1. Bradycardia (normal is 70-90 beats/min) or AV blocks.
      a. Treat with atropine 0.02-0.04 mg/kg or glycopyrrolate 0.001 mg/kg.[4]
      b. Administration of intravenous calcium-gluconate may be beneficial in foals with decreased myocardial contractility.
   2. Ventricular premature contractions may be treated with a bolus of Mg-sulfate and lidocaine 0.5-1 mg/kg slowly iv.
C. **Hypotension/Shock (Chapter 18)**
   1. Suggested to keep mean arterial pressure (MAP) above 60 mmHg (optimal is between 70-90 mmHg).
   2. Treat first by increasing fluids and decreasing plane of anesthesia.
   3. *Inotropes*: Dobutamine (2-5 ug/kg/min) produces dose dependent increase in heart rate, arterial blood pressure, and renal and splanchnic blood flow. Mix 50 mg dobutamine in 500 ml of saline to make 100 ug/ml solutions.
   4. V*asopressors*: Norepinephrine 0.1-1.5µg/kg/min and Vasopressin 0.25- 1.5mU/kg/min

5. Dopamine is not recommended as first line inotrope or vasopressor anymore.

References:

1. Klein, L.: Anesthesia for neonatal foals. <u>Vet Clin North Amer Equine Pract</u> 1:77-89, 1985.
2. Koterba, AM, Drummond, WA, Kosh, PC.: Intensive care in the neonatal foal. <u>Vet Clin N Am Equine Pract</u> 113-115, 1985.
3. Carter, SW, Robertson, SA, Steel, CJ, et al.: Cardiopulmonary effects of xylazine sedation in the foal. <u>Equine vet J</u> 22:384-388, 1990.
4. Martinez, EA.: Anesthetizing neonatal foals. <u>Vet Medicine</u>, Sept 1995: 879-892.
5. Taylor, PM.: Anesthesia of the foal. <u>Proc of the Fourteenth Bain-Fallon Memorial Lectures</u>, Sydney, Australia, 1992, p 59-65.
6. Doherty, T., Valverde, A.: <u>Manual of Equine Anesthesia and Analgesia</u>. Blackwell. UK. 2006
7. Steffy EP, et al.: Clinical investigations of halothane and isoflurane for induction and maintenance of foal anesthesia. <u>J Vet Pharmacol Therapy</u> 14:300-309, 1991.

Chapter 51 Sedation and Anesthesia

Table 1: Normal Physiologic Parameters in Anesthetized Neonatal Foals

Parameter	Normal Values*
Heart rate	60-90 beats/min
Respiratory rate	10-20 breaths/min
Systolic pressure	90-120 mm Hg, 82±7 mm Hg**
Mean arterial pressure	75-100 mm Hg, 60±6 mm Hg**
Diastolic pressure	55-90 mm Hg, 48±6 mm Hg**
Body temperature	100.5-101.5 F (38 to 38.5 C)
Arterial pH	7.25-7.45
P_aCO_2	40-60 torr
P_aO_2	100-350 torr
End-tidal CO_2	30-50 torr
Base excess	0±1 mEq/L
Packed cell volume	32-38%***
Total serum protein	5.8-7.0 g/dl***
Glucose	144-180 mg/dl*** (8-10 mmol/l)

* Except where noted, normal values are from Riebold, T.W.: Monitoring Equine anesthesia. Vet Clin North Am (Eq. Pract) 6:607-624;1990; Hubbell, JAE.:Monitoring. Eq Anes :Monitoring and Emergency Therapy (WW Muir; JAE Hubbell, eds) Mosby-Year Book, St. Louis, Mo., 1991; pp 153-179; and Dunlop, CI.: Anesthesia and sedation of foals. Vet Clin. North Am (Eq. Pract) 10:67-85;1994.

** Unpublished data from anesthetized neonatal foals (n=11) at the Veterinary Teaching Hospital, Texas A&M University, 1994.

CHAPTER 52
ULTRASONOGRAPHY OF THE FETUS AND THE NEONATE

I. TRANSABDOMINAL FETAL ULTRASOUND

A. Overview:
In many cases, the goal of transabdominal ultrasound in the pregnant mare is to document and monitor placental abnormalities. Mares with placentitis can be placed on appropriate antimicrobial therapy and ultrasound used to monitor treatment response. Although transrectal ultrasound is the technique of choice to diagnose ascending placentitis at the cervical star, infection can occur throughout the placenta and often requires a combination of transabdominal and transrectal ultrasound for accurate diagnosis. A normal transrectal ultrasound should not preclude a transabdominal ultrasound exam.

Ultrasound is also useful to evaluate fetal viability, ranging from assessing well-being and growth on serial exams to confirmation of fetal demise. Ultrasonographic confirmation of fetal death can be surprisingly difficult, especially if a long bone obscures visualization of the fetal heart. In such cases, prolonged absence of fetal activity throughout the exam may be interpreted as fetal death. Repeat assessment should always be performed and results considered in conjunction with other parameters such as fetal ECG and rectal palpation.

Transabdominal ultrasound can also be used to document twins in mid-gestation. If desired, ultrasound guided procedures can be performed to assist with fetal reduction.

B. Indications:
1. Vaginal discharge
2. Premature lactation/mammary development
3. Systemic disease
4. Recent colic surgery
5. Abdominal growth greater than stage of gestation, i.e. concern for twins or hydrops
6. Previous complicated pregnancy

C. Technique:

Patient:
1. Preparation - Clipping often necessary, especially in late gestation. Alcohol saturation is less optimal and is difficult to apply to ventral surfaces. Pressurized garden sprayer is useful for ventral saturation.
2. Positioning - Examiner should sit on same side as fetus to prevent shoulder fatigue.
3. Sedation - Often not necessary. If necessary, small doses of detomidine HCl (0.005-0.01 mg/kg IV)) can be used.

Equipment:
1. Transducer (fetal exam): 2-5 MHz curvilinear required
2. Transducer (placenta/fetal fluids): 4-6 MHz curvilinear (microconvex) is ideal. 5-10 MHz rectal linear or tendon format transducer may be adequate in thin mares or during mid-gestation.
3. Program: Select "deep" program for fetal exam (equine or large animal abdominal programs). For placental imaging, "superficial" program may be used if mare is thin or in mid-gestation. In late term, fat mares or in mares with significant ventral edema, a "deep" program may be necessary to image placenta and fetal fluids.
4. Scanning depth - 15-30 cm for fetal examination, depending on stage of gestation. 5-15 cm for placental/fetal fluid examination.

Procedure:
1. Initial goal - locate fetus.
   a. Place transducer on ventral abdomen in longitudinal plane with indicator oriented towards mare's head.
   b. Look for fetal ribs and rib shadows. Once fetus located, sit on same side of mare as fetus. Adjust depth to maximize fetal visualization.
2. Locate fetal heart - determine fetal positioning
   a. Most foals in late gestation are in cranial presentation. Heart will be seen in fetal thorax as probe is slid caudally on mare. Thorax tapers towards heart in cranial thoracic region (Figure 1).

b. If in caudal presentation, fetal thorax will taper towards heart as probe is slid cranially on mare (Figure 2).
c. Twins - Visualization of two separate fetal hearts and rib cages. Assessment most easily performed in mid gestation when fetuses are small and fetal fluids constitute larger percentage of uterus. In late gestation, assessment is difficult due to large fetal size. A singleton's heart can be seen over a large region of the mare's abdomen, leading to misinterpretation as 2 fetal hearts. In contrast, a 2nd fetus may be located dorsal to a visible fetus, out of range of the ultrasound machine's maximal depth.

3. Fetal Heart Rates (HR):
   a. Resting HR: Slide cursor into center of B-mode image of heart at any location and obtain M mode image. Image only needs to show 2-3 consecutive beats. Measure distance between heartbeats to calculate fetal HR with ultrasound machine software (Figure 3).
      i. Obtain 2-3 measurements
      ii. Normal HR decreases with increasing fetal age:
      iii. Month 6 of gestation: 113 ± 9.0 bpm (Bucca, et al 2005)
      iv. Month 7-9 range: 112 ± 11.2 to 91 ± 6.6 bpm, respectively (Bucca, et al 2005)
      v. Late gestation/month 12: 66.4 ± 6.5 bpm (Bucca, et al 2005); 74.6 ± 7.4 bpm (Reef, et al 1995)
      vi. Persistently elevated or persistently depressed fetal heart rates have been associated with poor fetal outcome
      vii. Hint: Utilizing ultrasound machine software to obtain HR values from M modes is more accurate than counting fetal heartbeats while scanning.
   b. Activity HR - M mode acquisition during actual fetal movement is difficult. Heart rarely remains

intersected by M mode cursor for sufficient length of time. Obtain immediate post-activity HR measurements instead (Figure 4). Values should be elevated relative to resting HR.

i. Hint: Obtain resting heart rates first, then continue with exam. Once fetal movement is detected, immediately return to heart to obtain "activity" HR.

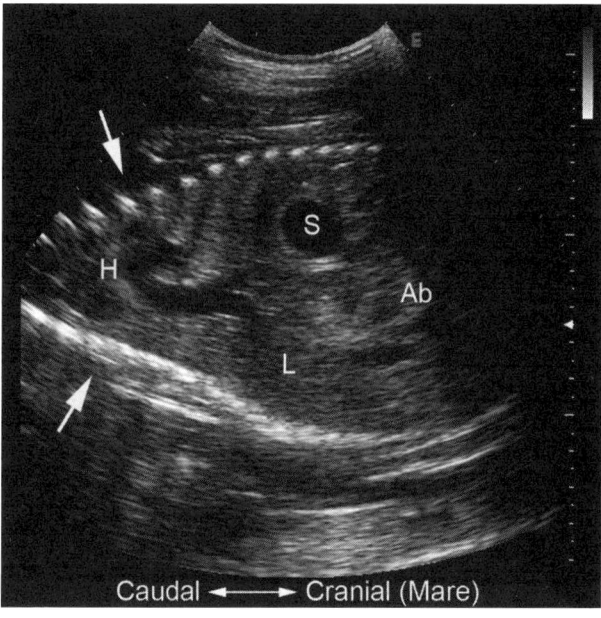

Figure 1: Fetus in cranial presentation. Fetal thorax (arrows) tapers caudally within mare's abdomen. H=heart, S=stomach, L=liver, Ab=fetal abdomen.

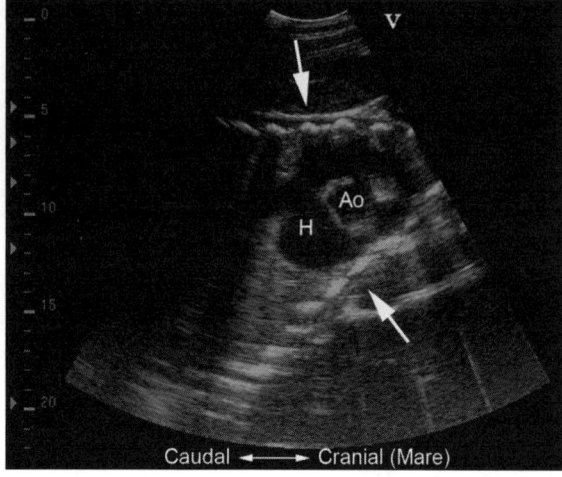

Figure 2: Fetus in caudal presentation. Fetal thorax (arrows) tapers cranially towards mare's head. H=heart, Ao=aorta.

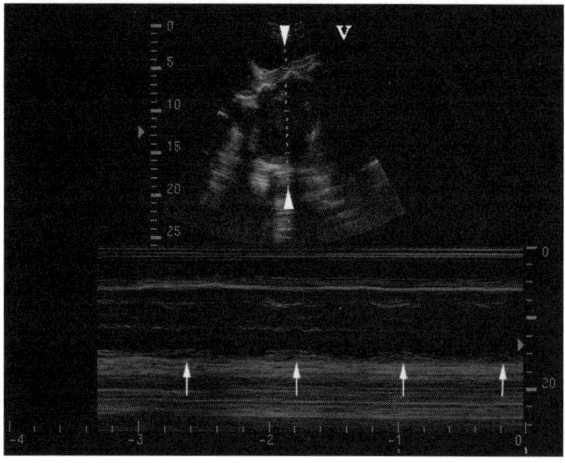

Figure 3: B mode image (top) showing cursor placement (arrowheads) within heart to obtain M mode image (bottom) in which 4 fetal heart beats can be seen (arrows). Heart rate calculated by ultrasound machine software after measuring distance between consecutive heart beats.

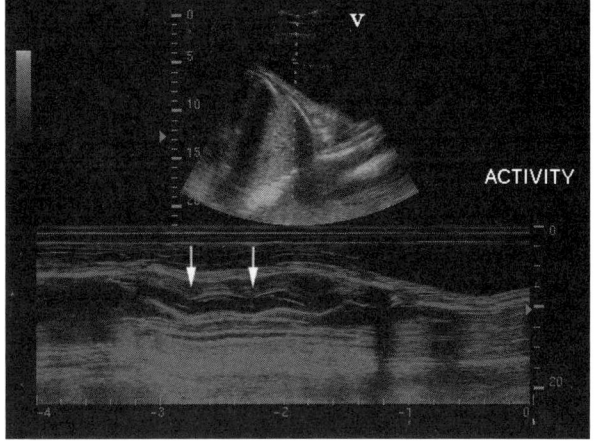

Figure 4: B/M mode image of fetal heart rate during activity. HR calculated from 2 consecutive heart beats (arrows) in M mode image. Heart not visible in B mode image due to fetal movement just before acquisition.

    4. Fetal Aorta:
        a. Echogenic circle (Figure 5) or 2 bright parallel lines (Figure 2) located in center of heart.
        b. Measure using "leading edge to leading edge" technique.
        c. Aortic diameter increases with fetal growth and should be approximately 10% of thoracic diameter.
            i. Month 6-9 range: 10.28 $\pm$ 1.7 mm to 18.19 $\pm$ 1.6 mm (Bucca et al, 2005)
            ii. Late gestation: 22.8 $\pm$ 2.15 mm (Reef et al, 1995)
            iii. Measurement most closely associated with birth weight. Lower than expected aortic diameter has been correlated with low birth weight.
    5. Thoracic diameter:
        a. Maximal diameter obtained at fetal diaphragm
        b. Diaphragm most visible in midgestation and becomes less apparent with fetal growth. Located at intersection of fetal lung and liver

(Figure 6). Fetal liver is less echogenic than fetal lung.
c. Measurements parallel diaphragm and extend beyond fetal ribs to include body wall. Measurements increase with gestational age.
d.

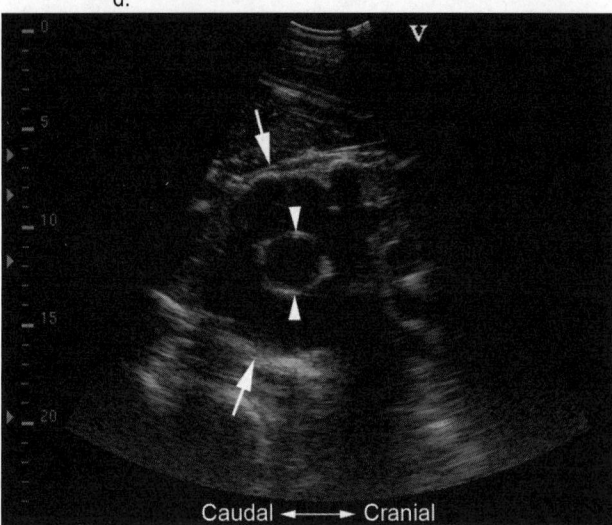

Figure 5: Circular appearance of aorta (arrowheads) located within center of fetal heart (arrows).

Chapter 52 Ultrasonography of the Fetus and the Neonate

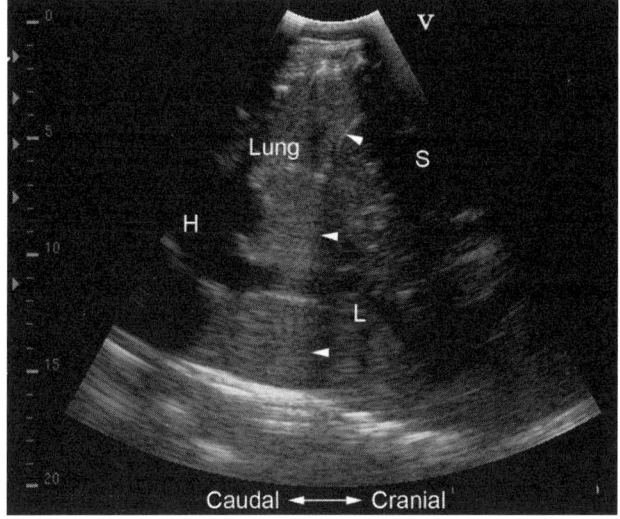

Figure 6: Fetal diaphragm (arrowheads) visualized between fetal liver (L) and lung. S=stomach, H=heart.

6. Allantoic and Amniotic Fluids - Evaluate vertical fluid depths to left and right of fetus. Locate and measure largest fluid pockets in cranial, mid and caudal quadrants on right and left sides, for a total of six quadrants.
   a. Allantoic fluid:
      i. Majority of visible fetal fluids. Located deep and adjacent to uteroplacental unit (Figure 7).
      ii. Measured fluid depths can vary substantially between quadrants. Seen in most quadrants, but may not be visible if fetus is laying directly on placenta (common in 1-2 quadrants).
      iii. Maximal allantoic fluid depths: Late gestation: 13.4 ± 4.4 cm (Reef, et al 1995)
      iv. Hippomane: Often visible within allantoic cavity. Is multilayered with a smooth elliptical shape (Figure 8).

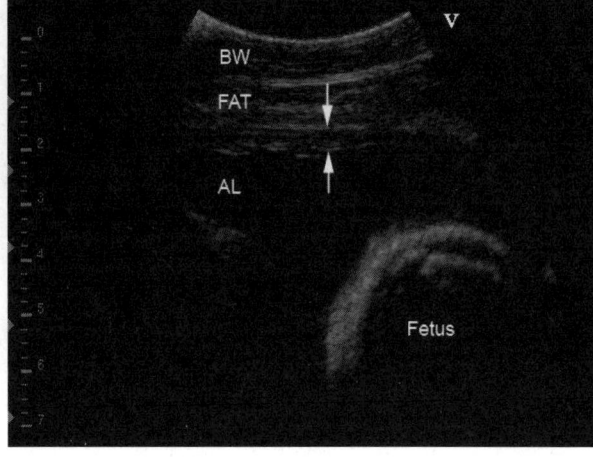

Figure 7: Allantoic fluid (Al) located deep and adjacent to uteroplacental unit (arrows). BW=body wall.

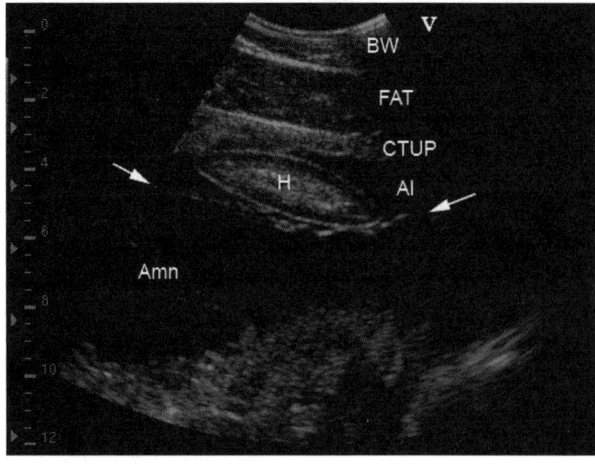

Figure 8: Hippomane (H) located within allantoic space (Al). Amniotic membrane (arrows) divides allantoic from amniotic (Amn) cavities. BW=body wall, CTUP=combined thickness of uteroplacental unit.

Chapter 52 Ultrasonography of the Fetus and the Neonate

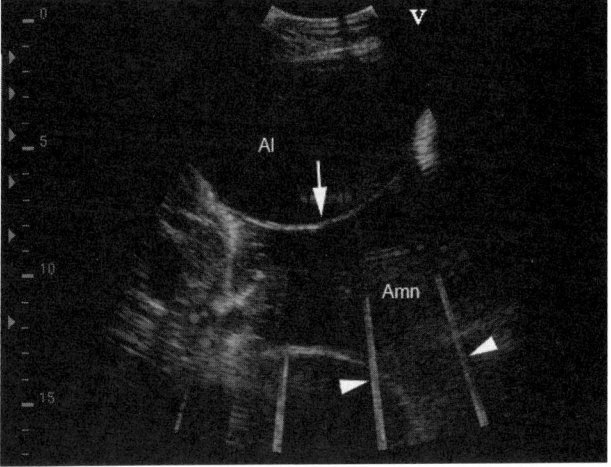

Figure 9: Normal allantoic (Al) and amniotic (Amn) fluids separated by thin amniotic membrane (arrow). Note "Herbie" reverberation artifact (arrowheads) created by scanning through large fluid quantity.

  b. Amniotic fluid:
    i. Differentiated from allantoic fluid by location deep to amniotic membrane (Figure 9). Amniotic membrane has a thin smooth linear appearance and moves freely with fetal movement.
    ii. Most easily seen in caudal quadrants. In other locations, amnion is often located adjacent to fetus, and amniotic fluid will not be visible.
    iii. Maximal amniotic fluid depths:
     • Late gestation: 7.9 ± 3.5 cm (Reef, et al 1995)
  c. Abnormalities/Variations:
    i. Debris: Echogenic particulate material floating within amniotic and/or allantoic fluid is common in normal foals, especially during fetal movement.
    ii. Herbie artifact (Figure 9): Common artifact created by scanning through large

quantities of fluid. Appearance differs between transducers and can be misinterpreted as debris.
   iii. Hydrops amnion and hydrops allantois have been reported and are recognized by grossly increased fluid depths. With the exception of one case report, both conditions are associated with fetal or perinatal death and can result in significant physical/health risk to the mare
   iv. Markedly decreased amniotic fluid depths have also been associated with fetal hypoxia and negative outcomes.
7. <u>Uteroplacental Unit</u>:
   a. Located deep to body wall and retroperitoneal fat layer; adjacent and superficial to allantoic fluid (Figure 10).
   b. Evaluation of entire visible portion of uteroplacental unit should be performed and measurements obtained from representative sites in each of six quadrants, i.e. left cranial, mid and caudal and right cranial, mid and caudal.
   c. Differentiation of layers of uteroplacental unit is not usually possible, and combined thickness measurements are used for assessment.
   d. Normal appearance:
      i. Combined thickness of uteroplacental unit (CTUP) can vary throughout gestation.
      ii. Normal mid-gestation CTUP measurements range from 5-10 mm.
      iii. In late gestation, CTUP tends to increase. Normal measurements range from 1.15 ± 0.24 cm (Reef, et al 1995)
      iv. Mild undulation of placenta adjacent to allantoic space is within normal limits.
      v. Non-fetal horn (Figure 11): Has a thickened appearance with increased folding in normal mares. Often confused with placentitis.

8. Abnormal:
    a. <u>Placentitis</u>: Increased uteroplacental thickness +/- increased placental folding (Figure 12). May appear edematous.
    b. <u>Placental separation</u>: Creates linear anechoic space between uterus and placenta. Can be differentiated from placental blood vessels by rotating the transducer 90 degrees (Figure 13). Small areas of separation have been seen in mares that delivered healthy foals. Large areas are considered significant.

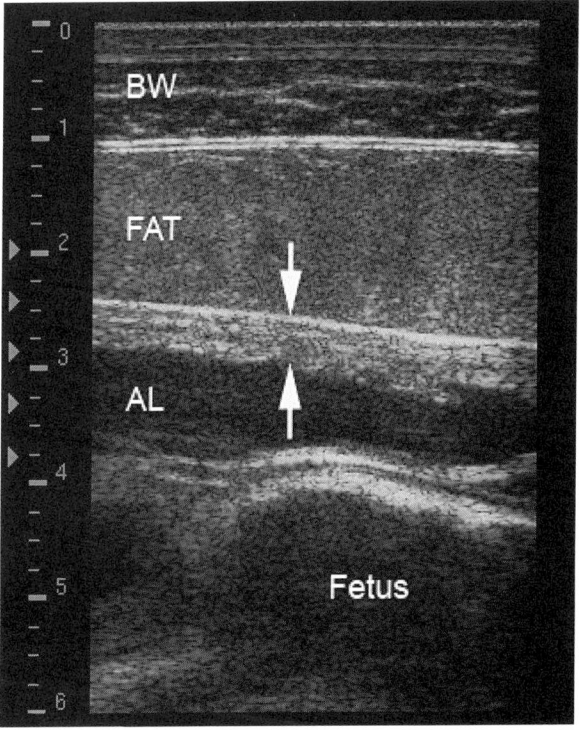

Figure 10: Normal appearance of uteroplacental unit (arrows) located deep to body wall (BW) and retroperitoneal fat layer. Al=allantoic fluid

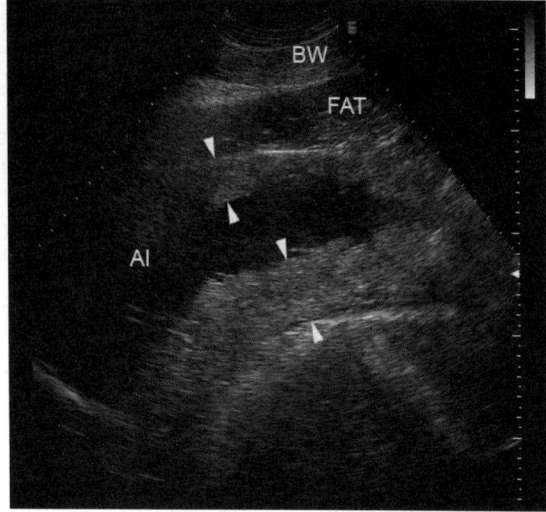

Figure 11: Normal appearance of nonfetal horn (arrowheads) with its thickened appearance compared to the fetal horn (Figs 7,10).

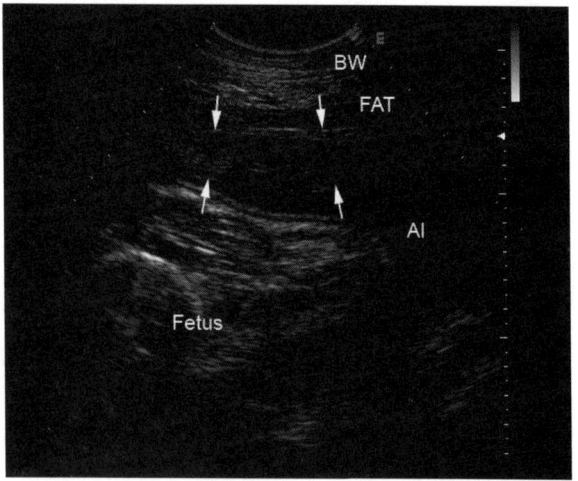

Figure 12: Abnormal appearance of uteroplacental unit showing increased thickness, placental edema and folding consistent with placentitis (arrows). BW=body wall, Al=allantoic fluid.

Chapter 52 Ultrasonography of the Fetus and the Neonate

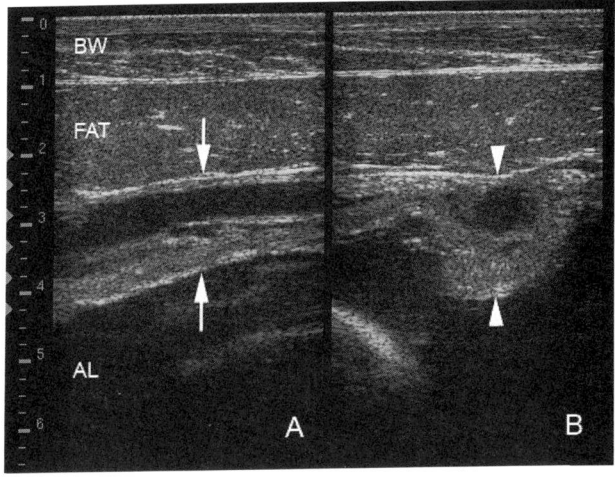

Figure 13: a) Longitudinal image of uteroplacental blood vessel (arrows). May be confused with placental separation. b) 90 degree rotation of transducer produces circular image, confirming blood vessel versus placental separation.

References:
1. Reef WB, Vaala WE, Worth LT, et al. Ultrasonographic evaluation of the fetus and intrauterine environment in healthy mares during late gestation. *Vet Radiol* 1995;36(6):533-541
2. Reef WB, Vaala WE, Worth LT, et al. Ultrasonographic assessment of fetal well-being during late gestation: development of an equine biophysical profile. *Equine Vet J.* 1996;38(3):200-208
3. Bucca S, Fogarty U, Collins A, et al. Assessment of feto-placental well-being in the mare from mid-gestation to term: Transrectal and transabdominal ultrasonographic features. *Theriogenology* 2005;64:542-557

II. UMBILICAL ULTRASOUND

A. **Overview:**
   The value of umbilical remnant ultrasound is well established, as it can readily diagnose infection in foals

without drainage from the umbilical stump or other palpable abnormalities. Additional sites of umbilical remnant infection can be detected in foals with visible stump abnormalities. Ultrasound can also identify the umbilicus as the source of infection in foals with sepsis, septic arthritis, pneumonia, etc.

Ultrasonographic measurements of umbilical structures are helpful to identify abnormal structures; however, infection may be present despite measurements within reference ranges. Abnormal luminal contents, thickening of arterial, venous and urachal walls and peristructural thickening or inflammation are other important indicators of infection.

B. Anatomy:
1. Umbilical vein: Extends along ventral midline from umbilical stump to liver. Becomes falciform ligament.
2. Umbilical arteries: Extend caudally from umbilical stump to right and left of bladder in caudal inguinal region. Become round ligaments of the bladder.
3. Urachus: Extends from umbilical stump caudally to apex of bladder. Located between the right and left umbilical arteries.

C. Indications:
1. Palpable enlargement and/or purulent drainage from umbilical stump
2. Patent urachus
3. ADR, FUO (fever of unknown origin), hyperfibrinogenemia
4. Septic arthritis/tenosynovitis
5. Pneumonia

D. Technique:
Patient:
1. Preparation: Clip 3-4" strip of hair from sternum to umbilical stump along ventral midline. Extend clipped area into right and left inguinal regions.
2. Positioning: Standing or lateral recumbency – both require adequate restraint
3. Sedation: Important for examiner safety. Butorphanol (DOSE mg/kg) added to Xylazine or Valium may help to decrease kicking.

Equipment:
1. Ideal transducer: 7-14 MHz linear ("tendon" probe)
2. Adequate transducer: Rectal linear
3. Useful transducer: 4-8 MHz curvilinear (microconvex). Small size of probe allows easier placement into inguinal region for evaluation of umbilical arteries.
4. Program: Select superficial program (i.e. tendon, musculoskeletal, vascular or small parts program - name of program will vary by machine)
5. Scanning depth: 3-5 cm
6. Orientation: Transverse views of all structures are most useful and easiest to obtain compared to longitudinal views.

E. **Umbilical Vein**

Procedure: Begin immediately cranial to umbilical stump, locate vein deep to linea alba (between rectus abdominus muscle bellies), follow vein cranially to liver along ventral midline. Measure the diameter cranial to umbilical stump, in midvein region and at liver.

Normal appearance: (Figure 14)
1. Diameter: cranial to stump = 0.61 ± 0.20 cm, midvein = 0.52 ± 0.19 cm, liver = 0.60 ± 0.19 cm (Reef & Collatos, 1988)
2. Thin walls with no to minimal anechoic luminal contents
3. Variation: Small amount of homogeneously hypoechoic contents can be present to 7-10 days of age (Figure 15). Typically represents blood clot formation but can also be seen with early infection. Recheck in 3-7 days if remain suspicious for infection

Abnormal appearance: Omphalophlebitis
1. Increased diameter measurements
2. Thickened walls (Figure 16)
3. Hyperechoic luminal contents (Figure 17)
4. Increased accumulation of echogenic, especially heterogeneous, material within lumen.

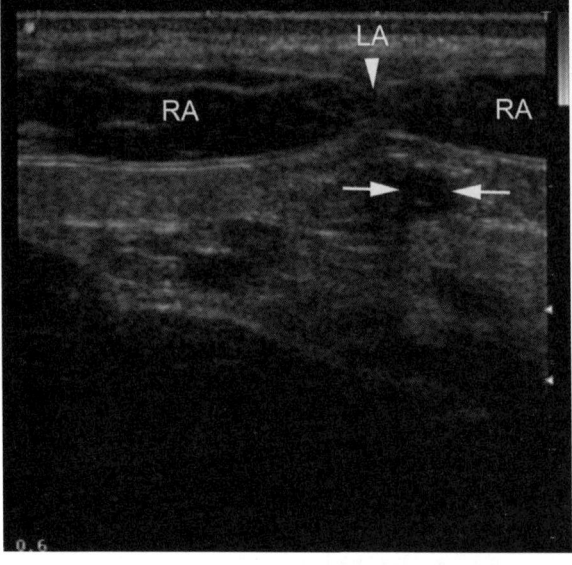

Figure 14: Normal umbilical vein (arrows) located deep and adjacent to rectus abdominus (RA) muscle bellies near linea albea (LA).

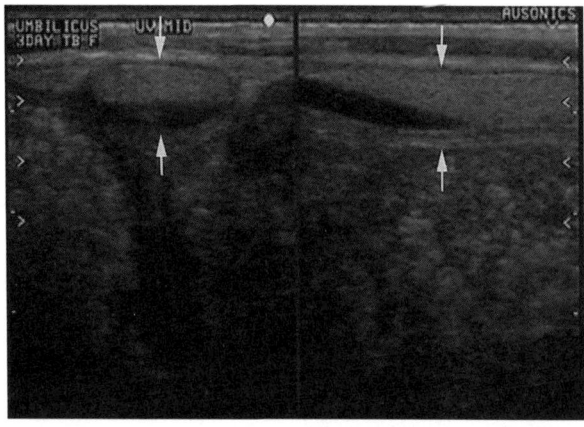

Figure 15: Blood clot formation within umbilical vein (arrows) in a 3-day-old foal. Thin walls support diagnosis of hematoma versus infection.

Chapter 52 Ultrasonography of the Fetus and the Neonate

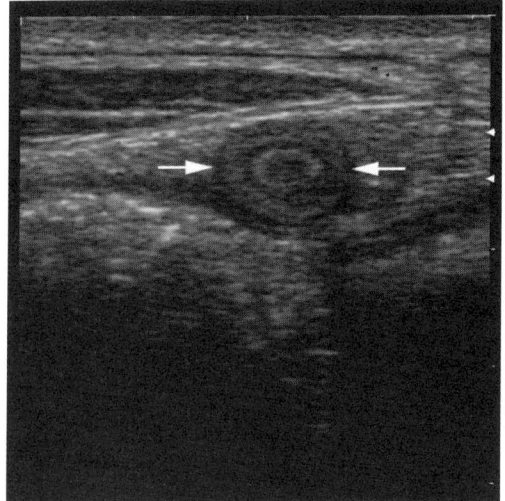

Figure 16: Abnormal umbilical vein (arrows) with increased wall thickness and abnormal luminal contents in a foal with omphalophlebitis.

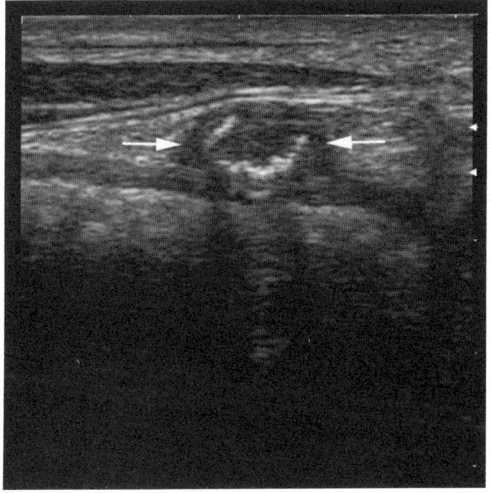

Figure 17: Abnormal umbilical vein (arrows) showing hyperechoic luminal contents in a foal with omphalophlebitis.

F. Umbilical Stump - "ET View"

Procedure: Place transducer immediately caudal to umbilical stump. Visualize urachus between right and left umbilical arteries (Figure 18). Follow urachus to bladder apex.

Normal appearance:
1. Combined diameters: 1.75 ± 0.37 cm (Reef & Collatos, 1988)
2. Thin walls of all structures. Minimal luminal contents.
3. Variation: Hypoechoic clot material within arteries is common to 7-10 days of age. Recheck if remain suspicious for infection.

Abnormal appearance:
1. Enlargement of entire structure or of individual structures
2. Thickened arterial and/or urachal walls. Periurachal or periarterial thickening (Figure 19).
3. Hyperechoic luminal contents (Figures 19).
4. Urachal abscess: Large accumulation of echogenic material within urachus (arrows, Figure 20).
5. Patent urachus: Anechoic space within urachal lumen (Fig 18). Patency may not be visible sonographically along length of urachus due to pressure from transducer

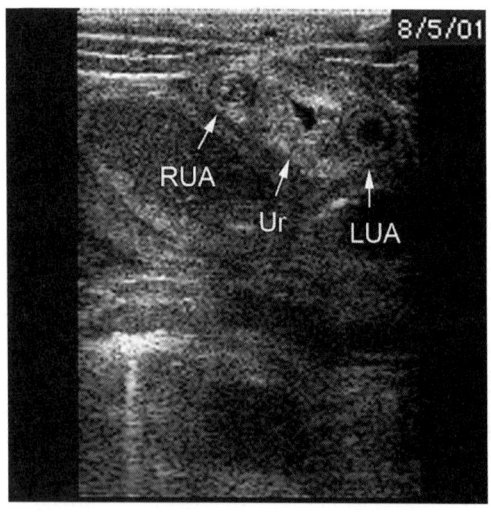

Figure 18: "ET" view showing left umbilical artery (LUA), right umbilical artery (RUA) and urachus (Ur) in a 4-day-old foal. Anechoic fluid within urachus is consistent with patency.

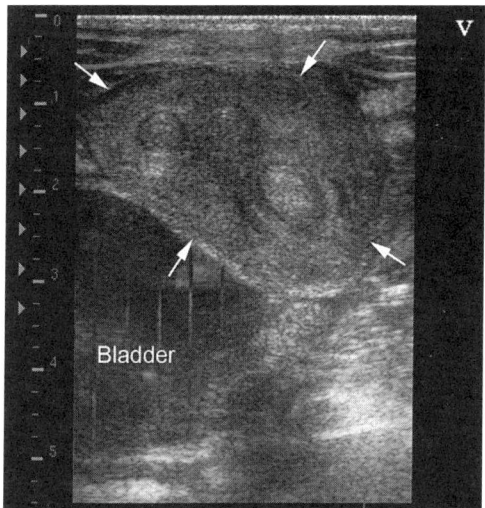

Figure 19: Marked periurachal/urachal inflammation with increased luminal contents of left and right umbilical arteries.

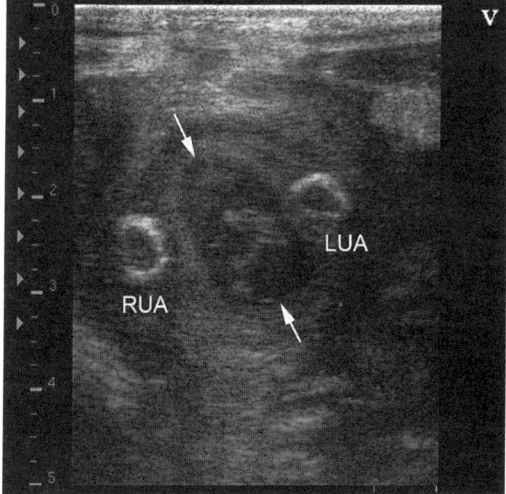

Figure 20: Urachal abscess (arrows) with left and right omphaloarteritis (hyperechoic luminal contents).

G. Umbilical Arteries

Procedure: From "ET View", follow each umbilical artery individually to right and left of bladder as far caudally as possible. Adequate restraint/control of hind limbs is most important for this portion of exam.

Normal appearance:
1. Diameter: 0.85 ± 0.21 cm (Reef & Collatos, 1988)
2. Thin walls with minimal to no luminal contents (Figure 21)
3. Variation: Hypoechoic clot material may be present to 7-10 days of age (Figure 22). Recheck in 3-7 days, if suspicious for infection.

Abnormal appearance: Omphaloarteritis
1. Increased diameter measurements
2. Hyperechoic luminal contents (Figure 23)
3. Thickened arterial walls (Figure 24)
4. Large accumulation of echogenic material within lumen is consistent with abscessation

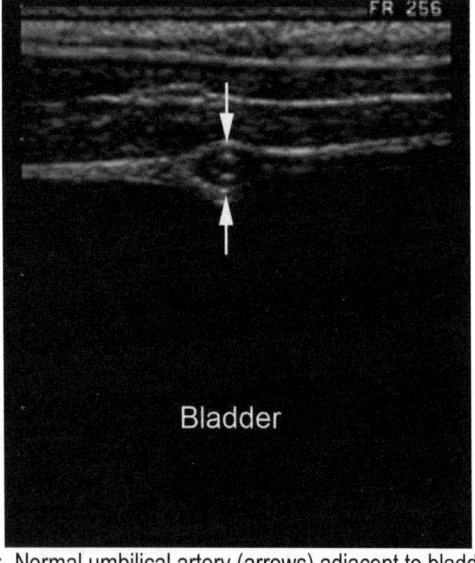

Figure 21: Normal umbilical artery (arrows) adjacent to bladder.

Chapter 52 Ultrasonography of the Fetus and the Neonate

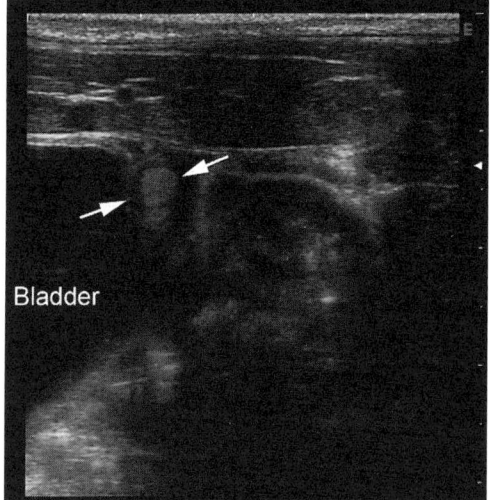

Figure 22: Hypoechoic luminal contents within left umbilical artery, consistent with blood clot formation.

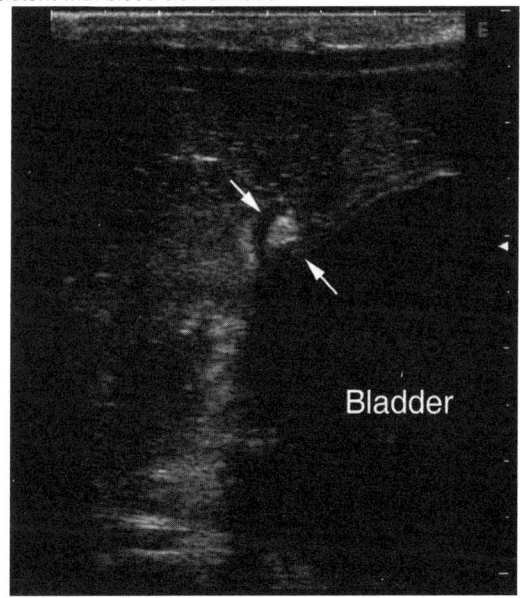

Figure 23: Hyperechoic luminal contents within right umbilical artery, consistent with infection/omphaloarteritis. (Image courtesy of Dr. Olga Seco)

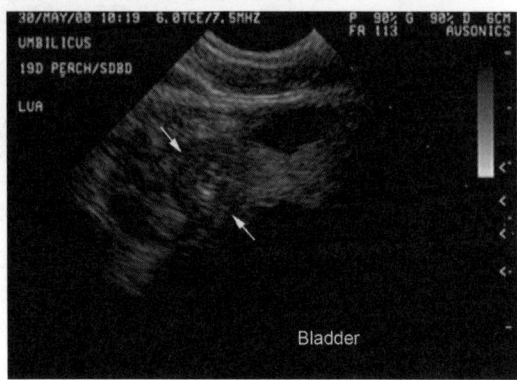

Figure 24: Hyperechoic luminal contents and increased wall thickness in a 19-day-old foal with omphaloarteritis of left umbilical artery.

References:
1. Reef VB, Collatos C. Ultrasonographic of umbilical structures in clinically normal foals. *Am J Vet Res* 1988;49(12):2143-2146
2. Reef VB, Collatos C, Spencer PA, et al. Clinical, ultrasonographic, and surgical findings in foals with umbilical remnant infections. *J Am Vet Med Assoc* 1989;195(1):69-72
3. Franklin RP, Ferrell EA. How to perform umbilical sonograms in the neonate. In *Proceedings. Am Assoc Equine Pract* 2002;48:261-265

III. THORACIC ULTRASOUND

A. Overview:
Thoracic ultrasound is the imaging modality of choice for the ambulatory practitioner. A thorough exam can be easily performed in the field with a standard ultrasound machine and a rectal transducer. Interpretation is relatively straightforward compared to other regions and often helps to clarify radiographic findings. While aerated lung may obscure pathology deep within the lung, most abnormalities are visible on ultrasound.

B. **Anatomy:**
   The equine lung field generally extends from the 3rd to 15th ICS, from the level of the tuber coxae dorsally to the point of the elbow ventrally.
C. **Indications:**
   1. ADR
   2. Fever of unknown origin
   3. Hyperfibrinogenemia
   4. Cough
   5. Nasal discharge
   6. Abnormal thoracic radiographic findings
D. **Technique**
   Patient:
   1. Preparation: Alcohol saturation. Clipping not necessary in most foals.
   2. Position: Standing preferred
   3. Sedation: Light, if necessary

   Equipment:
   1. Ideal transducer: 7-14 MHz linear (tendon), 5-10 MHz rectal linear
   2. Useful transducer: 4-8 MHz curvilinear (microconvex) - useful when increased penetration is necessary in foals with large areas of consolidation.
   3. Program selection: Majority of lung field is located within 1-5 cm of skin surface, and therefore any "superficial" program can be used in foals. If severe pathology requires an increased depth of penetration, use "abdomen" type program (small animal abdomen, equine abdomen) to enhance penetration and visualization.
   4. Scanning depth: 4-8cm if no consolidation is present; 10-15cm if have large areas of consolidation or severe effusion.

   Procedure:
   Orient transducer parallel to ribs in last (17th) ICS, slide transducer from dorsal to ventral to view entire pleural surface, making sure to image ventral lung margin. Repeat technique in each rib space.

   Normal appearance (Figure 25)
   1. Pleural surface (hyperechoic line deep to intercostal muscles) should be smooth and glide freely with

inspiration and expiration. Mild undulation as lung glides against ribs and intercostal muscles is normal.
2. Portion of image located deep to normal pleural surface is artifactual due to sound wave reflection by normally aerated lung.
3. Variation - Very small comet tails are normal, especially cranioventrally (Figure 26)

Abnormal appearance:
1. Comet tails: Diffuse small comet tails are suspicious for infection - recheck if clinical signs persist. Large comet tails are significant for infection and are often due to small areas of consolidation on pleural surface (Figure 27).
2. Consolidation (Figure 28, arrows): Cellular and/or fluid infiltrate allows penetration of ultrasound waves into pulmonary tissue. Consolidated lung is diffusely hypoechoic and may appear similar to liver ("hepatized lung"). Most commonly found in cranioventral lung field.
3. Pleural effusion: Relatively uncommon in foals. If present, will be found cranioventrally.
4. Abscessation: Most common in older foals (3-6 months) due to *Rhodococcus equi*. Uncommon in younger foals. Abscesses can appear similar to consolidation but are usually well demarcated (Figure 29). Older abscesses may show encapsulation.
5. Any combination of these findings may be present in foals with severe pneumonia or pleuropneumonia.

Chapter 52 Ultrasonography of the Fetus and the Neonate

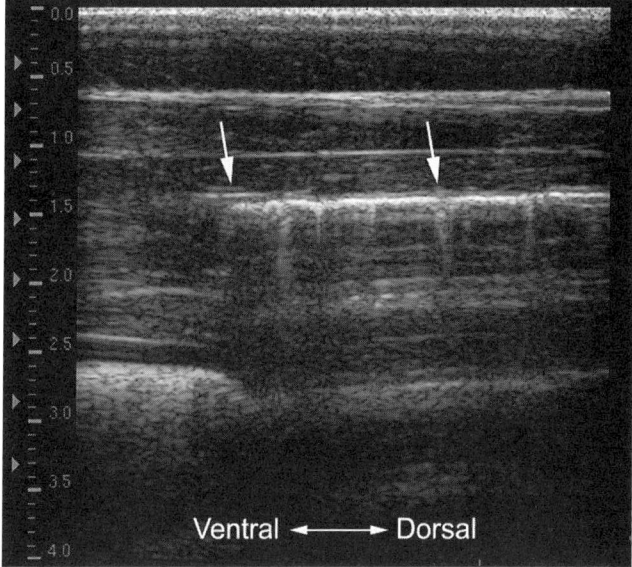

Figure 25: Normal pleural surface (arrows). Fine comet tails as shown in this image are within normal limits. Significance should be considered in conjunction with other clinical and ultrasonographic findings.

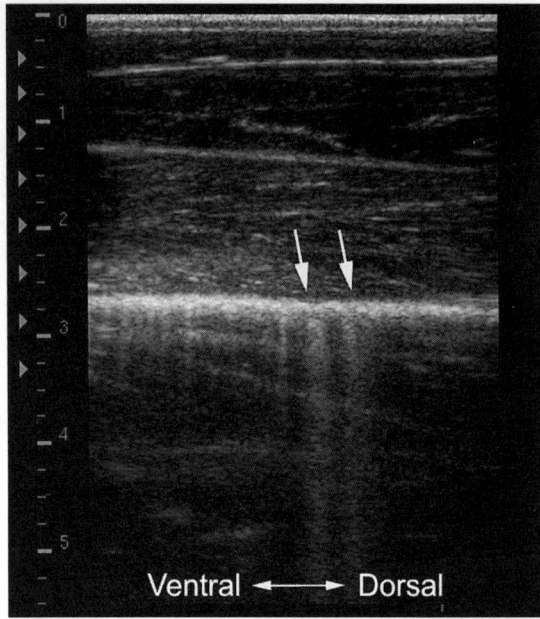

Figure 26: Occasional small comet tails (arrows) are a common finding in normal foals.

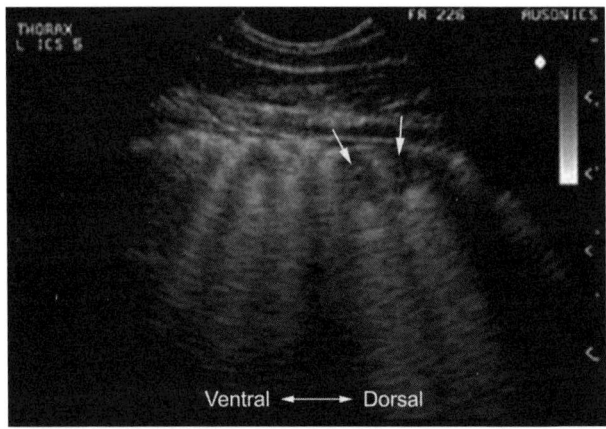

Figure 27: Multiple large comet tails with small areas of consolidation (arrows) are consistent with pneumonia.

Chapter 52 Ultrasonography of the Fetus and the Neonate

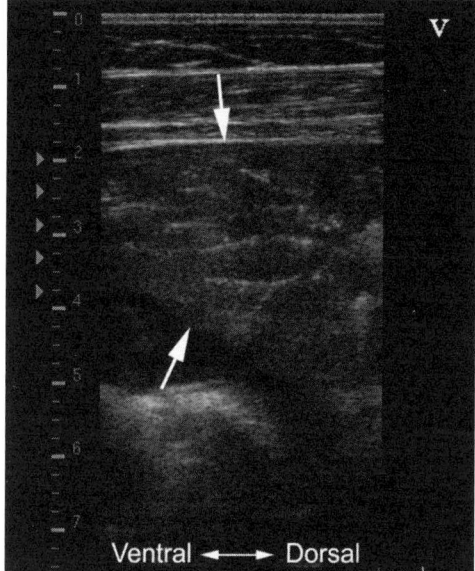

Figure 28: Cranioventral consolidation (arrows) in a foal with pneumonia. Note visible bronchial tree branching within the consolidated wedge of lung.

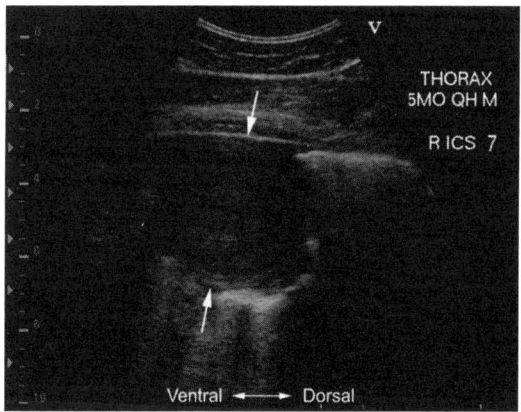

Figure 29: Well demarcated and encapsulated pulmonary abscess (arrows) in a 5-month-old foal with pneumonia due to *Rhodococcus equi*.

295

References:
1. Ramirez S, Lester GD, Robert GR. Diagnostic contribution of thoracic ultrasonography in 17 foals with *Rhodococcus equi* pneumonia. *Vet Radiol* 2004;45(2):172-176
2. Slovis NM, McCracken JL, Mundy G. How to use thoracic ultrasound to screen foals for *Rhodococcus equi* at affected farms. In Proceedings. *Am Assoc Equine Pract* 2005;51:274-278

IV. ABDOMINAL ULTRASOUND

A. Overview:
The use of abdominal ultrasound continues to increase in foals and adult horses alike, as more practitioners recognize its value beyond the acute abdomen. This portion of the chapter will focus on the most common ultrasonographic abnormalities to affect foals, including gastric distention, duodenitis, enteritis, intussusception, ileus, ruptured bladder and abscessation. Potential abnormalities are numerous, and a complete examination should be performed whenever possible.

B. Indications:
1. ADR
2. Fever of unknown origin
3. Hyperfibrinogenemia
4. Colic
5. Bruxism
6. Abdominal distention

C. Technique:
Patient:
1. Preparation: Alcohol saturation provides adequate visualization in most foals. Clipping the hair will improve image quality, especially in heavily coated foals.
2. Positioning: Exams should be performed in the standing position whenever possible. Small intestine abnormalities are common and are usually found on the ventrum due to their weight and dependent nature. Such abnormalities may be missed if foal is scanned in right, left or ventral recumbency.
3. Sedation: Light, if necessary

Equipment:
1. Ideal transducer: 4-8 MHz curvilinear (microconvex)
2. Adequate transducer: 2-5 MHz curvilinear (low frequency results in poorer resolution in neonates)
3. Adequate for some (superficial) abnormalities: 5-10 MHz rectal linear
4. Program selection: If using microconvex transducer, choose either small animal or equine abdominal program, depending on foal size.
5. Scanning depth: 5-15 cm, depending on structure being evaluated
6. Technique: Individual structures will be addressed below. For complete exam, evaluate entire paralumbar fossa/flank region, each ICS from ventral lung margin to costochondral junctions and entire ventrum from sternal to inguinal regions. Repeat for other side of abdomen.

D. **Common Ultrasonographic Findings:**

Duodenitis: Descending duodenum is seen in its fixed location ventral to the right kidney in the right 15-17th ICS (Figure 30) and deep to the right liver lobe in the right 11-15th ICS (Figure 31). Affected foals show an increased wall thickness (>3mm) and often present with clinical signs consistent with gastric ulceration. Distention and/or hypomotility may also be present. Gastroscopy can be negative in affected foals.

Enteritis: (Figure 32) Affected SI loops show an increased wall thickness (>3mm) and will be found in the dependent portion of the abdomen due to their increased weight (ventral if standing). Hypomotility with some degree of distention is usually present.

Intussusception: Nearly always found in dependent portion of abdomen (ventral if standing). Characteristic "target sign" formed by three layers of intussusception (Figure 33). Distention and hypomotility may be seen proximal to intussusception (Figure 34).

Gastric distention: Stomach is left sided structure seen in midthoracic intercostal spaces. A severely distended stomach has a large radius of curvature and is often visible to the last (17th) ICS (Figure 35). Fluid contents often visible ventrally.

Abscessation: Generally seen in older foals (3-6 months). Abscesses may be filled with hypoechoic fluid contents and have a well-defined capsule (Figure 36) or may be heterogeneous with poorly marginated borders (Figure 37). *Rhodococcus equi* abscesses can be quite large.

Ruptured Bladder: Most prominent feature is severe anechoic peritoneal effusion. A small spherical bladder may be seen due to residual urine contents. Bladder wall defect often not visible.

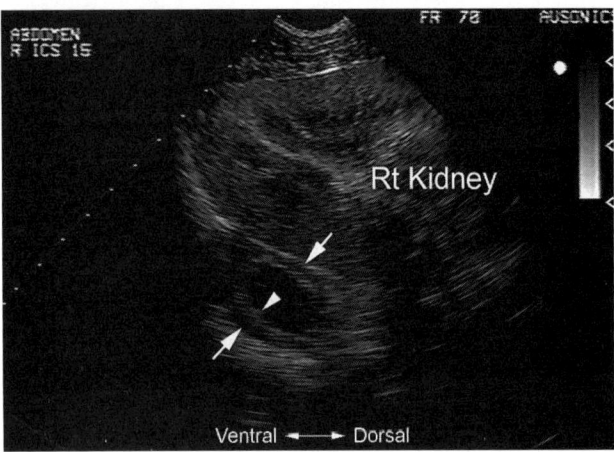

Figure 30: Location of descending duodenum (arrows) deep to right kidney in right caudal intercostal spaces. Wall thickness is increased (6-7 mm, arrowhead) in this foal with colic due to duodenitis.

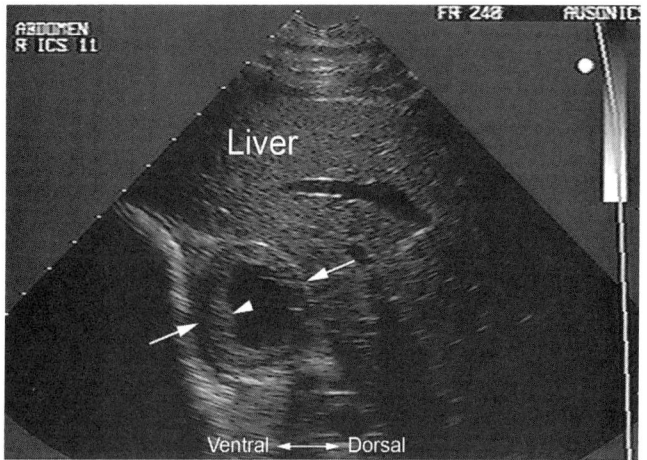

Figure 31: Location of descending duodenum (arrows) deep to right liver lobe in right mid intercostal spaces. Note the markedly increased wall thickness (arrowhead, 8-9 mm) in this foal with chronic duodenitis.

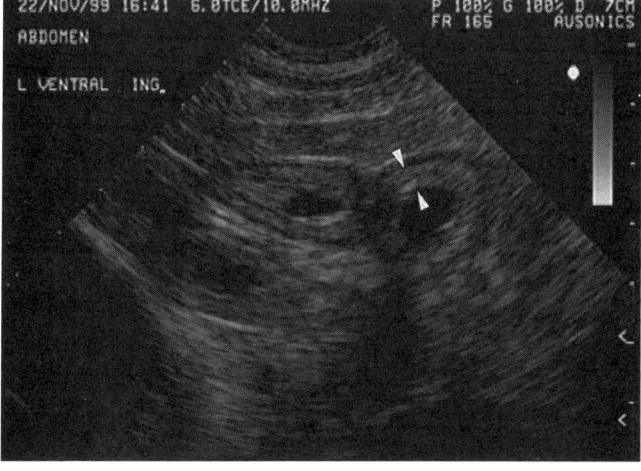

Figure 32: Multiple thickened small intestine loops (arrowheads) found in the ventral abdomen in a foal with diarrhea and chronic enteritis.

Chapter 52 Ultrasonography of the Fetus and the Neonate

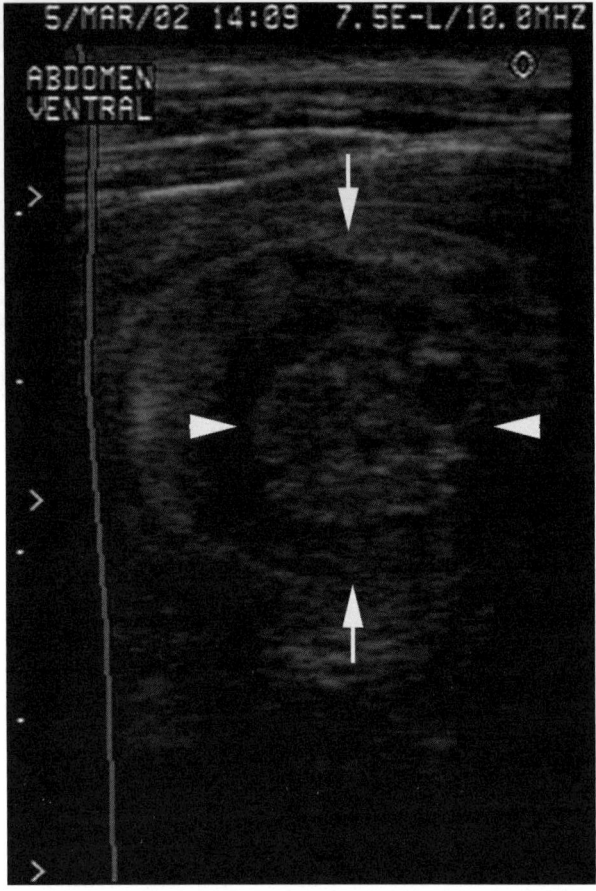

Figure 33: Small intestinal intussusception located in the ventral abdomen. The inner intussusceptum (arrowheads) is surrounded by the outer intussuscipiens (arrows). (Image provided courtesy of Dr. Olga Seco, University of Pennsylvania)

Chapter 52 Ultrasonography of the Fetus and the Neonate

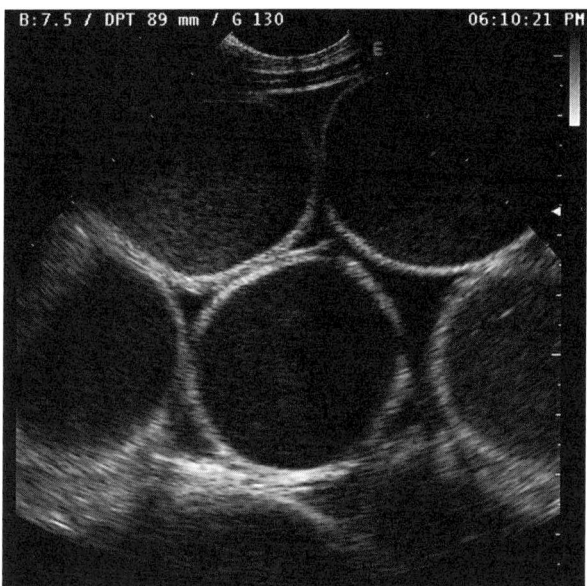

Figure 34: Severe small intestinal distention and ileus in a 2-week-old foal secondary to distal jejunal obstruction.

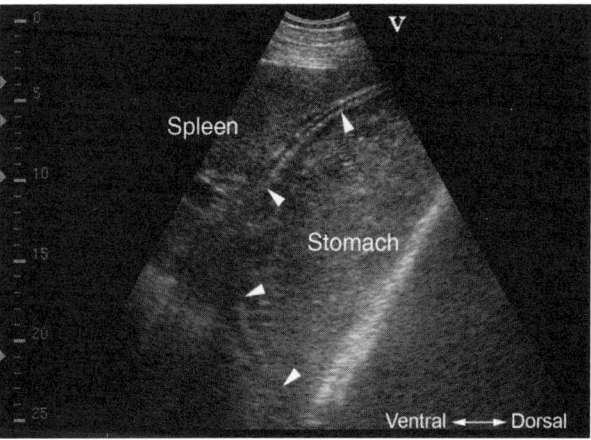

Figure 35: Gastric distention with increased ventral fluid accumulation. Note the large radius of curvature of the gastric wall (arrowheads) adjacent to the spleen.

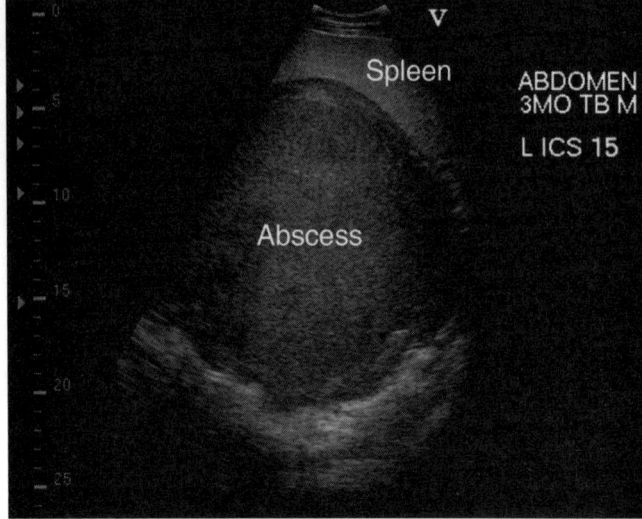

Figure 36: Large intra-abdominal *Rhodococcus equi* abscess located deep to the spleen. Note the homogeneous fluid contents and clear encapsulation compared to that in the similarly affected foal shown in Fig 37.

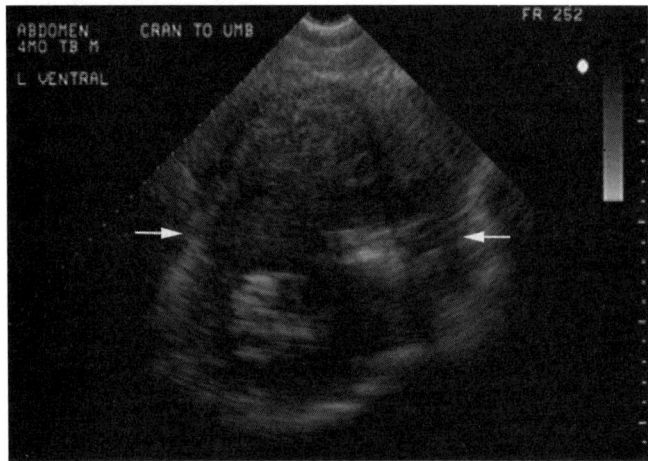

Figure 37: Large intra-abdominal *Rhodococcus equi* abscess (arrows) visualized from the ventral abdomen. Note heterogeneous appearance of abscess contents and absence of visible encapsulation, compared to Fig. 36.

References:
1. Porter MB, Ramirez S. Equine neonatal thoracic and abdominal ultrasonography. *Vet Clin North Am Equine Pract* 2005;21:407-429

V. MUSCULOSKELETAL IMAGING

A. Overview:
Evaluation for septic arthritis/tenosynovitis and/or septic physitis is the most common indication for musculoskeletal imaging in foals. Findings are often complementary to radiographs and may result in an earlier diagnosis of infection. Ultrasound has also been shown to be useful and superior to radiographs to diagnose rib fractures in foals.

B. Technique:
Clipping produces superior images. A high frequency linear transducer designed for musculoskeletal use is preferred. Depth settings: 3-8 cm, depending on structure being evaluated. Program selection: Superficial (musculoskeletal, tendon, small parts)

C. Ultrasonographic Findings:

Normal fetal cartilage/physes: Depending on joint/region being evaluated, foals have prominent cartilage layers due to normal juvenile incomplete ossification. Cartilage has hypoechoic to anechoic appearance and multiple pinpoint echoes that can easily be mistaken for cellular synovial fluid (Figure 38). In addition, the underlying subchondral bone is often irregular (Figure 39) and can be misinterpreted as osteomyelitis. Normal physes show a "V" shape in the bony surface deep to the cartilage layer.

Osteomyelitis: Affected bone may show a "fluffy" or thickened cortical surface with an overlying hypoechoic to anechoic layer (Figure 40). Chronic infection shows obvious bony destruction (Figure 41).

Septic synovial structures: While severe effusion can cause concern for sepsis (Figure 42), ultrasound more commonly reveals markedly thickened synovium with a lacey, edematous appearance (Figure 43). Ultrasound can aid with synoviocentesis in such foals to confirm infection.

Rib Fractures: Rib fractures occur with regularity in foals during parturition. While affected foals may appear clinically normal, fractures can penetrate vital structures, such as the lung and heart. Similar to other fractures, ultrasound will reveal step defects in the normally smooth bony surface (Figure 44). Local hemorrhage and/or muscle tearing can be present.

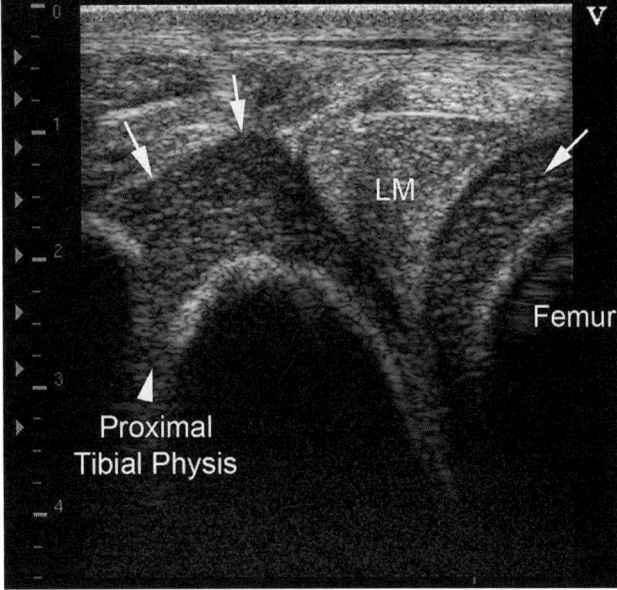

Figure 38: Normal appearance of lateral stifle in a 1-day-old foal. Note the thick cartilage layer (arrows) with its speckled appearance and the "V" shaped appearance of the proximal tibial physis. LM=lateral meniscus.

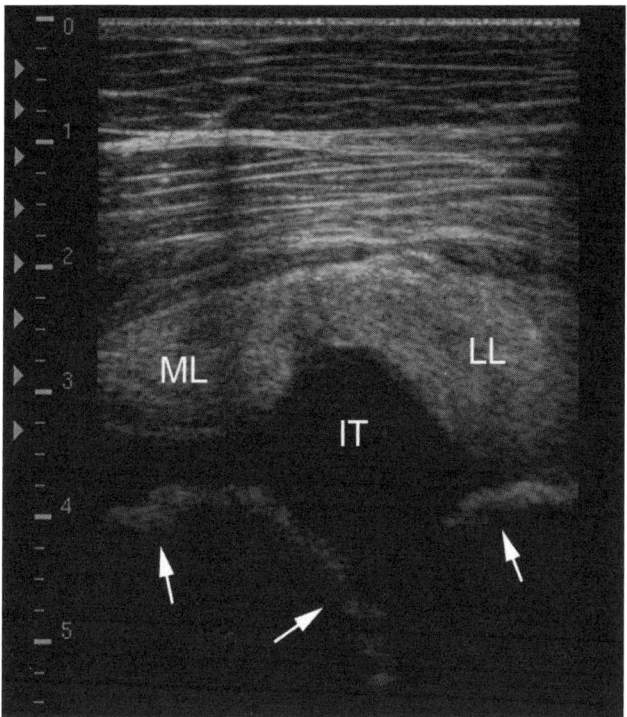

Figure 39: Normal appearance of medial and lateral lobes (ML,LL) of the biceps tendon and proximal humeral tubercles in a 4-month-old foal. Note the thick cartilage layer of the intermediate tubercle (IT) and the normal irregular contour of the subchondral bone (arrows)

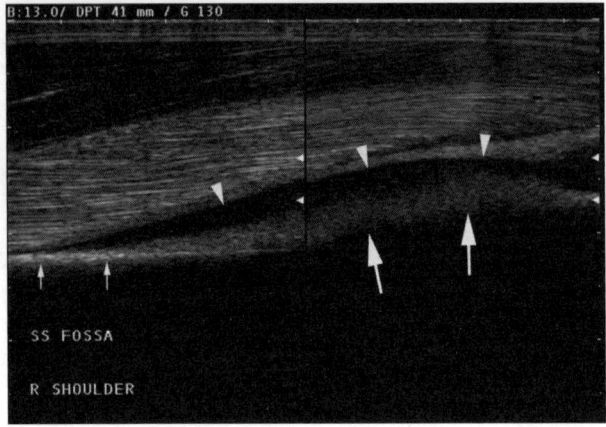

Figure 40: Osteomyelitis of the proximal scapula (supraspinous fossa) in a 6-week-old foal showing a thickened and fluffy periosteal/cortical surface (large arrows) with an overlying hypoechoic layer (arrowheads). Normal cortical surface is seen to the left (small arrows).

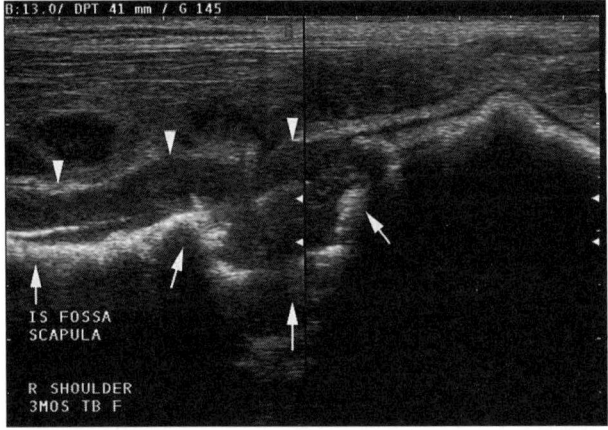

Figure 41: Chronic osteomyelitis of the proximal scapula (infraspinous fossa) in a 3-month-old foal due to *Rhodococcus equi* showing a large area of bony destruction (arrows) and a hypoechoic layer (arrowheads) overlying the abnormal bone.

Chapter 52 Ultrasonography of the Fetus and the Neonate

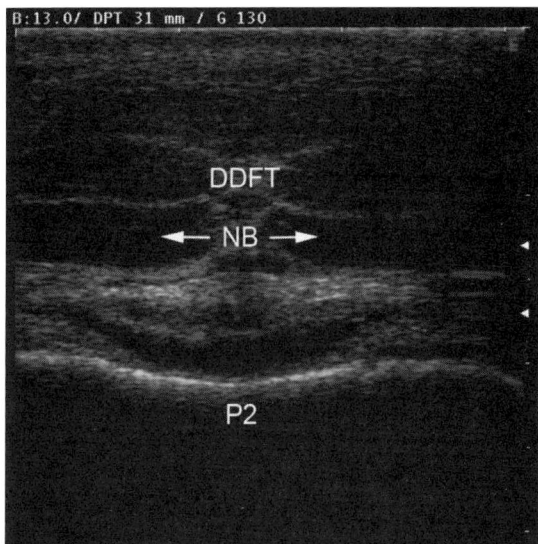

Figure 42: Nonseptic navicular bursitis (NB) with anechoic effusion and minimal synovial thickening. Image obtained proximal to navicular bone with transducer placed transversely between heelbulbs and directed towards toe. (DDFT=deep digital flexor tendon, P2=second phalanx)

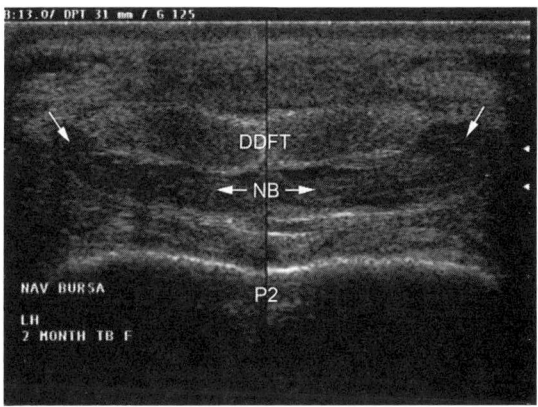

Figure 43: Septic navicular bursitis (NB) in a 2-month-old foal showing severe synovial thickening and minimal fluid pocketing. Image obtained as in Fig 42.

Chapter 52 Ultrasonography of the Fetus and the Neonate

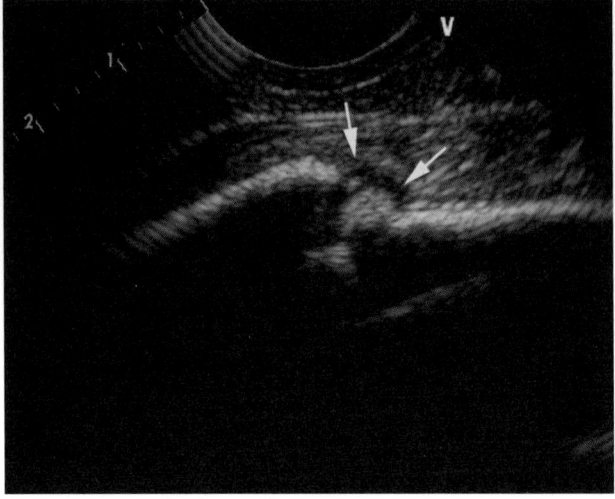

Figure 44: Rib fracture with a large step defect in the normally smooth bony surface (arrows). (Image provided courtesy of Dr. Johanna Reimer, Lexington, KY)

VI. ECHOCARDIOGRAPHY (PRACTICAL APPROACH) SEE ALSO CHAPTER 56:

A. **Overview:**
   This portion of the chapter will focus on congenital abnormalities most likely to be encountered in practice.
B. **Indications:**
   1. Murmurs other than those consistent with patent ductus arteriosus
   2. Foals with clinical signs of heart failure
C. **Technique:**
   Equipment:
   1. Ideal transducer: 2-5 MHz phased array
   2. Adequate transducer: 4-6 MHz curvilinear microconvex transducer in young foals. 3-5 MHz mechanical sector transducer can also be used, but detail resolution is typically suboptimal.
   3. Program: Equine cardiac program. If not available, use small animal cardiac or abdominal program.
   4. Depth: 10-20 cm

Chapter 52 Ultrasonography of the Fetus and the Neonate

Procedure:
1. Right parasternal views obtained from right 4th ICS. Three long axis views (right outflow, left outflow, four chamber) and three transverse views (aortic valve, mitral valve, left ventricle) should be obtained.
2. Left parasternal views are especially useful if mitral abnormalities are suspected.
3. While the structural defects discussed below can be seen with B mode imaging, color Doppler is required to determine the size and extent of shunts or regurgitant jets.

D. **Ventricular septal defects (VSD)**
1. Most common congenital abnormality
2. Auscultation - bilateral systolic murmur, usually loudest on right.
   a. Right sided murmur created by left to right shunt through VSD
   b. Left sided murmur loudest over pulmonic valve region (murmur of relative pulmonic stenosis).
   c. Accurate assessment of left sided point of maximal intensity is important to differentiate VSD from mitral insufficiency, in which case murmur is loudest in mitral to aortic valve region.
3. Subaortic defects most common. Best seen on left outflow tract view (long axis) as defect in membranous portion of septum just below aortic valve (Figure 45). On transverse views, best seen on aortic view as defect in aortic wall (Figure 46).
4. Affected foals should have normal life expectancy if:
   a. VSD measures less than 2.5cm in its widest dimension
   b. Peak shunt velocity is **greater** than 4 m/sec
   c. No aortic insufficiency or additional congenital abnormalities.
5. Tetralogy of fallot: Murmur will sound similar to VSD murmur, but left murmur is louder than right murmur. In addition to VSD, echocardiography will reveal pulmonic stenosis, overriding aorta and right ventricular hypertrophy.

E. **Atrial septal defects:**
1. Less commonly identified.

2. Best visualized on four chamber long axis view as defect in septum between left and right atria (Figure 47).
3. Should be differentiated from patent foramen ovale. PFO is common in normal foals and is best seen on four chamber view. Two membranous layers of PFO will be seen to open and close within interatrial septum (Figure 48).

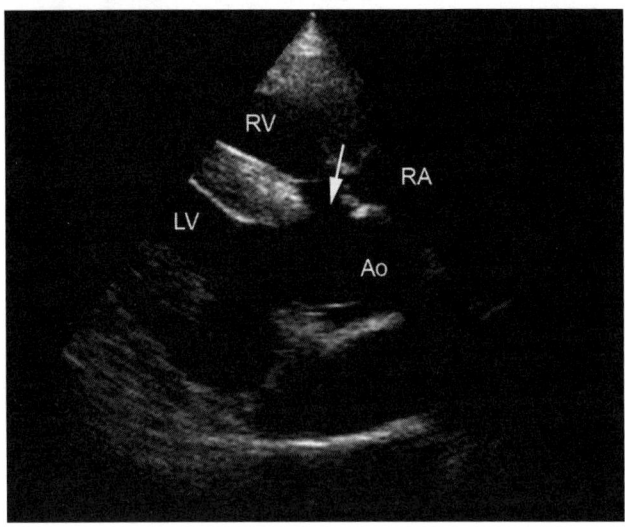

Figure 45: Left outflow tract view obtained from right parasternal window showing most common location of subaortic ventricular septal defect (arrow). RV=right ventricle, RA=right atrium, LV=left ventricle, Ao=aorta.

Chapter 52 Ultrasonography of the Fetus and the Neonate

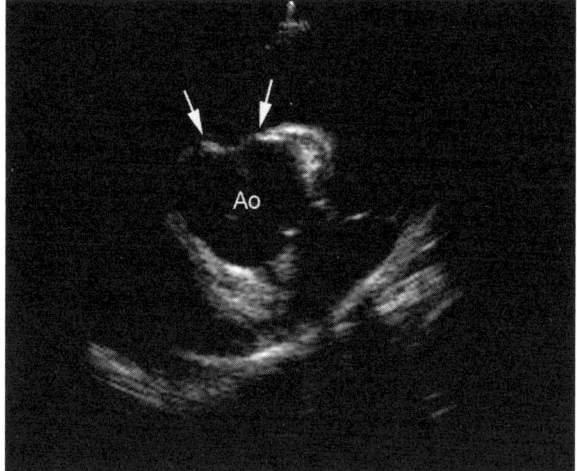

Figure 46: Transverse view of aortic valve obtained from right parasternal window showing subaortic VSD (arrows) seen in Fig 45.

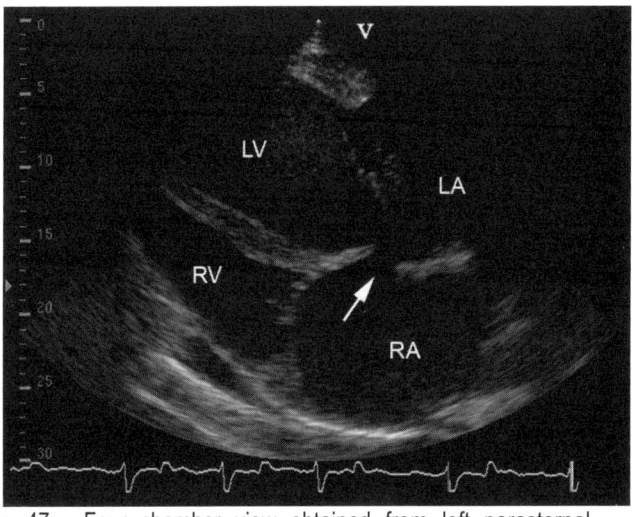

Figure 47: Four chamber view obtained from left parasternal window showing atrial septal defect (arrow). LV=left ventricle, LA=left atrium, RV=right ventricle, RA=right atrium.

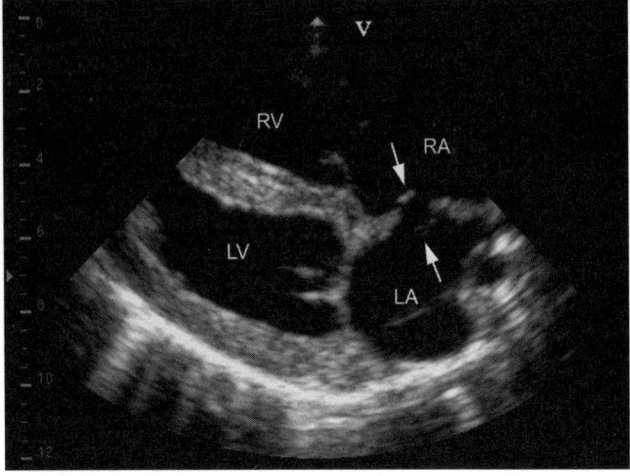

Figure 48: Four chamber view obtained from right parasternal window showing patent foramen ovale. Note the two visible layers of the foramen ovale (arrows).

References:
1. Bucca S, Fogarty U, Collins A, et al. Assessment of fetoplacental well-being in the mare from mid-gestation to term: Transrectal and transabdominal ultrasonographic features. *Theriogenology* 2005;64:542-557
2. Reef VB. Echocardiographic findings in horses with congenital cardiac disease. *Compend Contin Educ Pract* 1991;13(1):109-117
3. Reef VB. Evaluation of ventricular septal defects in horses using two-dimensional and Doppler echocardiography. *Equine Vet J Suppl* 19;1995:86-96

CHAPTER 53
THORACIC AND ABDOMINAL RADIOGRAPHY

Each clinic should obtain normal thoracic and abdominal films with their equipment in a 1 and 3 day old foal for reference.

I. THORACIC RADIOGRAPHY[1]

It has been difficult to adequately assess the neonatal foal's respiratory system with the standard techniques of auscultation and percussion. Ultrasound is a useful tool. Radiography can significantly aid in the detection of respiratory conditions, determination of therapy and in monitoring the response to therapy. Radiographic findings should be interpreted in a serial fashion whenever possible. Patterns seen tend to be overlapping amongst specific neonatal disorders.

  A. **Normal** - right lateral recumbency position.
  1. Exposure should allow penetration to clearly outline thoracic dorsal spinous process.[2]
  2. Examine rib borders and trabecular bone patterns for evidence of motion blurring.[2]
  3. Clear lung fields within 12 hours of birth.[2]
  4. Heart and pulmonary vasculation are well-defined without notable interstitial or bronchial pattern.[2]
  B. **Radiographic Patterns**
  1. Sites affected
     a. Caudal-ventral and cranial-ventral region abnormally can indicate pneumonia or edema.
     b. Both caudal-ventral and caudo-dorsal may indicate pneumonia, edema or atelectasis.
     c. Diffuse lung changes can be associated with septicemia (blood borne pneumonia), edema, atelectasis, viral pneumonia.
  2. Immature and septicemic foals.
     a. Diffuse marked interstitial pattern.
  3. Respiratory distress syndrome.
     a. Granular pattern progresses to complete pulmonary opacification with air bronchograms.
     b. Represents atelectasis and congestion.

C. Other thoracic radiograph findings
1. Fractured ribs, diaphragmatic hernia, pleural effusion, size of heart, vertebral fractures or osteomyelitis.

D. Techniques
1. **Portable analog, and portable digital DR and CR systems**
   up to 120 kVp (20-40 mA)
2. **Stationary hospital units**
   up to150 kVp (500 mA)
3. **Analog films / Digital Sensors**
   Size up to 17 inches
   Resolution for digital: up to 3 megapixels
4. **Standing** lateral view or right lateral recumbency - two views possible
   a. Cranial lung field
   b. Caudal lung field
5. **Ventrodorsal views** may be possible in young neonate
6. **Film focal distance** - 100 cm.
   a. In foals < 1 week old we have used 90 kVp, 10 MA with a time of 0.10 - 0.2 seconds (higher figure for cranial view).
   b. Larger machines 80 kVp and 5 MA.[2]

Each practice will have to develop their own technique chart based on their machines. Foals with higher respiratory rates are more difficult to obtain adequate quality films because of motion artifacts.

II. ABDOMINAL RADIOGRAPHS[1]

Standing lateral radiographs of the neonatal foal's abdomen provides added information when colic symptoms or abdominal distension is present. In general, foals have increased amounts of gas in the small and large intestine. Use radiographs in conjunction with clinical findings to make a diagnosis.

A. Normals (Plain standing left lateral films).[3]
1. Gas cap over fluid and ingesta in stomach.
2. Small collections of gas in the small intestine in the cranial and mid-central abdomen.

      a. Cannot easily identify individual loops to determine size in foals.
  3. Gas caps over fluid and ingesta in the cecum and large colon in the cauda dorsal abdomen.
      a. Cannot localize within a specific large intestine structure.
  4. Small amounts of gas in the small colon and ± gas in the rectum.

B. Obstructions - In general are characterized by markedly increased gas distension within the affected segments. Mechanical or functional ileus cannot be radiographically distinguished by plain films.

  1. **Gastric Distension** may be associated with:
      a. Gastric ulcers
      b. Pyloric stenosis
      c. When in combination with small intestine distension indicates small intestine obstruction.
  2. **Small Intestine**
      a. Distension of small intestine seen as multiple, tubular, gas filled loops with folding turns and vertical orientation in cranio-dorsal abdomen.
      b. Comparing width of a distended small bowel to the length of the lumbar vertebrae has been used to evaluate distension.
          i. A $\geq$ 1:1 ratio of small intestine width: lumbar vertebrae length has indicated distension.
      c. Distension causes are adhesions, volvulus, ileus, impactions, incarceration within mesodiverticular band, diaphragmatic hernia, large colon impaction, aganglionosis.
  3. **Large Intestine**
      a. Distension seen as large volumes of gas within markedly widened loops.
          i. With complete obstruction can fill entire abdomen with distended bowel.
          ii. Complete or long standing may produce secondary small intestine distension.

     b. Many foals with large intestine distension have impactions which may often be managed medically.
     c. Presence or absence of gas in the rectum not correlated with any abnormalities.
  4. **Gastrointestinal Rupture**
     a. Free peritoneal gas may be noted by increased visualization of kidney and serosa of intestine.
C. **Enteritis**
  1. **Foals often** present with abdominal pain.
  2. **Characterized** by an increased volume of gas accumulation throughout GI tract without discrete distended loops of intestine.
  3. **Laboratory work** often shows a degenerative left shift and peritoneal tap is often normal in enteritis.
  4. **Difficult** to distinguish enteritis and obstruction.
  5. **Diagnosis** is based on a combination of clinical signs, hematology, radiography, and response to therapy.
D. **Gastrointestinal Contrast Study**[4]
  1. **In foals** less than 14 days of age, fasted for 4 hours, a dose of 5 ml/kg of a 30% weight/volume barium suspension produces:
     a. Gastric emptying within 2 hours.[4]
     b. Barium transit time to transverse colon of approximately 3 hours.
  2. **Barium enemas** have aided the diagnosis of colonic atresia.
  3. **Obstructive disorders** due to strangulations or incarceration of a portion of bowel may be identified.
  4. **Retrograde contrast radiography**[5] (180 ml/foal up to 20 ml/kg of a 30% weight/volume barium sulfate suspension) has a 100% sensitivity and specificity for evaluating obstructions in the transverse and small colon. It is slightly less sensitive (86%) and specific (83%) to evaluate the entire large colon.[5] Small NGT or Harris flush enema tube (Seamless Hospital Products Co., Wallingford, CT) can be passed into rectum. Do not force or pump barium into the tube, allow passage by gravity flow (avoid rectal tear).

f. **Contrast cystography** for the detection of ruptured bladder. Use an aqueous based, organic, iodine solution via urethral catheterization.
E. Necrotizing enterocolitis[6]
1. Seen in foals less than 48 hours of age.
2. Intraluminal gaseous distension.
3. Pneumatosis intestinalis or intramural air.
   a. Produces a bubbly pattern
   b. Intramural air is seen as:
      i. Localized cystic collections
      ii. Diffuse linear strips
      iii. Ring-shaped areas of radiolucency
   c. Bowel perforation may appear as free gas in the abdominal cavity.

F. Techniques
1. **Standing lateral films**
   a. 26 inch FFD
   b. 90 or 100 KVP
   c. 10 MA
   d. 0.25 - 0.3 seconds
   e. Rare earth screens
   f. High speed film

References:
2. Butler, J., Colles, C., Dyson, S., Kold, S., Poulos, P.: <u>Clinical Radiology of the Horse</u>. Third edition. Blackwell. 2008.
3. Lamb, C.R., O'Callaghan, M.W., Paradis, M.R.: Thoracic radiography in the neonatal foal: A preliminary report. <u>Vet Radiol</u> 31:11-16, 1990.
3. Fisher, T.D., Kerr, L., O'Brien, T.R.: Abdominal radiography of the foal. <u>Vet Rad</u> 28, 1987.
4. Cambell, M.L., Ackerman, N., Peyton, L.C.: Radiographic gastrointestinal anatomy of the foal <u>Vet Rad</u> 25:194-204, 1984.
5. Fisher, T. Yarbrough, TY. Retrograde contrast radiography of the distal portions of the intestinal tract of foals. <u>J. Am. Vet. Med. Assoc.</u> 1995;207:734.
6. Cudd, T.A., Pauly, T.H.: Necrotizing enterocolitis in two equine neonates. <u>Compend Cont Educ Pract Vet</u> 88:88-92, 1987.

CHAPTER 54
NASOTRACHEAL INTUBATION

Endotracheal intubation is indicated whenever direct access to the lower airway is required.

I. TECHNIQUE OF INTRODUCTION[1,2]

A. **Open a sterile,** 55 cm long, 7 to 10 mm Bivona® silastic endotracheal tube.
B. **Inflate the cuff** with a 5-20 ml syringe (depending on the size of the cuff) and make sure that the cuff does not leak.
C. **Lubricate the cuff** and the end of the tube (but not the lumen) with sterile K-Y jelly.
D. **Gently pass the tube into the nasal** cavity along the ventromedial side of the canal. Gently rotate the tube counterclockwise and clockwise as it is advanced.
E. **If the tube meets an obstruction**, withdraw it slightly, rotate it 180° and re-advance it. Do not try to force the tube past the obstruction.
F. **If several attempts have failed** to pass through the nasal cavity, either try the other nostril or a smaller endotracheal tube.
G. **Once the endotracheal tube has passed into the nasopharynx** (as determined by a reduced resistance to further introduction of the tube) extend the foal's head and, while gently rotating the tube, introduce the tube into the larynx.
H. **Presence of the tube in the trachea** can be confirmed by feeling or listening to large volumes of air moving out of the tube during exhalation.
I. **If the tube passes instead into the esophagus**, withdraw it into the nasopharynx, rotate it 180°, place pressure with fingers on proximal esophagus to prevent entry and re-advance it.
J. **If the tube again does not pass into the larynx,** withdraw it, change the foal's head and neck position and re-insert it.
K. **If several positions and several attempts have failed**, visualize the larynx with a long laryngoscope blade and attempt to introduce the tube under direct visualization.

- L. **If this technique is also unsuccessful**, introduce a long, relatively stiff plastic stylet through the lumen of the tube and into the larynx. This stylet may then be used to guide the larger endotracheal tube into place.
- M. **If this technique also fails,** grasp the end of the tube (which can be visualized in the oropharynx) with a long forcep (which has been introduced through the mouth) and direct the end of the tube into the larynx.
- N. **The tube should be introduced far enough** so that the cuff is beyond the larynx and so that the tip of the tube is short of the thoracic inlet.
- O. **Apply tape to the tube, leave tag to allow** suturing to the nostril.
- P. **Tubes should be changed daily** because the lumen can accumulate material and plug airway.

II. TECHNIQUE FOR INFLATION OF THE CUFF[1,2]

- A. The cuff may need to be inflated during positive pressure ventilation to prevent unwanted leakage. The cuff is inflated during application of positive pressure to the airways and while listening to the air leak.
- B. The cuff should be inflated just to the point that it prevents the back-leak of air at the pressure being used. Any more pressure may cause damage to the tracheal wall which must, at all costs, be avoided.
- C. The cuff should be inflated with a syringe and the volume used should be recorded. The proper level of cuff inflation should be re-evaluated periodically and changes in the volume of air required to provide the seal should be noted.

References:
1. Magdesian, KG.: CPCR. VME-464. Lecture notes. UC Davis. 2010.
2. Corley KT, Axon JE.: Resuscitation and emergency management for neonatal foals. <u>Vet Clin North Am Equine Pract</u>. 2005 Aug;21(2):431-55.

CHAPTER 55
TRANSTRACHEAL ASPIRATION OR WASH

The transtracheal wash (TTW) can be used in equine neonates to obtain a lower respiratory tract specimen for culture, cytology, gram stain and chemical determination of surfactant.

I. MATERIALS REQUIRED

A. **Sterile gloves.**
B. **Prep materials** - razor, scrub, betadine, alcohol.
C. **Lidocaine** and 3 cc syringe, 22 gauge needle.
D. **Introducer needle and catheter**
   1. We use Medicut® 12 gauge - 2" with a sterile #5 French polypropylene canine urinary catheter.
E. **#15 blade.**
F. **Sterile Vacutainer®.**
   1. Transport media
   2. 12 cc syringe
   3. Non preservative sterile saline.

II. METHOD

A. **Palpate tracheal rings** at mid neck region.
B. **Prep area** – shave, 3 scrubs, betadine, alcohol.
C. **Local infiltration block** - 2% Lidocaine subcutaneously.
D. **Open kit and glove** (sterile).
E. **Provide restraint** of foal in standing or sternal position.
F. **Use stab incision** in skin with #15 blade.
G. **Immobilize trachea** with fingers on either side.
H. **Insert Medicut®** needle with plastic catheter cover between tracheal rings pointing slightly downward.
I. **Aspirate air** to verify needle is within the trachea.
J. **Remove needle** leaving plastic catheter in place.
K. **Thread sterile catheter** through Medicut® and down trachea.

1. When using canine urinary catheter, prior to procedure cut off distal end to allow better aspiration.
- L. **Attempt to aspirate fluid** - if cannot aspirate inject 10 cc sterile saline (non-preservative containing) and aspirate back while removing catheter slowly.
- M. **Remove catheter.**
- N. **Remove Medicut® plastic introducer** and place betadine gauze wrap around site.
- O. **Submit samples for analysis** - cytology, gram stain, culture.

III. TRACHEAL ASPIRATE

- A. **When gram stain only** is sufficient, pass nasotracheal tube and pass #5 French catheter into airway for aspirate.
  1. May be less stressful in compromised foals.

CHAPTER 56
ECHOCARDIOGRAPHY

There have been few studies of the normal echocardiogram of neonatal horses.[1,2] For more practical details go to Chapter 52.

I. **POTENTIAL INFORMATION** to be gained from the M-mode, two-dimensional (2D) or Doppler echocardiogram includes:

   A. **Cardiac anatomy**, including atrial and ventricular septa and walls, valves, and great vessels. Combined with IV injection of saline containing microbubbles, right-to-left intracardiac shunting disorders can be demonstrated - 2D is superior to M-mode for this purpose.
   B. **Cardiac chamber size** and wall thicknesses - M-mode is easier to measure and the technique is considered to be the gold standard of echocardiographic measurements.
   C. **Cardiac function** - combining measurements of wall thickness, systolic and diastolic chamber dimensions, and LV shortening fraction [SF% = (LVED- LVFES)/LVED X 100] allows evaluation of myocardial contractility and recognition of volume overload or pressure overload states.
   D. **Evaluation of blood flow** - Doppler echocardiography is the most accurate non-invasive means of velocity measurements.

II. **ECHOCARDIOGRAM OF THE NORMAL NEONATAL HORSE**

   A. **Normal M-mode echocardiographic** measurements reported in Thoroughbred and pony foals are shown in Tables 1-5.[1,2]
   B. **Normal 2D echocardiography** is now routinely performed in every neonatal ICU. Reproducible images can be obtained from both right and left intercostal transducer positions. Right intercostal long-axis views are useful for evaluating the right and left atria and ventricles, mitral, tricuspid and aortic valves, atrial and ventricular septa. Right intercostal short-axis views are useful for evaluating cardiac contractility in M-mode, evaluation of

the aortic and pulmonary arteries and semilunar valves. Left caudal intercostal long-axis and 4 chamber views are useful for evaluating both atria and ventricles, mitral and tricuspid valves, and atrial and ventricular septa. Left cranial intercostal short-axis views are useful for evaluating the aortic and pulmonic valves, pulmonary artery, ascending aorta and, in some cases, the ductus arteriosus.

C. **Doppler Echocardiography** [3, 4]

Doppler echocardiography is used for non-invasive blood flow evaluation of the heart and great vessels. It has several types: Continuous-wave (CW), Pulsed-wave (PW), and Color-flow (CF). CW Doppler is used to accurately determine peak velocities of blood flow. CF Doppler is a special form of pulsed wave Doppler, in which Doppler signals appear as color-coded pixels superimposing the 2D or the M-mode image within the Doppler window. The frequencies are color coded, and flow to the transducer appears as red, flow away from the transducer appears as blue. The lighter colors refer to higher velocities.

D. **Contrast Echocardiography** [3, 4]

Contrast echocardiography involves the creation of microbubbles in the circulation using injectable agents (carbon dioxide, 0.9% NaCl, 5% Dextrose, indocyane dye). These agents are usually mixed with the blood of the patient and injected back to a vein. The technique allows imaging the acoustic difference between the microbubbles and the patient's blood, and used to visualize, right to left shunts.

E. **Transesophageal Echocardiography.** [3,4]

Transesophageal Echocardiography (TEE) can be performed in foals with standard TEE transducers. The technique provides a superior visualization of the great vessels, and can be carried out when transthoracic approach failed to image a particular structure.

III. **ECHOCARDIOGRAPHIC EXAMINATION** can be useful in evaluating the following types of neonatal disorders[5]:

A. Congenital cardiac anomalies, including simple defects such as aortic or pulmonic stenosis, atrial or ventricular septal defects, mitral and tricuspid dysplasia, and complex or multiple defects. The severity of a pressure or volume overload state may be estimated by the degree of ventricular hypertrophy or dilation present.

B. Myocardial depression (decreased contractility), indicated by normal to increased LV end-diastolic and increased end-systolic dimension or volume, and resulting decreased fractional shortening (FS).

C. Hypovolemia, indicated by decreased atrial and ventricular diastolic dimension or volume.

D. Primary pulmonary/pleural disorders, in which serious cardiovascular disease can usually be confidently excluded as the cause of clinical signs.

E. Inflammatory processes within the heart or adjacent organs (endocarditis, pericarditis) can be evaluated.

F. Traumatic injuries (heart or great vessel lacerations, cardiac tamponade) can be imaged usually just immediately before death.

References:
1. Lombard, C.W., Evans, M., Martin, L., Tehrani, J.: Blood pressure, electrocardiogram and echocardiogram measurements in the growing pony foal. Equine Vet J 16:342-347, 1984.
2. Stewart, J.H., Rose, R.J., Barko, A.M.: Echocardiography in foals from birth to three months old. Equine Vet J 16:332-341, 1984.
3. Marr, C.: Cardiology of the Horse. Saunders. Philadelphia.1999
4. Reef, V. B.: Cardiovascular ultrasonography. in Reef, VB.(editor): Equine Diagnostic Ultrasound. pp. 215-273.Saunders, Philadelphia, 1997.
5. Voss, E: The Cardiovascular System in McAuliffe, SB. Slovis, NM (eds): Color Atlas of Diseases and Disorders of The Foal. 189-212. WB. Saunders. Philadelphia. 2008

Table 1: Left Ventricular end-diastolic (LVEDD) and end-systolic dimensions (LVESD), percentage diastolic change in dimension (% D) and right ventricular end-diastolic dimension (RVEDD) and posterior left ventricular wall thickness (PLVWT) (mean±sd) in 16 foals from birth to three months old. * $p<0.05$; ** $p<0.01$, *** $p<0.001$

Age	Body Weight (kg)	LVEDD (cm)	LVES (cm)	% D	RVEDD	LVPWT
Birth	45.13±8.61	6.04±0.64	4.58±0.38	24.31±6.47	2.19±0.61	0.54±0.06
60 mins	45.13±8.61	6.21±0.58	4.93±0.51	22.62±6.60	2.37±0.29	0.52±0.04
2 hrs	45.13±8.61	5.94±0.68	4.88±0.60	22.46±6.00	2.26±0.50	0.56±0.08
12 hrs	45.53±8.89	5.70±0.59*	4.76±0.57	19.54±3.59	2.23±0.50	0.54±0.07
24 hrs	46.96±8.98	5.81±0.53*	4.67±0.56	21.33±2.93	2.37±0.40	0.55±0.04
48 hrs	48.14±8.68	5.89±0.64	4.99±0.37**	22.77±4.82	2.79±0.51*	0.58±0.06
4 Days	51.19±9.04	6.19±0.74*	5.44±0.84***	18.61±3.76	2.46±0.88	0.61±0.04
7 Days	56.89±10.05	6.50±0.53**	5.50±0.41***	20.08±5.01	2.61±0.27	0.70±0.08*
14 Days	64.67+12.45	6.91±0.51**	6.00±0.14***	20.17±3.76	2.55±0.86*	0.84+0.10*
1 Month	80.66+13.67	7.40+0.65**	6.52+0.11***	16.25+1.77*	2.64+0.34*	1.28+0.14***
2 Months	96.48+12.96	7.45+0.71**	6.86+0.18***	18.18+4.51	2.90+0.09***	1.48+0.19***
3 Months	111.83+16.80	7.76+0.65**	6.92+0.88***	21.06+1.37	2.74+0.23***	1.58+0.16***

Table 2: Interventricular septum end diastolic thickness (IVST) and percentage septal systolic thickening, ratio of posterior left ventricular wall thickness to interventricular septal thickness (PLVWT/IVST) and mitral-septum (C-Septum) and mitral posterior left ventricular wall distance (C-PLVW) (mean ± sd) in 16 foals from birth to 3 months old. ** $p<0.05$; ** $p<0.01$; *** $p<0.001$ (n = 8)

Age	Body Weight (kg)	IVST (cm)	% Systolic thickening	C-Septum	C-PLVW	PLVWT/IVST
Birth	45.13±8.61	1.09±0.27	47.43±16.22	4.06±0.36	2.07±0.39	0.49±0.02
60 mins	45.13±8.61	1.08±0.22	51.92±19.81	4.08±0.58	2.34±0.46	0.48±0.03
2 hrs	45.13±8.61	1.10±0.08	57.20±16.00	4.30±0.33	2.15±0.33	0.51±0.04
12 hrs	45.53±8.89	1.30±0.16**	38.76±16.44**	3.74±0.46	2.32±0.24	0.42±0.04
24 hrs	46.96±8.98	1.27±0.25**	48.84±19.52	4.03±0.27	2.29±0.26	0.43±0.06
48 hrs	48.14±8.68	1.34±0.19**	47.12±12.20	3.86±0.50	2.24±0.47	0.43±0.05
4 Days	51.19±9.04	1.31±0.21**	45.10±13.55	4.56±0.62*	2.44±0.39	0.47±0.06
7 Days	56.89±10.05	1.35±0.23**	43.06±12.00	4.50±0.43*	2.47±0.38	0.52±0.07
14 Days	64.67±12.45	1.33±0.19**	41.82±14.64*	5.32±1.87**	2.75±0.52**	0.63±0.08*
1 Month	80.66±13.67	1.38±0.20***	36.12±13.67**	5.48±1.12**	3.16±0.62**	0.93±0.11***
2 Months	96.48±12.96	1.42±0.31***	41.05±12.87	5.97±0.08***	3.86±1.30***	1.01±0.13***
3 Months	111.83±16.80	1.46±0.09***	49.96±12.46	6.23±0.44***	3.96±0.11***	1.08±0.12***

Chapter 56 Echocardiography

Table 3: Heart rate and left ventricular systolic time intervals (mean±sd) in 12 foals from birth to three months old. * p<0.01; ** p<0.001, n = 8

Age	Heart rate (bpm)	EMS (msec)	LVET (msec)	LVPEP (msec)	LVPEP/ LVET	LVICT
Birth	104±16	317.41±80.51	260.6±46.80	31.20±11.14	0.12±0.02	7.00±1.60
60 min	97±17	333.87±67.61	272.8±44.71	32.74±10.45	0.12±0.03	7.79±2.39
2 hrs	75±11	351.80±65.23	292.8±59.90	29.20±10.76	0.10±0.03	9.22±2.59
12 hrs	87±12	336.17±31.09	294.1±37.67	41.17± 5.26	0.14±0.03	12.00±2.45*
24 hrs	91±15	336.54±36.76	303.07±69.84	48.49± 6.24*	0.16±0.02*	14.43±6.05*
4 days	84±18	305.23±46.61	259.36±35.35	45.87±10.04*	0.18±0.03*	23.08±5.47*
7 Days	88±27	312.00±55.48	260.07±47.10	51.93± 8.61**	0.20±0.04**	23.69±4.85**
14 Days	83±19	350.44±81.11	292.44±72.03	58.00±14.67**	0.20±0.03**	28.71±3.50**
1 Month	77±12	301.76±84.94	249.63±55.55*	52.13±15.04*	0.21±0.05**	32.40±6.88**
2 Months	70±13	432.75±66.38*	363.50±79.81**	69.25±12.31**	0.19±0.04*	31.60±3.51**
3 Months	69±13	409.75±71.81*	344.00±90.42*	65.75±10.09**	0.19±0.05*	33.20±4.11**

Table 4. Aortic root dimension (AoRD), left atrial dimension (LAD) and left atrial dimension/aortic root dimension ratio (LAD/AoRD) and body weight (mean ± sd) in 16 foals from birth to three months old.

Age	Bodyweight (kg)	AoRD (cm)	LAD (cm)	LAD/AoRD
Birth	45.13±8.61	3.09±0.29	3.33±0.98	1.08±0.34
60 min	45.13±8.61	2.86±0.30	3.23±0.75	1.13±0.30
2 hrs	45.13±8.61	2.84±0.31	3.02±0.54	1.06±0.21
12 hrs	45.53±8.89	3.39±0.28	3.22±0.73	0.95±0.28
24 hrs	46.96±8.98	3.70±0.25	3.01±0.70	0.81±0.15*
48 hrs	48.14±8.68	3.60±0.28	2.99±0.56	0.83±0.15
4 days	51.19±9.04	3.57±0.31	3.07±0.67	0.86± 0.17

CHAPTER 57
ELECTROCARDIOGRAPHY

I. POTENTIAL INFORMATION TO BE GAINED FROM THE ECG INCLUDES:

- **A.** Cardiac rate and rhythm - high sensitivity/specificity.
- **B.** Cardiac chamber enlargement - low sensitivity/ specificity.
- **C.** Ischemia, hypoxemia, electrolyte disorders and other extracardiac disorders - low sensitivity/specificity.

II. ECG OF THE NORMAL NEONATE

- **A.** Normal ECG values reported in thoroughbred and pony foals are shown in Tables 1 and 2 [1,2]. Like adult horses, there is considerable variability in the QRS morphology and frontal plane mean QRS electrical axis of foals. Although there is some individual tendency for the electrical axis to evolve from a cranial rightward to caudal leftward orientation over the first few months, this is extremely variable and of little clinical value in distinguishing foals with significant heart disease.
- **B.** Heart rate of neonatal horses varies from a relative bradycardia immediately after birth (65-70/min), to a relative tachycardia during the period of initial activity (120-130/min), to a resting heart rate of about 90-100/min in the first few days up to 2 weeks. Thereafter, heart rate gradually declines toward adult levels over several months.

III. CARDIAC ENLARGEMENT

- **A.** The P wave is usually positive or biphasic in leads I, II, III, and aVF. P waves greater than 0.4 mV or wider than 60 msec may indicate left and/or right atrial enlargement.
- **B.** The QRS complex is quite variable and may be positive or negative in each limb lead, but is usually less than 1.5 mV in amplitude. QRS duration greater than 60 msec or amplitudes greater than 2 mV are probably abnormal and may indicate ventricular enlargement. With LV enlargement the QRS complexes tend to become mainly positive in leads I, II, aVF, and left precordial leads. With

concentric RV hypertrophy the QRS complexes may be mainly negative in these leads.

IV. CARDIAC ARRHYTHMIAS AND CONDUCTION DISORDERS[3]

A. **The normal cardiac rhythm** of foals is a sinus rhythm with minimal sinus arrhythmia.

B. **Second degree AV block**, which is commonly found in adult horses, is usually not present in foals. Escape beats due to atrioventricular dissociation are also uncommon in foals.

C. **Cardiac arrhythmia** recognition requires an ECG, usually using lead II or a base-apex lead to facilitate identification of P waves and QRS complexes.

D. **Premature contractions**: supraventricular (atrial and junctional) premature beats are marked by a premature, but normal or near normal QRS complex, often but not always proceeded by an altered P wave. Ventricular premature beats are marked by a premature, wide and aberrant QRS complex not preceded by a P wave, but followed by a compensatory pause, with the next P wave occurring at the expected time.

E. **Tachycardia:** Sinus tachycardia is marked by normal complexes, including P waves, and often by periods of acceleration or deceleration. Atrial tachycardia is a type of supraventricular tachycardia characterized by a rapid ectopic atrial rhythm (sustained premature atrial complexes, PAC) and a normal QRS complex, with regular R-R intervals indicating a lack of direct involvement of the AV node. Atrial flutter is uncommon in foals and is characterized by abnormal atrial re-entry activity with distinct and continuous flutter waves (up to 300-400/min), normal QRS complexes (size, shape, frequency), but irregular R-R intervals. It may progress to atrial fibrillation. Atrial fibrillation is marked by absence of P-waves, variable baseline fibrillation waves, and normal QRS complexes with irregular R-R intervals (See Chapter 17). Supraventricular tachycardia (atrial or junctional in origin) is marked by normal or near normal QRS complexes, P waves (when visible) differently shaped from P waves associated with initial pacemaker, and little variation in rate unless it is intermittent. AV nodal and junctional tachycardias have not been extensively studied in horses although they usually are characterized by a normal P-wave followed by a narrow or wide QRS. Ventricular tachycardia (VT) can be uniform or multiform depending on the shape of QRS complexes. VT is marked by wide, aberrant QRS complexes, capture or fusion beats, and AV dissociation. Torsades de pointes (twist of point) is a unique form of multiform ventricular tachyarrhythmia, where the electric axis of the heart and the shape of waves are rapidly changing. Ventricular fibrillation is the end stage of ventricular tachyarrhythmias and is characterized by the absence of P and T-waves and wide, low amplitude fibrillation waves as well as significant decrease in cardiac output followed by fainting, syncope, seizure and death.

F. Bradycardia: Sinus bradycardia is marked by normal complexes occurring at a slow rate. Causes include hypothermia, hyperkalemia, and other cardiac and extracardiac disorders. Other types of consistent or intermittent bradycardia include sinoatrial arrest, marked by a pause in the rhythm without P waves, and second or third degree AV block, marked by one or more nonconducted P waves between QRS complexes. Evaluation and management of these rhythm disorders should follow guidelines discussed in other texts.

References:
1. Rossdale, P.D.: Clinical studies on the newborn thoroughbred foal. II. Heart rate, auscultation and electrocardiogram. Brit Vet J 123:521-532, 1967.
2. Lombard, C.W., Evans, M., Martin, L., Tehrani, J.: Blood pressure, electrocardiogram and echocardiogram measurements in the growing pony foal. Equine Vet J 16:342-347, 1984.
3. Marr C.: Cardiology of the Horse. Saunders. Philadelphia. 1999.

Table 1: Lead II ECG values in 30 Thoroughbred Foals Reproduced from Ref. 1 with permission.

	P - P	Q - T	P amplitude	Q(-ve)	R(+ve)
Mean (sec) ±SD	0.613 ±0.2269	0.3053 ±0.0203	1.916± 0.7083	3.08±n/a	2.88±n/a
Range (min.-max.)	0.44 - 0.76	0.28 - 0.36	1-4	0-11.5	0-14

Table 2: Electrocardiogram measurements of 12 pony foals

** Significantly different ($P<0.05$). Values are given as mean ± sd. MEA= Mean electrical axis. Reproduced from Ref. 2 with permission.

Age days	Heart rate (bpm)	PR	QRS	QT	MEA Frontal Plane	# Observations
1	106± 17	0.11± 0.01	0.057± 0.005	0.30± 0.02	209±126	10
7	111± 18	0.11± 0.01	0.051± 0.009	0.27± 0.03**	263± 40	11
14	100± 11	0.11± 0.01	0.05±0.005**	0.29± 0.04	275 ± 41	11
21	110± 10	0.11±0.01	0.046± 0.011**	0.26± 0.02**	281± 23	8
30	103± 14	0.11± 0.01	0.046±0.007**	0.26± 0.04**	290± 20	9
60	77± 9**	0.13± 0.01**	0.05± 0.009	0.32± 0.05	263± 40	8
90	67± 9**	0.15± 0.01**	0.066± 0.007**	0.35± 0.02**	290± 36	8

CHAPTER 58
NASOGASTRIC INTUBATION

I. INDICATIONS

A. Administration of fluids and milk to foals with a depressed suck reflex.
B. To check for fluid or gas distention in the stomach of painful, bloated or weak foals.

II. TECHNIQUES

A. Tube Selection
1. Sterile Kaslow® size 18 french 48 inch tube (American Pharmaceal Co., American Hospital Supply).
2. Harris® Enema Tube - 24 french, 60 inches (American Hospital Supply).
3. Nutrifoal ®- foal enteral feeding tube, 12 french, 45 inches, (Ross Laboratories - Distributed by W.A. Butler, Co., 800-282-3148 or Columbus Service: 800-282-1073).
4. Mila® Nasogastric Feeding tubes - non-irritating radiopaque polyurethane material with stylet. Available sizes (5Fr-18Fr, 55-240cm (22 inches-100 inches). Tubes are length adjustable. www.milaint.com
5. Cook® Clearview Nasogastric Feeding Tube 10Fr-150cm (60inches). www.cookgroup.com
6. Silicon stomach feeding tube. 6mmx150cm. Jorgensen Laboratories. www.jorvet.com

B. Method of passing tube
1. Warm the tube to room temperature in water.
2. Measure the tube next to the foal to determine the length required to gain entrance to the stomach. (Distal 2/3's of chest; approximately the 12-14th intercostal space). Mark the tube with tape.
3. Lubricate the end with K-Y jelly.
4. Pass the tube in the ventral nasal meatus.

5. Advance the tube when swallowing occurs. Rotate the tube or push air through the tube to aid swallowing if necessary.
6. Verify the tube is in the esophagus by all these methods.
   a. Increased resistance.
   b. Visualization of distension on the left side of the neck.
   c. Palpation of the tube in the neck area when moving it back and forth.
7. Pass the tube into the stomach.
8. Check for reflux by putting water into the tube and aspirating back.
9. Administer fluids or milk.

C. Method for passing small and flexible tubes
1. These tubes are small diameter and are very well tolerated by foals.
2. Tube can be left in place and foal can still nurse the mare and be tube fed supplemental milk.
3. We use these tubes in convalescing foals that need additional milk or fluids and can still try to nurse mare.
4. Because the tube is small and flexible - can chill the tube in freezer to stiffen it up for passage or use a guide wire.
   a. May need to check position radiographically.
5. I prefer to measure length required to get into stomach, cut any excess length off distal end. Pass tube until proximal end is within the nostril. Suture it directly to nostril. Foal cannot rub tube and can still easily nurse.
6. This tube comes with a feeding system containing a 3 liter bag and coupling that fits into the end of the stomach tube. Nutrifoal pouch with pre-attached flexiflo gravity feeding set - Ross Laboratories - Distributed by W.A. Butler - 800-282-3148.

III. LEAVING THE TUBE IN PLACE

A. Use the smallest tube possible.
B. Flush the tube with clean water and cap with syringe or plug.

- **C.** Remove tube from stomach to distal esophagus.
- **D.** Place tape on tube (dry spot) adjacent to false nostril leaving a flap. Secure tape to tube with superglue or suture (otherwise, when tape is wet, tube slips). Suture a 1" piece of folded tape to the false nostril. Tie the two tape ends in place with suture to secure the tube in place.
    1. Alternately, tape tube to halter.
    2. Secure tube as described.
- **E.** Larger tubes may be kept in place for 48 to 72 hours. Change to other nostril if irritation, nasal discharge, bleeding or signs of pain occur. Small tubes can be in place for 7-10 days.
- **F.** Fluids, milk or liquid medication should be given with the foal's head up to allow gravity flow into the stomach. If cardia spasm occurs, the tube should be placed in the stomach for each feeding and re-secured in the distal esophagus at the end of the feeding.

CHAPTER 59
BLOOD CULTURE

I. **MATERIALS NEEDED**

   A. Sterile gloves.
   B. Prep materials - razor, scrub, Betadine, alcohol.
   C. 20 cc syringe.
   D. 2-19 gauge needles.

   Blood culture broth - tryptase soy or brain heart infusion broth with agar for anaerobic cultures.

   SPS (Sodium Polyanethol Sulphate) anticoagulant for aerobic culture (Becton Dickinson & Co., Cockeysville, Maryland), (Septi-Chek, Roche Laboratories, Nutley, NJ).

   If blood culture medium is not readily available, the sample can be transferred in a yellow top tube containing anticoagulant citrate (ACD).

II. **METHOD**

   A. Restraint of foal.
   B. Sterile prep of shaved area over jugular vein.
   C. Glove and aspirate 20 cc of blood into syringe with 19 gauge needle from jugular or peripheral vein.
   D. Remove needle and replace with a new 19 gauge needle.
   E. Wipe top of blood culture bottle with 2% iodine.
   F. Inject 5-7 cc into each of two bottles.
   G. Repeat in 1 or 2 hours up to 3-4 collections if clinical signs allow, before antimicrobial therapy is initiated.
   H. If already on antibiotics, take cultures prior to the next scheduled administration of antimicrobials.

III. **INTERPRETATION**[1-4]

   A. Growth in both bottles is significant.
   B. Negative blood cultures do not rule out septicemia. Over 50% of foals with *E. coli* septicemia have negative blood cultures.[1]

C. Organisms found most commonly are *E. coli, Actinobacillus spp, Klebsiella pneumoniae, Pseudomonas sp, Citrobacter spp, Enterobacter spp, Salmonella* and gram-positive organisms such as Streptococcus, Staphylococcus, Enterococcus.

References:
1. Wilson, W.D. and Madigan, J.E.: Comparison of bacteriologic culture of blood and necropsy specimens for determining the cause of foal septicemia: 47 cases (1978-1987). <u>JAVMA</u> 195:1759-1763, 1989.
2. Sanchez LC, Giguère S, Lester GD: Factors associated with survival of neonatal foals with bacteremia and racing performance of surviving Thoroughbreds: 423 cases. (1982-2007). <u>J Am Vet Med Assoc</u> 2008. Nov1;233(9):1446-52.
3. Russell CM, Axon JE, Blishen A, Begg AP.: Blood culture isolates and antimicrobial sensitivities from 427 critically ill neonatal foals. <u>Aust Vet J</u>. 2008 Jul;86(7):266 71.
4. Vaala WE., House JK., Lester GD.: Neonatal Infection in Smith BP. (ed.): <u>Large Animal Internal Medicine.</u> 4th edition. 281-292. WB. Saunders. Philadelphia. 2008.

CHAPTER 60
CEREBROSPINAL FLUID COLLECTION

The lumbosacral (LS) site provides a representative sample of CSF and can be done in the standing or recumbent foal. An atlantooccipital (AO) tap can also be done if the foal does not have increased intracranial pressure. Normal intracranial pressure in healthy neonatal foals is reported between 2-15mmHg[1]. Certain anesthetics (ketamine) may also increase intracranial pressure. Definitive signs of increased intracranial pressure in the foal are not known.

I. MATERIALS REQUIRED

- **A.** LS: 3 inch 20 gauge spinal needle; AO: 20 gauge, 1.5-2 inch disposable.
- **B.** Sterile prep materials, surgical gloves.
- **C.** Diazepam or midazolam for sedation.
- **D.** Lidocaine, 25 gauge needle and 3 cc syringe.
- **E.** 6 cc syringe for aspiration.
- **F.** Sterile Vacutainer® for collection.

II. LUMBOSACRAL TECHNIQUE

- **A.** Standing foals restrained by tail or rump and chest; or down in lateral recumbency.
- **B.** Sedation - may aid restraint.
- **C.** Have the foal stand with equal weight on rear limbs.
- **D.** Locate caudal edge of L-6, mid portion of tuber sacrale and spine of sacral vertebrae.
- **E.** Palpate depression posterior to L-6 and just cranial to a line connecting the mid portion of the two tuber sacrale.
- **F.** Prep area - shave, scrub, alcohol, Betadine.
- **G.** Local bleb of anesthesia in skin over site.
- **H.** Maintain needle in vertical plane with assistance from "spotter".
- **I.** Penetrate skin, fascia, interarcuate ligament, dura mater, arachnoid membrane.
- **J.** Remove stylet and aspirate at various levels; if no fluid aspirated, replace stylet and advance needle until meet bone.

- **K.** A "pop" with brisk contractive movement of the foal indicates penetration into subarachnoid space.
- **L.** Remove stylet, if CSF is blood tinged, draw first 2-3 cc in syringe and discard if fluid becomes clearer and save next 5 cc.
- **M.** Gently draw 5 cc for protein, cytology, Gram stain, culture, - compress jugular veins to increase CSF pressure and flow into syringe.
- **N.** Replace stylet and withdraw needle.
- **O.** If hit bone remove and re-direct.
- **P.** Frank blood in needle indicates have deviated off midline into venous sinus - remove, change needle and redirect.

III. ATLANTOOCCIPITAL SITE TECHNIQUE

- **A.** Need dependable immobilization – **Caution:** if penetrate too deeply permanent spinal cord damage may result.
- **B.** General anesthesia preferred immobilization. Others have used 2-5 mg Diazepam- Valium ® IV in semi-comatose foals and control of foal's legs and head in lateral recumbency.
- **C.** Head should be at right angle to the neck.
- **D.** Landmarks are point of intersection of an imaginary line between cranial borders of the wings of the atlas and midline.
- **E.** Prep the site by shaving and scrub.
- **F.** A palpable depression at the site is usually noted.
- **G.** Position and insert a 20 gauge 1.5 inch disposable needle directed at the mandible.
- **H.** Slowly advance and check for fluid. A change in resistance at a depth of 1-1.5 inches occurs on entry into the subarachnoid space.
- **I.** Fluid will drain from the hub of the needle in droplets.
- **J.** If a steady stream of clear fluid under pressure is seen, remove needle immediately as brain herniation may occur causing permanent damage.
- **K.** Penetrating too deeply may damage the spinal cord.
- **L.** Normally collect 3-6 cc of CSF.

IV. NORMAL EQUINE NEONATAL CSF [2,3,4]

A. Total protein - 145 mg/dl ± 50.
  1. Biuret method.
  2. Use your laboratory normal values due to different methods.
B. Albumin 81 mg/dl ± 13.
C. Globulin 64 mg/dl ± 15.
D. Color - clear.
E. Creatine Kinase (CK) - 15.2 ± 9.2 IU/liter.
  1. Extreme variation may be seen.
  2. Does not correlate with serum levels.
F. White blood cell total - < 20/ul.
G. Red blood cell total - variable usually <200/ul.
H. Glucose 30-70mg/dl
I. Sodium: 140-150 mEq/l
J. Potassium: 2.5-3.5 mEq/l

V. INTERPRETATION[5,6]

A. Elevated proteins (>70 mg/dl), WBC (>7-10/ul) and increased neutrophils suggest infection.
B. Gram stain for organism - intracellular indicates infection.
C. Increased protein, xanthochromia may indicate spinal hemorrhage or vasculitis.
D. Glucose lower than 80% of blood glucose may suggest infection - this has not been determined in foals.
E. Increased protein and increase in small and large mononuclear cells suggests viral infection.
F. CSF analysis within normal parameters does not rule out septic meningitis. However, a positive finding indicates significant involvement and a poor prognosis[7].

Decreased buffering capacity of the CSF in foals compared to adults can cause rapid acid-base disturbances in the brain[8].

References:
1. Kortz GD, Madigan JE, Goetzman BW, Durando M. Intracranial pressure and cerebral perfusion pressure in clinically normal equine neonates. Am J Vet Res. 1995 Oct;56(10):1351-5.

2. Rossdale P.D., Cash R.S.G., Leadon D.P., et al.: Biochemical constituents of cerebrospinal fluid in premature and term foals. Equine Vet J 14:134-138, 1982.
3. Rossdale P.D., Falk M., Jeffcott L.B., Palmer A.C., et al.: A preliminary investigation of cerebrospinal fluid in the newborn foal as an aid to the study of cerebral damage. J Reprod Fert Suppl 27:593 -599, 1979.
4. Andrews FM, Geiser DR, Sommardahl CS, Green EM, Provenza M.: Albumin quotient, IgG concentration, and IgG index determinations in cerebrospinal fluid of neonatal foals. Am J Vet Res. 1994 Jun;55(6):741-5.
5. Adams R., Mayhew I.G.: Neurologic diseases. Neonatal Equine Disease Vet Clin, North Amer 209-234,1985.
6. Mayhew IG: Large Animal Neurology. Second edition. Wiley-Blackwell. UK. 2009
7. Toth B, Aleman M, Nogradi, N. Madigan JE: Meningitis in horses. 27 cases. 1987-2010. J. Am Vet Med Assoc, 240(5);580-7, 2012
8. Geiser DR, Andrews FM, Rohrbach BW, Provenza MK.:Cerebrospinal fluid acid-base status during normocapnia and acute hypercapnia in equine neonates. Am J Vet Res. 1996 Oct;57 (10):1483-7.

CHAPTER 61
PLACEMENT AND MANAGEMENT OF INTRAVASCULAR CATHETERS

I. **PLACEMENT**[1,2]

A. **Venous**
   1. Sites include jugular, cephalic, saphenous and lateral thoracic veins. Jugular veins are the easiest to access therefore is the most commonly used peripherial veins in equine neonate.
   2. Catheter selection
   a) Teflon catheters are not recommended and should be avoided for intravenous or intraarterial use unless no other type of catheter is available. They carry high risk for thrombosis and catheter induced sepsis.
   b) Polyurethane IV catheters with single, double or triple lumen (Mila®, Arrow®, Cook®, Jorvet®) with a guidewire or peel away introducers can be used in a size of 4-7FR X 5-10" (12-25cm).
   c) Clip or shave site.
   d) Surgical scrub and prep with alcohol and povidone iodine.
   e) Inject lidocaine over jugular and sterile part of field.
   f) Use sterile technique including sterile single or double gloves.
   g) Perforate skin with large gauge needle or Size 11 scalpel blade first.
   h) If vein is collpased or not visible and venous preparation is necessary, use sterile technique and blunt dissection.
   i) Place introducer needle in jugular vein.
   j) A J-wire is placed in the vein through the needle and the needle is removed.
   k) The actual catheter is threaded over the J- wire and down into jugular vein and wire removed.
   l) Suture or superglue catheter to skin in 4-5 points.
       i. Sutures: Attach T-port® if it is not included to the catheter set. If T-ports® are not available, attach an I.V. extension set to the catheter. Cap the open end of the extension set with an

       infusion plug. Making injections or drawing samples through the T-port® or extension set rather than directly from the catheter will prolong the life of the catheter. Place two simple interrupted sutures through the skin and around the T-port®. One suture should be on each side of the extension arm of the T-port®. The catheter and T-port® should lie in a straight line parallel to the vein.
   ii. Glue: Attach T-Port® and PRN® infusion plug or I.V. set to catheter. Tighten with hemostat. Apply tincture of benzoin to skin. Apply cyanoacrylate (Superglue®) and press catheter to skin.
   iii. Tape: Catheters in the cephalic or saphenous veins may be secured by placing a strip of adhesive tape, Vetwrap®, or Elasticon® sticky side up under the catheter and infusion plug then folding the tape over the catheter (back on itself) and continuing around the leg. The skin should be dried before applying tape.

m) Catheter can be used for up to 2-3 weeks.

n) Silicone elastomer catheters (Mila®, Braun®, Arrow®, Cook®) with single or double lumen (60cmX5-7Fr) have minimal thrombogenicity and can be left in a central vein for up to 30+ days.

B. Arterial
   1. Sites include metatarsal, facial and femoral arteries.

a) Catheter selection: 20 or 22 ga, 1.25" to 2.5" Mila®, Arrow® or Jorvet® polyurethane over-the-needle catheters. 18 or 20 ga. catheters may also be used in the femoral artery.

b) Although placement of the over the wire catheters into the arteries requires lots of practice they are usually not indicated unless long term direct blood-pressure measurements are performed.

   2. Preparation, placement and securing as for venous catheters.

Chapter 61 Placement and Management of Intravascular Catheter

II. MANAGEMENT[1,2]

A. Dressings
   1. Apply povidone iodine ointment at insertion site.
   2. Cover dry 4" X 4" gauze sponges with povidone ointment and wrap entire neck or limb with gauze and elastic tape.
B. Manipulation of Catheter
   1. Should be minimized. Avoid disconnecting the system once it has been established, e.g. when moving patient or taking blood samples.
   2. Use sterile technique. Swab injection ports with alcohol before using.
   3. Change all infusion sets and fluid containers every 24-48 hours.
   Flush catheters QID with 2-3 mls of sterile isotonic fluid containing 10U/ml of heparin.
C. Changing Intervals
   1. Change catheter sites depending on the catheter type, or sooner if there is evidence of inflammation or loss of catheter integrity. Remove all intravascular catheters as soon as therapeutically possible. These steps should help minimize catheter-related infections.

References:
1. Spurlock, S.L., Spurlock, G.H., Parker, G, et al.: Long term jugular vein catheterization in horses. JAVMA 196:425-430, 1990.
2. Hardy, J.: Critical Care in Reed, S. M., Bayly, W. M., Sellon, D. C. (eds.): Equine Internal Medicine, 2nd Edition 273-288. WB. Saunders, St. Louis, 2004

CHAPTER 62
BLOOD SAMPLING TECHNIQUES

I. VENOUS SAMPLES

A. **Sites** include jugular, cephalic and saphenous veins.
B. **Equipment:** needles, syringes, blood collection tubes, alcohol and/or povidone iodine Betadine® gauze and tape.
C. **Technique**
   1. Prepare site with alcohol and/or povidone iodine (Betadine®) (for blood cultures shave site and do complete sterile prep, Chapter 59).
   2. Use smallest needle practical.
   3. After obtaining sample apply firm, steady pressure to puncture site using gauze pledget secured with tape or held by hand.

II. ARTERIAL SAMPLES FOR BLOOD GAS ANALYSIS

A. Sites include facial, greater metatarsal, femoral and transverse facial arteries. (See Figure 1).
B. Equipment: heparinized 3 cc syringe, 25 gauge needle, rubber stopper, ice water bath, alcohol and povidone (Betadine), gauze and tape.
C. Technique: Squeeze all the heparin out of the syringe so it is just in the hub.
   1. Prepare site - (may be shaved).
   2. Use two fingers to palpate the artery. Start nearly perpendicular with needle on syringe.
   3. After penetrating the skin and wall of artery, slowly advance or withdraw the needle until blood is obtained.
   4. Tap air bubbles out of syringe, insert needle into a rubber stopper like a vacutainer top and place sample in ice water bath.
   5. Apply firm pressure to puncture site for 2-5 minutes.
   6. A 2.5 -3 cc volume of blood is adequate.
   7. Record body temperature and submit to lab with sample.
      a. Sample is stable in ice water for 6 hours.

III. ARTERIAL OR VENOUS SAMPLES FROM INDWELLING CATHETERS

A. Equipment: needles (20 gauge or smaller), syringes, blood collection tubes, heparinized saline.
B. Technique
1. If a stopcock or clamp is not present on the catheter extension use a hemostat to clamp the line while changing syringes or draw blood through injection cap.
2. Slowly withdraw about 5 cc of blood into heparinized syringe (volume depends on size and length of catheter).
3. Withdraw blood samples.
4. Replace blood drawn in 2, if blood sampling is frequent.
5. Flush catheter with heparinized saline.
C. Solutions previously flowing through catheter may alter some laboratory values
D. This technique may contribute to venous thrombosis.

Figure 1: Sites for arterial blood gas sampling in the neonatal foal.

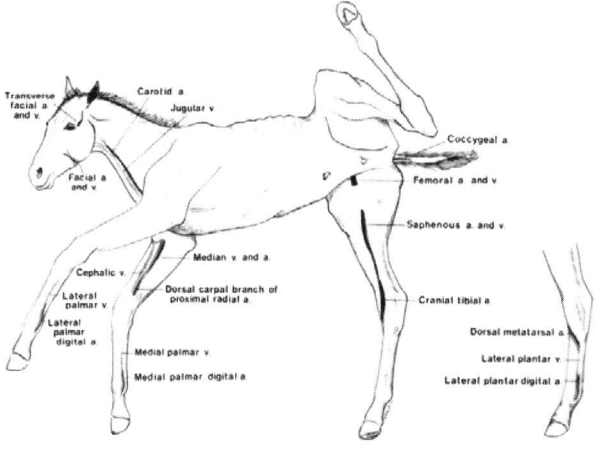

CHAPTER 63
BLOOD COLLECTION AND ADMINISTRATION

I. INDICATIONS

A. Conditions causing red cell destruction such as NI or immune mediated hemolytic anemia or significant blood loss.
B. Since PCV may remain "falsely" elevated with acute blood loss the criteria for transfusion with acute severe blood loss are different than those for chronic blood loss.
C. Acute blood loss with PCV <20% may indicate need for whole blood transfusion.
D. Acute decline of PCV continuously to 12% or less.

II. TRANSFUSED RED CELL HALF LIFE IN NEONATAL FOALS[3]

A. Studies have indicated longer half life (5.5 days) than adult horses (<4 day survival).
B. Autologous RBC had half life of 11.7 days.
C. Foal's dam or unrelated gelding both had same half life 5.5 days.

III. VOLUME OF BLOOD TO USE

A. Goal of transfusion of neonates is not to replace all lost RBC but to keep foal alive until bone marrow makes cells.
B. Half life of transfused cells should allow time for marrow to respond in NI cases.
C. Replace 20-40% of estimated blood loss with blood transfusion.
D. Administer so as to prevent volume overload in neonates. Usually a 0.5-1 liter/hr is a reasonable rate if shock is not present using a 50% solution of red cells.
E. Previous NI treatments have described 1-4 liters of whole blood suspension.
F. The greater the volume infused, the higher the likelihood for the development of hepatopathies secondary to iron toxicosis.

G. If blood products are not readily available, synthetic oxygen carrying substances can be used (Oxyglobin®, Biopure™) in a dose of 5-7.5ml/kg. The treatment is usually effective for 24 hours.

IV. BLOOD TYPE AND CROSS MATCH

A. Unknown Donor: Collect 10 ml yellow top ACD tube and 10 ml red top tube from recipient and donor.
  1. Submit to serology lab for major and minor cross match.
  2. Preferred donor is negative for blood groups A, Q, C and contains no anti-erythrocyte antibodies.
  3. If blood type unknown, may need to perform unmatched transfusion and watch for immediate reaction. May sensitize foal to later transfusion reactions or in females to producing NI foals. EC - Compared to being dead that's not so bad; if urgently needs blood give it.
  4. A rapid test (15 min.) was evaluated using anti-RBC sera and has been proven to be effective for detection of Aa, and Ca antigens[5].

B. **COLLECTION**[4]
  1. **Materials**
     a. 10 gauge X 3 inch angiocath.
     b. #15 scalpel blade.
     c. Surgical gloves.
     d. Blood collection set.
     e. Blood bags (trauma liners) or bottles.
     f. Evacuation chamber for blood bags.
     g. Vacuum pump.
     h. ACD solution 100 ml/liter blood.
     i. 60 cc syringe.
     j. 3 inch teat cannula.
     k. Blood administration set.
  2. **Technique**
     a. Using syringe and teat cannula, put 200 ml of ACD solution into each 2 liter blood bag. (100 ml ACD/liter).
     b. Surgically prep the skin overlying jugular vein and block with lidocaine.

c. Place the bag with ACD into the evacuation chamber connecting the bag to the chamber and the chamber to the pump.
d. Connect one end of transfer set to the adaptor (keep other end sterile).
e. With sugical gloves on, catheterize the jugular (10 ga X 3"). Be sure to first cut the skin with a scalpel blade to help overcome skin resistance. Attach blood collection set to catheter.
f. Turn on pump, set to 4-5 mmHg negative pressure.
g. Keep the jugular held off.
h. Ensure the blood and ACD are mixing well.
i. When the bag is full:
    i. Stop the pump.
    ii. Remove the adaptor from the full bag and insert into the next ACD bag (DO NOT contaminate the connector or remove the transfer set). Close the bag to atmosphere.
j. If 4 liters or more of whole blood is taken from the donor, replace this volume with LRS.
k. Wash in cold water all material having any contact with blood.
l. To simplify this, consider purchasing a blood collection kit from Veterinary Dynamics Inc and keeping it on hand with instructions and all connections needed. 800-654-9743 or 805-434-3840.

C ADVERSE REACTIONS
1. Severe anaphylaxis may occur - treat with epinephrine and NSAID and antihistamines.
2. Mild reactions may need to slow administration rate.
3. Consider pre-transfusion medication with flunixin, antihistamine and/or short acting steroid.
4. With cross matching should have fewer problems.

D. HANDLING[4]
1. Sodium citrate is the preferred anticoagulant for immediate use; blood:sodium citrate: 9:1.
2. Heparin should not be used when transfusing > 1 liter of blood as bleeding problems could arise with its use in larger volumes.

3. Most whole blood is used immediately; if not, anticoagulant storage medium is required.
   a. ACD - 3 week storage in humans.
   b. CPDA-1 (citrate-phosphate-dextrose-adenine); popular in human medicine.
   c. Bacterial contamination can preclude any storage.
   d. Commercial CPDA-1 bags have been shown to be the most suitable for storage[6].
4. Plastic containers, i.e., bags, do not activate Factor XII or platelets, do not injure RBCs, are unbreakable, store easily.
5. Whole blood or packed RBCs should be refrigerated at 4°C if not used immediately.

E. ADMINISTRATION
1. As for plasma. In-line filters must be used to remove clots.
2. In foals with neonatal isoerythrolysis (NI):
   a. Exchange transfusion with blood from suitable donor. See NI (Chapter 35) for method.
   b. Washed RBCs suspended in isotonic saline (0.9%) 50:50.
   c. Alternately, foal's dam, gelding, Shetland pony (have a low incidence of A and Q alloantigens) may be suitable donors.
   d. Watch the foal for adverse reactions. If noticed, stop the IV drip and evaluate respiration, circulation and treat accordingly.

References:
1. Smith, JE, Dever, M, Smith, J, DeBowes, RM.: Post-transfusion survival of Cr-labeled erythrocytes in neonatal foals. J Vet Int Med 6:183-185, 1992.
2. Owens SD, Snipes J, Magdesian KG, Christopher MM.: Evaluation of a rapid agglutination method for detection of equine red cell surface antigens (Ca and Aa) as part of pretransfusion testing. Vet Clin Pathol. 2008 Mar;37(1):49-56.
3. Librach,F.: Blood collection methods. In: Manual of Equine Neonatal Medicine 2nd Ed. 1991.

4. Mudge MC, Macdonald MH, Owens SD, Tablin F.: Comparison of 4 blood storage methods in a protocol for equine preoperative autologous donation. Vet Surg. 2004 Sep-Oct;33(5):475-86.

CHAPTER 64
RESTRAINT AND HANDLING OF FOALS

I. **NORMAL FOALS**

  A. Holding the foal.
  1. Foals should not be restrained by their heads with halters as we do with adult horses. For holding and moving neonates we place an adult horse halter upside down and attach through front legs and buckle under thorax and use as a harness that controls the mid-section of the foal. See Figure 1.

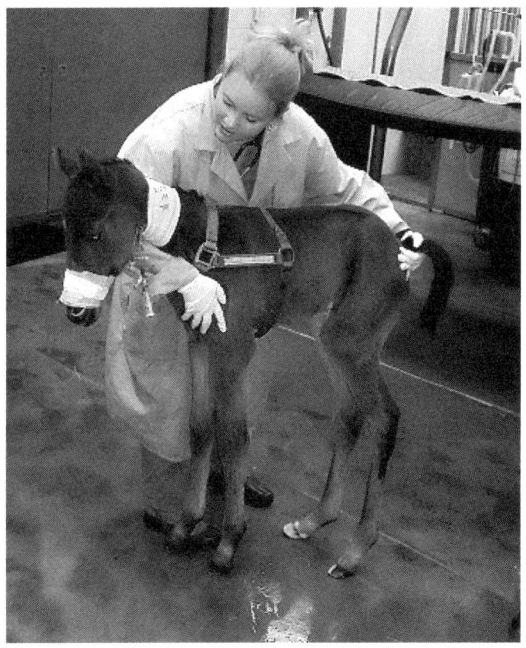

Figure 1: Use of an adult horse halter upside down as a foal harness.

2. For short procedures the foal can be placed up against a stall wall or corner and restrained with hand around chest and other arm around rump or if needed grasping the tail.
3. Flopping reaction of foals occurs when pressure is applied to body and foal will sink to the ground and suddenly arouse with pressure being decreased on the body.
4. For prolonged procedures in foals less than 1 week old consider placing foal in lateral recumbency using the Madigan Squeeze Induced Somulence method[1] (see below).

B. Placing in lateral recumbency for brief procedure
   1. EC: Perform this after allowing the foal nursing access to mare so it is full.
      a. The foal is restrained by placing the arms around the neck area and rump and holding the tail
      b. The right forearm of the handler is placed against the head of the foal, and the head is folded back toward the rump area while pressure is applied to the rear quarters with the other arm
      c. The foal leans backward and sags toward the handler, becoming recumbent
      d. Without releasing any pressure, the foal is allowed to sag to the ground and is kept in the folded position until completely recumbent and relaxed.
      e. The front legs are then grasped with the right hand, and the forearm is placed on the neck area. The rear legs are held with the left hand
      f. The foal is held steady in this position until it is blindfolded and struggling stops.

C. NEW METHOD[1,2] Restraint for procedures 20 minutes – foals <7 days

   SQUEEZE INDUCED SOMULENCE: this method puts the foal into a sleep state, lowers heart rate, slows breathing, raises endorphin levels and raises pain threshold (see Manual of Neonatal Foal web site for video).

Briefly, using a cotton rope, place a loop around the foals neck with non-slip bowline knot. A half hitch is placed twice over the thorax and rope is held with tension from behind the foal and the foal lays down and goes to sleep (Figure 2). Keep tension on foal. Be careful, just asleep not anesthetized but easier to do procedures such as ultrasound of umbilicus, glue on shoe, treat an eye, suture a wound (with local anesthetic) etc.

Figure 2: Foal in somnolent recumbent state following application of Madigan Squeeze Induced Somulence method.

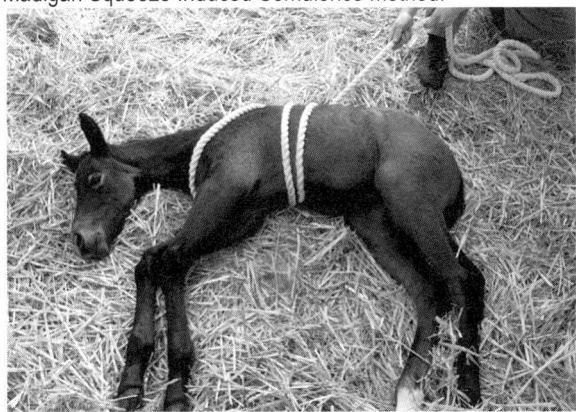

D. Moving the Foal
1. Do not allow foals to run loose. We prefer to harness with the halter as described above and have 1 person lead mare and 1 handle the foal.

E. General Comments
1. Foals have a short attention span so have everything arranged and ready prior to restraint efforts.
2. Don't over restrain for routine exams etc. Over handling foals can lead to pressure related patent urachus problems where urine is forced through involuting urachus
3. Let foals settle in between activities
4. Keep the mare as close to the foal as possible - during the first 14 days that means within a foot or two of the foal.

II. CRITICAL CARE ENVIRONMENT

A. Physical restraint
1. We rely heavily on human bodies to provide restraint and protection for tractable and intractable foals.
   a. Lateral recumbency with the down eye protected.
   b. Head and legs restrained.
   c. Violently thrashing foals may require another person at foal's hindquarters.
   d. Foal bed or platform is helpful to place catheters, etc.
   e. When sternal recumbency of the severely depressed foal is required, heavy wedge-shaped blocks or bags may be placed at shoulders and hips to maintain this position.
   f. Standing immobilization.

B. Chemical restraint
1. For restraining purposes Diazepam (Valium) 0.05-0.1 mg/kg IV initial dose has been helpful.
2. Xylazine should not be used in a compromised foal. See Sedation (Chapter 51).
3. Phenobarbital 5-20 mg/kg slowly IV over 20 minutes - provides longer term sedation.

C. Where to put foal in need of critical care
1. The advantage of mare and foal in a stall:
   a. Preservation of the maternal-foal bond.
   b. Allow intermittent nursing of the mare.
   c. Minimizes restraint and continuous presence of an attendant.
2. The disadvantages of mare and foal in a stall:
   a. Unsanitary.
   b. Variable temperature, humidity (lacks thermoneutrality).
   c. Poor lighting.
   d. Easily inhaled/swallowed bedding.
   e. Poor maternal cooperation.
   f. Difficult to hang continuous IV fluids.
3. Provide an environment which minimizes potential for self-inflicted trauma.
   a. Prevention of decubital and corneal ulcers.

b. Allows frequent change of foal's position and maintenance of sternal position.
c. Minimizes injury from thrashing and seizures.
d. Prevention of urine scalding in the down foal.
e. Prevention of development of patent urachus, reported to be a common complication in the down foal.
f. Management of premature/dysmature bone and connective tissue and resulting angular limb deformities.
g. The foal should be removed from a foal table and intensive care setting as soon as possible to encourage the foal to develop into a functioning horse, suckle, stand, walk and attach to the dam or a nurse mare.

References:
1. Toth B, Aleman M, Brosnan RJ, Dickinson PJ, Conley AJ, Stanley SD, Nogradi N, Williams CD, Madigan JE. Squeeze induced somulence in neonatal foals. Proceedings of AAEP, 2011.
2. Toth B, Aleman M, Brosnan RJ, Dickinson PJ, Conley AJ, Stanley SD, Nogradi N, Williams CD, Madigan JE. Squeeze induced somulence in neonatal foals. Am J. Vet Res 73(12) 1881-9, 2012.

CHAPTER 65
BIOSECURITY FOR NEONATAL UNITS

Written biosecurity measures should be in place for neonatal care units. See references for sources of current information on veterinary hospital biosecurity. The immune system of the compromised neonatal foal is less functional than adult horses. Therefore an effort should be made to keep the ill foal in the cleanest environment possible. Adequate temperature control, clean dry bedding with washable surfaces is desired. Nosocomial infections in neonatal ICUs have included fungal, salmonella sp, clostridium difficile, cryptosporidia sp, and viral agents.

I. **Handwashing** is the simplest and most effective means of prevention. It is absolutely necessary prior to handling the foal.

II. **Gloves** worn by anyone handling the foal is also a cost effective ways of infection prevention.

III. **Plastic booties** or **rubber boots with foot bath** prior to entering neonatal ICU is recommended.

IV. **Foot baths** before entering NICU and at individual stalls inside NICU (bleach 4oz/gallon or Tek-trol 1/2oz/gal) have been suggested.

V. **Surgery wraps** or **gowns** are recommended in some cases before entering a stall at Neonatal ICU.

VI. **Clean, disinfected blankets, pillows and pillowcases** are desirable at neonatal ICU. On site laundry is essential due to frequent turnover of reusable materials.

VII. **Disinfection**

   A. Neonatal ICU should be designed to allow the removal of all equipment and complete disinfection of floors, walls, doors, counter tops, and foal table following the completion of a case before a unit is available for another foal.

B. Some clinics uses Tek-trol® (www.bio-tekusa.com), a phenolic disinfectant which is effective against all type of infective agents including highly resistant Clostridium spores.

C. Prevention of nosocomial infection is paramount to the success of a NICU.

D. General procedure for disinfecting the stall.
   1. Remove all bedding from the stall and sweep clean.
   2. Soak the walls with an anionic detergent solution that will loosen the cracked, dried organic matter.
   3. Wash the surfaces with a scrub brush or with pressure washer.
   4. Repeat steps 1, 2, 3 as long as needed to clean thoroughly.
   5. Spray the disinfectant and be sure to allow to air dry.
   6. Repeat disinfectant application and allow to completely dry.
   7. Bed the stall
   8. Repeat after each patient.
   9. Dirt floor stalls and stalls built from wooden material do not disinfect very well.
   10. Consult suggested biosecurity protocols available on the web for adaptation to your circumstances.[1,2]

References:
1. California Department of Food and Ag. 2012 web site. http://www.cdfa.ca.gov/ahfss/animal_health/equine_biosecurity.html A new updated equine biosecurity information and booklet for download. Also check out the 2012 web site for equine and farm biosecurity from Canada.
2. Dwyer, RM.: Rotaviral diarrhea outbreaks in foals: Recommended Controls and management. Vet. Med. 86:198-202. 1991.

CHAPTER 66
RESPIRATORY THERAPEUTICS

The goal of physical therapy is to facilitate the mobilization and removal of secretions from the respiratory tract and to improve ventilation and oxygenating efficiency of the lungs. Premature and term foals dramatically improve the efficiency of their respiratory function by merely moving from lateral recumbency to sternal or standing position. Blood oxygen levels may increase by as much as 40 mmHg with this body position change.

I. POSTURAL DRAINAGE

   A. The foals should be positioned so that secretions may gravitate from the involved peripheral airways to the larger central airways where they can be coughed or aspirated out of the respiratory tract. The foal's position should be alternated frequently (at least every 2 hours) to facilitate drainage.
   B. Recumbent patients without lung disease should be kept sternal. If in lateral position rotate the foal every 1-2 hours to minimize secretion accumulation and small airway and alveolar collapse in dependent regions of the lung. Every attempt should be made to keep the foal in sternal position.

II. DEEP BREATHING AND EARLY AMBULATION

   A. Deep breathing maximizes alveolar inflation and minimizes small airway and alveolar collapse.
   B. Encourage early ambulation which may improve deep breathing and postural drainage.
   C. Deep breathing may be inhibited by narcotic drugs and heavy sedation, restrictive thoracic or abdominal bandages, pleural or peritoneal space-occupying lesions, or neuromuscular weakness.

III. CHEST PERCUSSION AND VIBRATION (COUPAGE)

   A. Percussion and vibration are used to mechanically dislodge secretions from the smaller airways.

B. Percussion is a rapid series (200 or more per minute) of sharp thumps to the chest wall made with cupped hands with the fingers closed.
1. Do not slap the skin with the flat of the hand since this maximizes skin trauma and minimizes chest wall and lung vibration.
2. The air compression between the cupped hand and the chest wall generates the desirable vibrational energy which is transmitted to the underlying lung parenchyma.

IV. SYSTEMIC HYDRATION

A. A well hydrated foal is of paramount importance in the liquefaction of airway secretions. Airway nebulization therapy has minimal beneficial effect in a dehydrated patient.

V. AIRWAY HYDRATION

A. Mucosal drying predisposes to decreased mucous clearance, tracheal inflammation and infection, and epithelial damage.
B. The airways may be hydrated by either increasing the humidity of the inspired air or by the introduction of particulate water droplets into the inhaled air stream.
C. The water content of air produced by unheated humidifiers is between 10 and 20 mg/L and should be sufficient to prevent mucosal drying in endotracheally intubated patients with a normal respiratory tract.
D. The water content of air produced by direct installation of water into the respiratory tract (5 ml every 1-2 hours) and by unheated nebulizers varies between 15 and 30 mg/L and should be sufficient to prevent mucosal drying in endotracheally intubated foals with normal respiratory tracts or nonexudative diseases.
E. Heated humidifiers and nebulizers generate mist densities of 25-45 and 40-50 mg/L, respectively, and should be very effective in preventing mucosal drying in endotracheally intubated or tracheotomized foals and in providing some liquefaction of airway exudates.

F. If exudate liquefaction is the primary goal of the nebulization therapy, the very high mist densities associated with ultrasonic nebulizers should be used.
G. Large bore tubing with few angled joints should conduct air from the nebulizer to the foal to minimize impaction of water droplets on the walls of the conducting tubing.
H. When heated humidifiers and nebulizers are used, excess water will condense on the walls of the conducting tubing as the air cools on the way to the foal. Water which has accumulated in the conducting tubing may occlude airflow if not periodically drained.
I. Distilled water should be used if the primary objective is the prevention of surface drying. Saline should be used if liquefaction of thick airway secretions and the stimulation of coughing is the primary objective.
J. The heavier the mist density and the smaller the particulate size, the further into the respiratory tract the aerosol will be deposited.
K. Humidification therapy, when utilized, should be applied continuously. Nebulization therapy, particularly those forms associated with higher mist and water densities, should be administered at intervals throughout the day, but not continuously in order to avoid the deleterious effects of excess airway water; 10 to 30 minutes every 2 to 4 hours.
L. Water reservoirs and nebulization equipment support growth of microorganisms and aerosolized water droplets are capable of carrying these microorganisms into the depth of the lung.
  1. Nebulization equiment and delivery systems should be sterilized prior to each use and should be completely changed everty 24-48 hours.
  2. Only sterile solutions should be used in the nebulization reservoirs.
  3. Water accumulating in the conducting tubing should not be drained back into the reservoir in case it has become contaminated.
  4. Prophylactic antibiotics in the nebulizer reservoir are not indicated.

VI. NEBULIZED MEDICANTS

A. The most useful nebulized medicant is water. It prevents surface drying, soothes inflamed tissue, and liquifies thickened secretions. Few medicants liquify respiratory secretions more effectively than saline alone.

B. N-acetylcysteine (Mucomyst®. Mead Johnson) is effective in liquefying thickened mucus and also has some effect on purulent exudates.
1. The agent has an unpleasant sulfur odor, is a local tissue irritant, especially in high concentrations, and has been associated with stomatitis, nausea, and bronchospasm in humans.
2. It inactivates penicillin-type antibiotics.
3. Acetylcysteine is not deleteriously affected by nebulization, with either plastic or glass jet, or ultrasonic nebulizers, but should not be placed in heated nebulizers, or in contact with iron, copper, or rubber.
4. Nebulize 3-10 ml of a 10% solution 3-4 times daily; or instill 0.25-2.0 ml directly into the airway as often as hourly.

C. Aerosolized proteolytic enzymes (Varidase®, Lederle; Varizyme®, Cyanamid; Elase®, Parke-Davis) (combinations of streptokinase, streptodornase and fibrinolysin) may be beneficial in the treatment of viscous infectious exudates which contain large amounts of DNA, protein, and calcium.
1. Deoxyribonuclease depolymerizes DNA protein present in degenerating leukocytes and tissue cells.
2. Streptokinase activates intrinsic plasminogen within fibrin deposits.
3. Proteolytic enzymes are associated with a high incidence of pyrogenic and hypersensitivity reactions in humans and are irritating to normal tissues.
4. Their usefulness is limited to less than one week due to the development of inhibiting antibodies.
5. For persistent thick exudates, for which saline alone has been ineffective, nebulize 50,000 – 100,000 units of deoxyribonuclease in 2.5 ml of water 1-4 times daily.

D. Mucus is less viscous in an alkaline medium and a 1-2% solution of sodium bicarbonate in combination with another carrier may have some beneficial effects.

E. A 25-50% solution of ethyl alcohol decreases the surface tension of airway froth and may have some usefulness in frothy pulmonary edema.

F. Oral potassium iodide (Fleming®; Eli Lilly) 4-10 mg/kg 3-4 times daily) and some volatile oils (camphor, anise, lemon, and nutmeg) may increase bronchial gland secretory activity and decrease secretion viscosity.

G. $Beta_2$ receptor stimulating sympathomimetics cause bronchial and arterial relaxation.

1. Traditional sympathomimetics are often associated with the development of tolerance to the bronchodilating activity (epinephrine, isoproterenol, phenylephrine, ephedrine); an occasionally severe bronchoconstrictive rebound (epinephrine, isoproterenol, phenylephrine); exhibit a short duration of action and are ineffective by the oral route (epinephrine, isoproterenol); and may cause hypoxemia due to increased pulmonary ventilation/perfusion and maldistribution (isoproterenol), and tachycardia.

2. There is little reason to use the more generally acting sympathomimetics now that more selective $beta_2$ receptor stimulants have been developed.

3. The $beta_2$ receptor stimulants (terbutaline, isoetharine, albuterol, metaproterenol) are very potent bronchodilators when administered orally, subcutaneously, intravenously, or by aerosol. Minimal tolerance develops to the bronchodilating activity but good tolerance develops to the induced skeletal muscle tremors.

    a. Compared to the traditional sympathomimetics, these agents are longer lasting, are not usually associated with palpitations, marked tachycardia or hypertension.

    b. Suggested <u>nebulization</u> doses of bronchodilator drugs:

Albuterol	0.001-0.01 mg/kg q 6-8 hrs
Terbutaline	0.001-0.007 mg/kg q 4-6 hrs
Metaproterenol	0.10-0.30 mg/kg q 3-4 hrs

- **H.** Inhalational glucocorticoids
- **I.** Diuretics
- **J.** Antibiotics

CHAPTER 67
POSITIVE PRESSURE VENTILATION

Outcomes have greatly improved with this therapy in foals. A commitment must be made for a prolonged and expensive course of therapy prior to initiating PPV in foals. With central causes of hypoventilation we have avoided PPV by administering I.V. doxapram to foals with hypercapnia and hypoxemia (Chapter 13).

Positive pressure ventilation (PPV) is indicated whenever a patient is not ventilating adequately as might occur in central nervous system or neuromuscular disorders, loss of rigidity of the chest wall or open pneumonia. A closed pneumothorax is a specific contraindication to the use of PPV. PPV may be useful in foals with moderate to severe pulmonary parenchymal disease that cannot properly oxygenate blood because of small airway and alveolar collapse in hyaline membrane disease of premature foals.

I. GENERAL PRINCIPLES OF POSITIVE PRESSURE VENTILATION

   A. The amount of pressure to apply to the proximal airways for ventilation of normal lungs is about 20 cm H_2O. Apply just enough pressure to achieve a full and adequate tidal volume; additional pressure is not necessary and may deleteriously affect intrathoracic blood flow. It is often necessary to increase the peak airway pressure above 20 cm H_2O for lungs that exhibit reduced compliance due to parenchymal disease.
   B. Inspiration should last only as long as is necessary to achieve a full and adequate tidal volume; a longer inspiratory phase is not necessary and may induce inordinate impairment of thoracic blood flow. In normal lungs an inspiratory time of 1.0 - 1.5 seconds is usually sufficient.
   C. The tidal volume is determined by the airway pressure and the inspiratory time. The tidal volume should range between 10 and 20 ml/kg.
   E. Minute ventilation is the product of tidal volume and breathing frequency and should be 150-250 ml/kg/min.

F. Once the initial ventilator settings are established the patient should be evaluated clinically and, if available, by laboratory analysis of tidal volume, minute ventilation, and arterial blood oxygen and carbon dioxide to verify an acceptable patient response and the absence of any untoward effects.
   1. If the response is less than desirable the ventilator settings should be altered in an appropriate manner.
   2. If the patient begins to fight the ventilator or breathe at a rate faster than the ventilator, check for inappropriate ventilator settings, ventilator malfunction, or soda lime exhaustion. Ascertain that pre-existing conditions have not been worsened by the ventilation procedure (e.g., pneumothorax, hypotension).

II. END-EXPIRATORY PRESSURE

A. Indications
   1. Some lungs are so severely diseased that standard ventilator settings are not sufficient to restore acceptable blood oxygenation. Higher airway pressures and longer inspiratory times improve alveolar ventilation and are useful up to the point at which they cause inordinate impairment of venous return and cardiac output. The application of positive airway pressure during the exhalation phase of the breathing cycle enhances transpulmonary pressure and helps prevent small airway and alveolar collapse without impairing intrathoracic blood flow. Airway - alveolar units which do not collapse between breaths are better ventilated on the subsequent breath.

B. Methods
   1. Expiratory resistance may be applied by attaching a narrow apertured device to the exhalation port of the ventilator or patient circuit. Exhalation is retarded and mean airway pressure is increased, however, airway pressure will still decrease to atmospheric.
   2. A positive end-expiratory pressure (PEEP) plateau may be achieved utilizing a corrugated breathing tube leading from the pressure relief value or exhalation port of the ventilator to an underwater

position in a partially filled bottle. The depth to which the end of the tube is positioned determines the airway pressure at the end of exhalation. Commercial PEEP valves are also available.
3. Continuous positive airway pressure (CPAP) is a control variable on new ventilators which allows the patient to breathe spontaneously between cycles of the ventilator, while maintaining airway pressure at a preset level during the duration of the spontaneous breath. The inspiratory cycle of the ventilator is independently regulated.
   a. Optimal end-expiratory pressure is often in the range of 5-15 cm H_2O.
4. Optimal end-expiratory pressure is determined as:
   a. Settings which alleviate the clinical signs of hypoxemia while causing minimal diminution of measured blood pressure or palpated pulse quality in a peripheral artery; or
   b. Settings which generate an arterial partial pressure of oxygen (PaO_2) of at least 60 mmHg with an arterial partial pressure of carbon dioxide $PaCO_2$ of between 30 and 40 mmHg, and an inspired oxygen concentration of less than 50 to 60%, with less than about a 20% decrease in arterial blood pressure or cardiac output; or
   c. Settings which generate the highest oxygen availability (cardiac output x arterial oxygen content); or
   d. By settings which generate the highest mixed venous PO_2. Mixed venous PO_2 reflects the overall adequacy of oxygen delivery to the tissues compared to oxygen consumption.

III. MANAGEMENT OF A FOAL RECEIVING CONTINUOUS VENTILATORY SUPPORT

A. Minimize trauma to the trachea by the tube.
   1. Avoid traction or torsion on the tube by the foal or the ventilator circuit.

Chapter 67 Positive Pressure Ventilation

- **B. Minimize trauma to the trachea by the cuff.**
    1. Inflate the cuff carefully with the minimal occlusive volume and record the volume.
- **C.** Emergency intubation and tracheal suction equipment should be readily available.
- **D.** Maintain airway humidity and patient hydration.
- **E.** Carefully suction the trachea every 2-3 hours as necessary. If the suctioning procedure fails to collect any secretions consider that airway humidification procedures may not be adequate.
- **F.** Weigh foal daily and avoid overhydration.
- **G.** Consider nasogastric tube or TPN for nutritional support.
- **H.** Re-evaluate ventilator function and the foal's response to the therapy frequently throughout the day.

CHAPTER 68
TRACHEAL SUCTIONING

If the foal is unable to generate an effective cough or if coughing is ineffective at removing airway secretions, they may be removed by tracheal suctioning. This procedure is not without risk. Aseptic techniques and short time intervals are required. Cardiac arrhythmias may occur.

I. PRESSURES

   A. Safest pressure ranges for suction equipment range between 60 and 150 mmHg. The lowest pressure and flow rate that will effectively aspirate secretions from the airway should be used.

II. CATHETERS

   A. Suction catheters should be soft and flexible in order to minimize epithelial trauma during suctioning, and long enough to pass the end of the endotracheal tube.
   B. Suction catheters should have more than one hole in their tip to prevent excessive attraction of the catheter to the tracheal wall. When this occurs an epithelial plug is sucked into the hole and it is likely to be ripped away when the catheter is withdrawn.
   C. The suction catheter should have as large a lumen as possible to facilitate the removal of thick secretions.
   D. The outside diameter of the catheter should be no larger than 50% of the inside diameter of the smallest portion of the airway through which the catheter is placed.
      1. The air which is suctioned through the catheter comes from the room and must be able to flow freely down along the outside of the catheter. If this does not occur excessive reductions in intrapulmonary pressure will occur which increase the magnitude of the small airway and alveolar collapse.
   E. The suction catheter should have a proximal thumb hole so that suction can be applied in a controlled manner.
   F. The tracheal suctioning procedure must be aseptic to prevent contamination of the lower respiratory tract.

1. Trauma may be secondary to excessive manipulation of the catheter within the trachea or excessive attraction of the catheter to the tracheal wall.

III. TECHNIQUE OF TRACHEAL SUCTIONING

A. The airway should be well humidified, either by nebulization or by the direct installation of 2-5 ml of saline, immediately prior to the suctioning procedure.
B. If the foal is not receiving continuous oxygen, supplemental pre-oxygenation may help minimize suctioning-induced hypoxemia.
C. Mobilization of peripheral secretions to the central airways by postural drainage and percussion just prior to suctioning may improve the results of the suctioning procedure.
D. Gently insert the sterile catheter into the trachea as far as it will advance (without applying suction) with a sterile-gloved hand.
E. Suction is applied while the catheter is removed. The negative pressure should not be applied to the airway for more than a total of **10 seconds** to minimize the development of airway collapse and hypoxemia.
F. The catheter is withdrawn with a winding motion of the hand.
G. The suctioning procedure should cease immediately if excessive patient discomfort or restlessness, or changes in cardiac or respiratory rhythm occur.
H. The foal should be manually hyperinflated with 100% O_2 following the suctioning procedure to alleviate small airway collapse and hypoxemia.
I. The foal should breathe an enriched oxygen mixture for several minutes following the procedure.
J. The entire procedure may be repeated several times at each interval if necessary and should be repeated at approximately 2 hour intervals or sooner if secretions accumulate more rapidly.

CHAPTER 69
HOW TO PREVENT THE LEADING CAUSE OF DEATH IN NEONATAL FOALS: OPINION

The leading cause of illness in neonatal foals upon admission in our clinic is bacterial infection (septicemia due predominantly to mixed infection with gram positive and gram negative organisms). The second leading cause of problems are related to birth asphyxia. These two conditions have been listed by Kentucky foal post mortem studies as the leading cause of death. This is despite a number of studies indicating passive transfer failure and low serum IgG are the cause of most of these neonatal deaths.

However, a number of people have begun to question that low IgG is the sole cause of this problems. Additionally, our efforts to raise IgG by various means seem to have not eliminated the problem of septicemia over the last 10-15 years. Well conducted studies such as Balwin et al. (1991) have indicated that low IgG per se is not a health risk factor and several studies have indicated that foals with only 200 mg/dl IgG at 24 hours of age don't get sick on some farms.

Leo Jeffcott (1974) demonstrated the indiscriminate active absorption of large molecules by the "open" gut shortly after birth. Unfortunately this avenue as a potential major route of exposure of the foal to pathogens has been overlooked. Specialized cells line the newborn gut and will non-specifically ingest various large molecular weight compounds (via pinocytosis) and not just immunoglobulin. Additionally, the lack of tight junctions between gut barrier cells allowed >70,000 MW molecules to freely pass into the lymphatics and circulate between cells. When these cells are used up, the gut assumes its normal structure and no further absorption of large molecules can take place.

Early on in foal medicine the umbilicus was considered the route of infection for most foals with septicemia and septic arthritis. Numerous studies have shown the umbilicus is not involved in the majority of foal septicemias. We developed the hypothesis that delayed gut closure and exposure to bacteria during udder seeking or due to delayed feeding or nursing and subsequent environmental licking or ingestion of bacteria by the newborn foal is the risk factor

Chapter 69 How to Prevent The Leading Cause of Death in Neonatal Foals-Opinion

and source of bacteria for most septicemias in foals. Early administration or ingestion of colostrum may be associated with reduced illness in foals because of early (rapid) gut closure and prevention of absorption of bacteria across the gut wall. Thus a foal with high IgG could be a marker for wellbeing based on rapid and early feeding prior to bacterial access to the foal across the open gut. Additionally, this would explain healthy foals that stood and nursed vigorously but did not become ill despite low serum IgG. Delayed nursing and early exposure to pathogens (prior to any colostrum) are the key factors in risk of infection in this hypothesis.

This means that conditions that may be associated with delayed gut closure, such as neonatal maladjustment syndrome (birth hypoxic encephalopathy), prematurity, dystocia, musculoskeletal problems, weak at birth foals, twins, would have significant incidences of septicemia, which they certainly do. Good management for preventing infections are clean stalls, clean mares, factors that aid early ingestion of colostrum and short term post birth antibiotics in the newborn.

II. METHOD FOR PREVENTING SEPTICEMIA

A. Keep the mare in facilities in which foaling will take place to allow production of antibodies to pathogens within the area. Clean foaling stalls twice daily and disinfect stalls prior to use. Wash the mare before foaling.

B. Immediately following delivery prevent the foal from contacting the mare until steps C and D are completed.

C. Wash the mare after foaling with large volumes of soap and water to remove bacteria around the perineum, udder and rear quarters where the foal may lick during udder seeking. Dry the mare.

D. Milk the mares cleaned mammary gland of 2-4 oz of colostrum (preferably greater than 1060 specific gravity) and bottle feed the foal, prior to the foal rising, upon obtaining a suck reflex. Use colostrum from colostrum bank if necessary.

E. If the foal is weak, tube feed the foal within 1 hour of birth with 6-8 oz of colostrum or, if none available, use mare milk replacer or, if none available, use cow's milk. In

F. In any foals without an observed birth and for foalings in an unclean area without the above precautions, I recommend veterinarians prescribe and begin antibiotic therapy within 8 hrs of birth and treat for 48 to 72 hours only. Longer treatment may produce antibiotic resistance and should be reserved for ill foals. The choice of antibiotic therapy will vary with the area. Post birth antibiotics have been a routine part of management on stud farms in the UK for the past 40 years and the incidence of sepsis is much lower than the United States.

orphan foals continue feeding from a bottle or pan until 10% of body weight is fed. Feed when the foal is hungry.

For those of you concerned about aminoglycoside antibiotics in foals, monitor serum creatinine or urinalysis if you so desire. I find aminoglycosides safe in foals that are kept hydrated; that is most important. In a bright, alert foal receiving short term antibiotics, this should be no trouble.

These are my opinions. Keep doing what works for you. If bacterial infections in neonates are a problem, consider these observations.

References:
1. Cohen, N. Causes of and farm management factors associated with disease and death in foals. JAVMA 124:1644-1651, 1994
2. McGuire TC, Crawford, TB, Hallowell AL et al: Failure of colostral immunoglobulin transfer as an explanation for most infections and deaths of neonatal foals. JAVMA 170: 1302-1304, 1977
3. McGuire TC, Poppie MJ, Banks, KL: Hypogamma-globulinemia predisposing to infection in foals. JAVMA 166:71-75.
4. Rossdale, P. Modern concepts of neonatal disease in foals. Equine Vet J 4:117-128, 1972
5. Koterba, AM, Brewer, BD, Tarplee FA. Clinical and clinicopathological characteristics of the septicaemic neonatal foal: review of 38 cases. Equine Vet J 16:376-383, 1984.
6. Baldwin, JL, Cooper, WL, Vanderwall, DK, Erb, HN. Prevalence (treatment days) and severity of illness in

hypogammagloubilinemic and normagammmaglobulinemic foals. <u>JAVMA</u> 198:423-428, 1991.
7. Walker RL; Madigan JE; Hird DW; Case JT; Villanueva MR; Bogenrief DS. An outbreak of equine neonatal salmonellosis. <u>J Vet Diag Invest</u>, 3(3):223-7, 1991.
8. Walker, RL, de Peralta, TL, Villanueva MR, Snipes KP, Madigan JE, Hird DW, Kasten, RW. Genotypic and phenotypic analysis of Salmonella strains associated with an outbreak of equine neonatal salmonellosis. <u>Vet Microbiology</u> 43:143-150, 1995.
9. Stoneham, S. The incidence of neonatal septicemia in a selected population of thoroughbred foals in Newmarket, England (1989-1994). <u>The Dorothy Russell Havemeyer Foundation: Neonatal Septicemia Workshop</u>. Westminster, Ma and Tufts University, N Grafton Ma.
10. Jeffcott, LB. Studies on Passive Immunity in the Foal II: The absorption of 125-Labeled PVP (polyvinyl pyrrolidone) by the Neonatal Intestine. <u>J Comp Path</u> 84:279-289, 1974.
11. Jeffcott, LB. Passive immunity and its transfer with special reference to the horse. <u>Biological Reviews</u>, 47:439-464, 1972
12. Jeffcott, LB. Immune passive transfer to foals: Sixty years on. <u>Equine Vet J.</u> 17:162-163, 1985.

CHAPTER 70
GUIDELINES FOR DRUG USE
IN EQUINE NEONATES

There are several important differences between neonates and adults in the way drugs are absorbed, distributed, metabolized and eliminated from the body.[1,2] Consequently, dosage regimens used for drugs in adult horses may not be appropriate for use in neonatal foals. With regard to drug administration, it does appear that normal equine neonates are more mature than neonates of many other species and that maturation after birth occurs more rapidly. Considerable maturation occurs in foals within the first 3 or 4 days of life and many metabolic and excretory processes are relatively mature by 1 week. Thereafter, maturation continues for many months but, in most respects, foals of > 1 month of age handle drugs in a manner similar to adults.

I. DIFFERENCES BETWEEN EQUINE NEONATES AND ADULTS IMPORTANT IN DRUG THERAPY:

A. **Comparatively larger ECF volume in foals** means most drugs have a larger volume of distribution. Thus, for equivalent doses, plasma concentrations of some drugs will be lower than in adults. This does not necessarily mean that tissue levels are lower or that the dose needs to be increased, since other features of distribution and elimination also influence drug concentrations.

B. **Lower plasma protein in neonates** means that a greater proportion of drugs which are highly bound to plasma protein, e.g. penicillin G, sulfonamides, trimethoprim, and phenylbutazone, are present in the circulation in the unbound (active) form.

C. **The hepatic metabolic pathways** (oxidation, reduction, hydrolysis and conjugation) are not fully functional at birth and are impaired further in premature foals. Thus drugs which undergo complete or partial hepatic metabolism prior to excretion may experience delayed elimination, especially during the first 3 or 4 days of life.
Examples include chloramphenicol, trimethoprim, sulfonamides, phenobarbital, phenytoin, and theophylline. Maturation of hepatic function to near adult capacity

occurs rapidly in term foals during the first 7 to 14 days of life.

D. **Renal excretion** is the principal process of elimination for most polar drugs (e.g. penicillins and aminoglycosides) and the majority of drug metabolites. The renal excretory mechanisms of glomerular filtration, tubular secretion and tubular reabsorption are relatively more mature in foals than in neonates of many other species. While not fully mature at birth, renal excretory mechanisms in foals mature rapidly during the first week of life.

E. **Premature foals** may have retarded maturation of their drug metabolizing and excreting mechanisms.

F. **Absorbable drugs administered orally** are generally better in neonates than in adults. The resultant serum concentrations of drugs such as ampicillin, amoxicillin, trimethorpim and sulfonamides tend to be higher[3,4]. This effect is especially marked during the first 24-48 hours and can be used to advantage therapeutically. However, enhanced absorption also has the potential to enhance toxicity, particularly when clearance mechansism are also immature.

G. **Neonates have a poorly developed blood-brain barrier**. This may be useful when treating meningitis but can pose problems when selecting doses for CNS depressants (e.g. barbiturates, xylazine).

H. **Neonates have a lower content of body fat** so there is less sequestration of lipid-soluble drugs. This can lead to higher plasma concentrations and more profound effects, e.g. with barbiturates.

II. **ANTIBIOTICS:**[5-8]

A. **Almost all systemic neonatal bacterial infections** involve gram-negative (often enteric) organisms, with or without accompanying gram-positive organisms. (The opposite is usually the case in adults).

B. **Septicemic foals deteriorate rapidly**. Antibiotic treatment should be started as soon as cultures have been collected and later modified, if necessary, after culture and susceptibility results are available. Front line antibiotics should have excellent activity against gram-negative bacteria and specific combination therapy is rational to broaden the spectrum. The most useful antibiotics for initiating treatment of suspected or confirmed sepsis are the aminoglycosides, e.g. amikacin or gentamicin, in combination with penicillin G, ampicillin, ticarcillin or a cephalosporin antibiotic. Depending on the susceptibility of bacterial isolates, other antibiotics which may prove useful include trimethoprim/sulfonamide, 3rd-generation cephalosporins, or ticarcillin/clavulanic acid.

C. **Bactericidal drugs are preferred** because neonates have suboptimal defense mechanisms and most infected foals have total or partial failure of passive transfer of colostral antibodies.

D. **The disease process** can interfere with drug absorption, therefore parenteral routes should be used in systemically ill foals - the IV route is preferred initially.

E. **Avoid** using antimicrobials which require extensive hepatic metabolism prior to excretion (e.g., chloramphenicol, erythromycin) especially in systemically ill foals with impaired liver function, and in premature foals.

F. **Use drugs** which are excreted unchanged in urine, e.g. penicillins, aminoglycosides[10,11], cephalosporins or those which undergo only limited hepatic metabolism, e.g. trimethoprim/sulfonamide.[9]

   1. Aminoglycosides, especially amikacin and gentamicin are very useful drugs because of their activity against gram negative bacteria. They have been used for 14 days or more at standard doses in normally hydrated foals without apparent problems but they are potentially nephrotoxic. The following precautions should be taken:
      a. In patients with renal disease, alternative antibiotics should be used if possible. If aminoglycosides are used the dosage interval should be adjusted (lengthened) according to measured peak and trough plasma concentrations.
      b. Ensure patients are adequately hydrated (dehydration enhances toxicity).
      c. Monitor urine for evidence of tubular damage - proteinuria, casts, RBC, (1+ proteinuria normal in newborn foals for 2-3 days).

Chapter 70 Guidelines for Drug Use in Equine Neonates

2. Current Dosing Regimens for Aminoglycosides[10-15]
   a. A once daily dosing regimen for aminoglycosides is more effective and often less nephrotoxic than the older lower dose, multiple dosing protocols in man and other species. Efficacy of aminoglycosides such as gentamicin or amikacin is concentration dependent. The magnitude of initial serum concentrations and area-under-the serum concentration vs. time curve (AUC) are more important in bacterial killing and in determining a post-antibiotic effect than is the duration that concentrations remain above the MIC of microbes. In adult horses, such a dosing regimen (6.6 mg/kg q 24 h) with gentamicin has been shown to produce significantly higher peak serum concentrations and AUC as compared to standard dosing protocols (2.2 mg/kg q 8 hr). Similar peaks and pharmacokinetics consistent with increased efficacy were determined in a study involving 21 mg/kg of amikacin administered once daily to neonatal foals for 10 days.
   b. Nephrotoxicity was not observed after a 10 day course of once daily administered gentamicin in adults and amikacin in neonatal foals. A retrospective study also showed that hospitalized neonatal foals had optimal pharmacokinetics of amikacin when administered at a dose of 20-25 mg/kg once daily, based on therapeutic drug monitoring.
   c. Therapeutic drug monitoring (TDM) ensures dosing intervals and quantities that are both safe and effective. TDM entails measuring serum concentrations of aminoglycosides from two serum samples, one obtained one hour after administration (after the distribution phase is complete) and a second obtained before the next dosing. In the case of once daily therapy, this second sample should be obtained 4-8 hours after dosing. Peak and trough concentrations can then be obtained. Target trough concentrations are minimum target

concentrations to minimize the risk for nephrotoxicity, and are ≤ 1 ug/ml and ≤ 4 ug/ml for gentamicin and amikacin, respectively. Target peak concentrations should be a minimum of > 10 ug/ml and 14 ug/ml for gentamicin and amikacin, respectively.

d. Patients on aminoglycoside therapy should be monitored for signs of nephrotoxicity, especially if hypovolemia or reduced renal perfusion is suspected. Serum concentrations of creatinine and blood urea nitrogen can be used, however urine indices (urine specific gravity, urinalysis, fractional excretions) are more sensitive and will detect toxicity earlier.

e. When on IV fluids: Just as therapeutic drug monitoring is important for patients with lowered volumes of distribution (dehydration, hypovolemia) to ensure safety, it is similarly important for those patients with increased volumes and clearance, such as those on intravenous fluid therapy, to ensure adequate peaks.

f. Intraosseous therapy of aminoglycosides has been shown to closely approximate the pharmacokinetics of these drugs given intravenously, and is a viable alternative route for patients where venous access is limited.[12]

References:

1. Baggot, J.D., Short, C.R.: Drug disposition in the neonatal animal with particular reference to the foal. Equine Vet J 16(4):364-367, 1984.
2. Vaala, W.E.: Aspects of pharmacology in the neonatal foal. Vet Clin N Am (Eq. Pract) 1(1):51-75, 1985.
3. Brown, M.P., Gronwall, R., Kroll, W.R., and Beal C.: Ampicillin trihydrate in foals: serum concentrations and clearance after a single oral dose. Equine Vet J 16:371-373, 1984.

Chapter 70 Guidelines for Drug Use in Equine Neonates

4. Love, D.N., Rose, R.J., Martin, I.C.A. and Bailey, M.: Serum levels of amoxycillin following its oral administration to Thoroughbred foals. Equine Vet J 13:53-55, 1981.
5. Wilson, W.D., Spensley, M.S. and Adamson, P.J.W.: Considerations for the selection of antibiotics in equine neonates. In: Proc 6th Annual ACVIM 6:628-634, 1988.
6. Carter, G.K., and Brown, S.A.: Use of antibiotics in foals. In: Proc 32nd Annual Conv of AAEP 32:209-221, 1986.
7. Sojka, J.E., and Brown, S.A.: Pharmacokinetic adjustment of gentamicin dosing in septic horses. J Am Vet Med Assoc 189:784-789, 1986.
8. Caprile, K.A. and Short, C.R.: Pharmacologic considerations in drug therapy in foals. Vet Clin N Am (Equine Pract) 3:123-144, 1987.
9. Adland-Davenport, P., Brown, M.P., Robinson, J.D. and Derendorf, H.C.: Pharmacokinetics of amikacin in critically ill neonatal foals treated for presumed or confirmed sepsis. Equine Vet J 22:18-22, 1990.
10. Zhanel GC, Pharm D, Ariano RE. Once daily aminoglycoside dosing:maintained efficacy with reduced nephrotoxicity? Renal Failure 1992; 14 (1): 1-9.
11. Brown, M.P., McCartney, J.H., Gronwall, R. and Houston, A.E.: Pharmacokinetics of trimethoprim-sulfamethoxazole in two-day-old foals after a single intravenous injection. Equine Vet J 22:51-53, 1990.
12. Golenz MR, Wilson, WD, Carlson GP, et al. Effect of route of administration and age on the pharmacokinetics of amikacin adminsitered by the intravenous and intraosseous routes to 3 and 5-day-old foals. Equine Vet J 1994; 26(5): 367-373.
13. Godber LM, Walker RD, Stein GE, et al. Pharmacokinetics, nephrotoxicosis, and in vitro antibacterial activity associated with single versus multiple (three times) daily gentamicin treatments in horses. Am J Vet Res 1995; 56 (5):613-618.
14. Magdesian KG, Hogan PM, Brumbaugh Gw, Bernard WV, Chaffin MK, Cohen ND. Pharmacokinetics of gentamicin administered once daily by the intravenous and intramuscular routes in horses. Proc. 40th AAEP convention. 1994: 115-116.
15. McFarlane D, Papich M, Brehaus B, Gaffney D, and M Wichtel. Pharmacokinetics of amikacin sulfate in sick and healthy foals. Abs in The Journal of Veterinary Emergency and Critical Care. 1996 6 (2) 120.

Antibiotic Doses Commonly Used in Neonatal Foals[1,2]

DRUG	DOSE	FREQUENCY
Penicillin G, K	20,000-40,000 iu/kg	QID
Penicillin G, Na	20,000-40,000 iu/kg	QID
Penicillin G, Procaine	22,000 iu/kg	BID
Ampicillin, Na	20 (10-50) mg/kg	TID or QID
Ampicillin trihydrate	20 mg/kg	TID
Amoxicillin trihydrate	20-30 mg/kg	TID or QID
Oxacillin	25-50 mg/kg	TID or QID
Amikacin sulfate	7 mg/kg or 10 mg/kg or 21 mg/kg	BID or TID / BID / Q24 h
Gentamicin sulfate	2.2 mg/kg or 3.3 mg/kg or 6.6 mg/kg	BID or TID / BID / Q 24 h
TMP/sulfa	5 mg/kg	BID or TID

CHAPTER 71
DRUG FORMULARY - EQUINE NEONATE

DRUG	TRADE NAME	INDICATION
Acteazolamide	Diamox	HYPP, hyperkalemia
ACTH (aqueous)	Cortrosyn	ACTH-test
ACTH (depot)	Adrenomone	Premature foals
Acyclovir	Zovirax	Herpes virus infection
Albuterol	Proventil	bronchodilator
Allopurinol	Zyloprim	prevention of free radical formation
Amikacin	Amiglyde	aminoglycoside
Aminocaproic acid	Amikar	Anti-hemorrhage, blocks plasminogen
Aminophylline	Theophylline	respiratory distress
Amiodarone	Cordarone	refractory ventricular arrhythmias

Chapter 71 Drug Formulary – Equine Neonate

DOSE	FREQ.	ROUTE	REMARKS
2-4 mg/kg	q6-12h	PO	
0.1 ug/kg	Once	IV,IM	
0.25-0.4 mg/foal	12 h	IM	See chapter on Prematurity for more options
10-20 mg/kg	q6h	PO	Poor oral bioavailability
2 puffs/foal	q4h	inhaler	Tachycardia may occur
40 mg/kg	Once	PO	Experimental. Do not use prior to 24 hr of age
20-25 mg/kg	q24h	IV	Monitor kidney parameters
10-70 mg/kg	q6-12 hr	IV slowly	
3-5 mg/kg	12 hr	IV	If assay available, maintain plasma concentrations of a 5-20µg/ml. Levels may increase when on highly protein bound drugs
4-7 mg/kg	12 hr	PO	
5-7 mg/kg	IV		Hypothyroidism reported in humans

Chapter 71 Drug Formulary – Equine Neonate

DRUG	TRADENAME	INDICATION
Amoxicillin	Amoxil	β-lactam antibiotic
Ampicillin	Amp-equine	β-lactam antibiotic
Atropine SO$_4$	Bradycardia	Bronchoconstriction
Azathioprine	Imuran	immunosuppressant
Azithromycin	Zithromax	macrolide antibiotic
Barium sulfate		x-ray contrast
Beclomethasone	Beclovent	inhalational steroid
Bethanecol	Urecholine	Bladder atony, GI prokinetic
Bismuth-subsalicylate	Peptobismol	Gastritis, diarrhea, enteritis
Bretylium	Tosylate	ventricular fibrillation
Butylscopolamine	Buscopan	spasmolytic
Butorphanol	Stadol, Torbugesic	Analgesia

Chapter 71 Drug Formulary – Equine Neonate

DOSE	FREQ.	ROUTE	REMARKS
10-30 mg/kg	8-12 h	PO	
11-22 mg/kg	8-12 h	IV	
0.01-0.04 mg/kg	Once	IM,IV	Use if bradyarrhythmia, bronchoconstriction present. Can cause ileus
1-3 mg/kg	q24h	PO	If glucocorticoids failed
10 mg/kg	q24h	PO	Can cause diarrhea, hyperthermia
3 mg/kg		PO	Do not use if leakage may occur
1-2 ug/kg, 1-4 puffs	q12-24hr	inhaler	
GI: 0.025mg/kg Bladder atony: 0.07mg/kg	q8hr q8hr	SC PO	Sweating, colic may occur with larger doses
4.5 ml/kg	q4-12hr	PO, via NGT	Causes dark feces
5-10 mg/kg	every 5-10 min	IV	Do not exceed 30-35 mg/kg
0.2-0.3 mg/kg	q8hr		May cause tachycardia Blocks neostigmine
0.01-0.1 mg/kg 0.0237mg/kg/min	q4 hr, as a CRI	IV, IM IV	Ataxia, tremor may occur. Increases feeding.

Chapter 71 Drug Formulary – Equine Neonate

DRUG	TRADENAME	INDICATION
Ca-EDTA		Lead toxicity, chelator, corneal ulcer
Caffeine	No-Doz	Respiratory stimulant
Calcium borogluconate		Hypocalcaemia
Cefazolin	Ancef	1st gen. cephalosporin
Cefepime	Axepime	4th gen. cephalosporin
Cefquinome	Cefaguard	4th gen cephalosporin
Cefotaxime	Claforan	3rd gen. cephalosporin
Ceftazidime	Fortaz	3rd gen. cephalosporin
Ceftiofur	Naxcel	3rd gen. cephalosporin
Ceftriaxone	Rocephine	3rd gen. cephalosporin
Cephalexine	Keflex	1st gen. cephalosporin
Cephalothin	Keflin	1st gen. cephalosporin
Chloramphenicol	Chloromycetin	Antibiotic
Charcoal	(activated)	Diarrhea, toxin absorbtion
Ciprofloxacin	Cipram	Flouroquinolone

DOSE	FREQ.	ROUTE	REMARKS
0.2 ml/eye	q4h	Topical	inhibits proteolytic enzyme activity
10 mg/kg initial 2.5mg/kg	q12 h	PO	for "dummy foals" with hypoventilation
150-250mg/kg (0.5-2 ml/kg 23% solution)	q12h	IV slowly	Do not mix with bicarbonate
15-20 mg/kg	q6-q8h	IV	Gram+ activity.
11 mg/kg	q8h	IV	High potency, costly
1-1.5 mg/kg	q24h	IV	Broad spectrum.
20-40 mg/kg	q6-q8h	IV	Coslty, broad spectrum.
20-50 mg/kg	q6h-q12h	IV	Broad spectrum, expensive.
4.4-10 mg/kg	q12hr	IV, SC, IM	Higher dose for young foals (<1-3 months).
25-50 mg/kg	q12h	IV	Broad spectrum antibiotic.
25mg/kg	q6h	PO	Gram+ spectrum
20 mg/kg	q6h	IV, IM	Gram+ spectrum
25 mg/kg 44-50 mg/kg	q6h q6-q8h	IV PO	Wear gloves, human aplastic anemia concern
1-2 oz/45 kg		PO	mix with warm water via NGT.
5mg/kg	q24h	IV	Maybe cause cartilage damage

DRUG	TRADENAME	INDICATION
Clarithromycin	Biaxin	Macrolide antibiotic.
Clenbuterol	Ventipulmin	Bronchodilator.
Dexamethasone	Azium - SP, Dex-A-Vet	Anti-inflammatory.
Desferrioxyamine		Iron toxicity.
Detomidine	Dormosedan	Sedation, analgesia.
Dextran	Gentran	Synthetic colloid.
Dextrose		Hypoglycaemia, hyperkalemia.
Diazepam	Valium	Seizures, sedation, appetite stimulant.
Digoxin	Lanoxin	Cardiac failure, supraventricular arrhythmias.
Di-Trioctahedral smecticide	Biosponge	GI absorbent.
Diphenylhydramine	Benadryl	Antihistamine.
Dipyrone	Dipyrone, Novin	Colic, pyrexia.
Dobutamine		Hypotension (shock).
Dopamine		Hypotension (shock). Anuric acute renal failure

Chapter 71 Drug Formulary – Equine Neonate

DOSE	FREQ.	ROUTE	REMARKS
10mg/kg	q24h	PO	may cause diarrhea, hyperthermia
0.8 µg/kg	12 hr	PO	
0.05-0.2 mg/kg	q12-24 hr	IV	SID dosing in the morning
10 mg/kg	q12hr	IV	May be useful in NI
0.005-0.04mg	as needed	IV	High doses for IM only, cause ileus.
2.5-10 ml/kg	q48hr	IV	Concern w/ Coagulopathies.
2.5-8 mg/kg/min	as CRI	IV	Monitor blood glucose
0.05-0.2 mg/kg	q4hrs	IV	Respiratory depression
0.0022-0.0077 mg/kg	q12h	IV	Can cause depression, colic, AV-block
60 ml/foal	q4-12hr	PO	
0.5-2 mg/kg	Q12-24hr	IV, IM	Hypotension.
10-20 mg	q12-q24hr	IV	May cause GI ulcers
2-10 µg/kg/min	as a CRI	IV	Use as infusion after correcting hypovolemia
1-10 µg/kg/min	as a CRI	IV	Dilute it to 400 µg/ml in saline Incompatible with alkaline solutions

Chapter 71 Drug Formulary – Equine Neonate

DRUG	TRADENAME	INDICATION
Doxapram HCl	Dopram-V	Respiratory stimulant.
Doxycycline	Vibramycin	Antibiotic.
Doxylamine	A-H solution	Antihistamine.
Enalapril	Vasotec	ACE blocker.
Enilconazole		Antifungal
Enrofloxacin	Baytril	Fluoroquinolone.
Epinephrine		Rescuscitation. Anaphylaxis
Erythromycin		Macrolide antibiotic, GI prokinetic
Famotidine	Pepcid	H_2blocker, GI ulceration
Fenbendazole	Panacur	Anthelminthic, fibrinolytic
Fentanyl patch	Duragesic	Opioid analgesic
Firocoxib	Equioxx	COX-2 blocker, NSAID
Fluconazole	Diflucan	Antifungal
Flunixin-meglumine	Banamine	Anti-inflammatory Endotoxemia, Colic
Furosemide	Lasix	Promoting diuresis
Gabapentin	Neurontin	Neuropathic pain
Gentamicin	Gentocin	Aminoglycoside

Chapter 71 Drug Formulary – Equine Neonate

DOSE	FREQ.	ROUTE	REMARKS
0.2-0.5 mg/kg 0.01-0.05 mg/kg/min		IV	If mechanical ventilation is not possible
5-10 mg/kg	q12h	PO	Can cause diarrhea!
0.5 mg/kg	q12h	IV	Hypotension risk
0.25-0.5mg/kg	12-24h	PO	
0.2% solution	q12-q24h	topical	Minimal systemic absorption
5-10 mg/kg	q24h	IV, PO	may cause cartilage damage
0.01-0.02 mg/kg		IV, SC	Supplied as 1:1:000 (0.01-0.02 ml/kg)- give 1 ml/foal
Antibiotic: 25 mg/kg Prokinetic: 1 mg/kg	q8h	PO IV in 1 hour	Diarrhea, fever may occur
2-4 mg/kg 0.2-0.5 mg/kg	q8h q8h	PO IV	
5-10 mg/kg	once or q24h for 5d	PO	High dose is larvicidal. Widespread cyathostomin resistance.
0.02-0.04mg/kg/h		dermal patch	Change every 48-72hrs!
0.1 mg/kg	q24h	PO	Less GI side effects
15 mg/kg then 5mg/kg	q24h	PO	Monitor liver enzymes
0.25-1.5 mg/kg	q6-q24h	IV	Monitor kidney function and GI side effects
0.25-2mg/kg	q4-q12h	IV	Monitor K^+ levels
13-20 mg/kg	q12-q24h	PO	May interact with opioids
6.6-10 mg/kg	q24h	IV	Monitor kidney values Can measure peak and trough levels

Chapter 71 Drug Formulary – Equine Neonate

DRUG	TRADENAME	INDICATION
Heparin		DIC, hyperlipemia, antithrombosis, adhesion prevention
Heparin Dalteparin Enoxaparin	Fragmin, Lovenox,	Anti-inflammatory anticoagulant, (low molecular weight)
Hetastrach	Hespan	Synthetic colloid, hypoproteinemia
Hydroxizine	Atarax	Antihistamine
Hyaluronate sodium	Legend	Chondroprotectant
Hydralazine	Apresoline	Vasodilator, heart failure
Hypertonic saline		Hypovolemic shock
Imipenem	Primaxin	Antibiotic
Insulin	Humulin	Hyperglycemia, hyperkalemia, hyperlipemia
Interferon alpha		Allergic airway disease
Iohexol	Omnipaque	Myelography, intraarticular and intravenous contrast
Ipratropium	Atrovent	bronchodilator
Itraconazole	Sporanox	antifungal
Ivermectin	Eqvalan	anthelminthic
Kaolin-Pectin	Kaopectate	Enteritis, diarrhea

Chapter 71 Drug Formulary – Equine Neonate

DOSE	FREQ.	ROUTE	REMARKS
20-100U/kg	q8-12h	IV, SC	monitor PCV
50-100U/kg 40-80U/kg	q24 q24	SQ SQ	Expensive
2-10 ml/kg	q24	IV	Large doses may alter coagulation
1 mg/kg	q12h	PO	counteracts with epinephrine
20 mg (1/2 vial)	q7 days	IV	Can be used with PSGAGs.
0.5-1.5 mg/kg	q12h	PO	
1-4 ml/kg	once	IV	Do not exceed sodium level 150 mEq/l
5-15 mg/kg	q6hr	IV slowly	Broad spectrum, costly
Protamine-Zn: 0.1U/kg Regular: 0.0011-0.01 U/kg/min	q12-24SC CRI		Monitor K^+ and Glucose
0.1-0.2 U/kg	q24hr	PO	
Myelograpy: 10-40 ml IV or IA: 5-20 ml			Use the same volume as volume of CSF drained
1-3 ug/kg	q8h	inhalation	Combine with a B_2-agonist
5 mg/kg	q24h	PO	Monitor liver enzymes
0.02 mg/kg		PO	can cause colic
4-8 ml/kg	q12h	PO	

DRUG	TRADENAME	INDICATION
Kefoprofen	Ketofen	Anti-inflammatory, NSAID
Ketamine	Vetalar	Short-acting anesthesia
Ketoconazole	Nizoral	Antifungal
Lactase		Lactose digestion
Lactulose		Liver failure, hyperammonemia
Lidocaine	Xylocaine-- Without epinephrine	Antiarrhythmic, anti-inflammatory, GI-prokinetic
Loperamide	Immodium	Diarrhea
Magnesium sulfate 50%		Ventricular tachyarrhythmia, Hypomagnesemia, Reperfusion injury, Neonatal maladjustment
Mannan-oligosaccharides	Bio-Mos	Prebiotic, energy source for microbial flora
Mannitol		CNS trauma/edema

Chapter 71 Drug Formulary – Equine Neonate

DOSE	FREQ	ROUTE	REMARKS
2 mg/kg	q12-24h	IV	Use with caution. Avoid using >5 days! Can induce GI ulcers and renal papillary necrosis!
Anesthesia 1.5-2.0 mg/kg	Once	IV	Pre-dose with xylazine or diazepam
Analgesia: 0.01-0.04 mg/kg/min	CRI	IV	Analgesia,
5-10 mg/kg	q12	PO	Monitor liver enzymes!
1500-3000U/kg	q6h	PO	
0.2-0.4ml/kg	q8hr	rectum	
3 mg/kg/h	as a CRI	IV	Individual sensitivity! Seizures may occur! Adjust dose in hypoalbuminemia!
VTach: 0.,25 mg/kg IV bolus slowly, then 0.5 mg/kg/min CRI		IV	
5-15 ml/foal	q6hr	PO	Can enhance toxin absorption!
Maladjustment 20 mg/kg then 25 mg/kg/hr	Slow CRI	IV	Monitor serum levels! Both ionized and total!
		IV	
Vtach: 2—4 mg/kg/min CRI		IV	
100-200 mg/kg	q6-8h	PO	
0.2-0.8 g/kg q4h	q2-4h	IV bolus over 20 minutes	Measure osmolality: (Max 330 mOsm/l). Warm up

DRUG	TRADENAME	INDICATION
Methocarbamol	Robaxin	Muscle relaxant
Metoclopramide	Reglan	Ileus. Gastric emptying disorders
Methyl-prednisolone	Solu-Medrol	Anti-inflammatory
Metronidazole	Flagyl	Antibiotic, Anti-protozoal
Midazolam	Versed	Anxiolytic, anti-convulsant
Mineral Oil		Colic, Meconium impaction
Misoprostol	Cytotec	GI ulceration
Morphine		Analgesic
Naloxone		Opioid antagonist, Shock, Mal-adjustment, hemorrhage
Neostigmine	Prostigmine	Ileus
Neupogen		Persistent leukopenia

Chapter 71 Drug Formulary – Equine Neonate

DOSE	FREQ.	ROUTE	REMARKS
40-60 mg/kg	q12h	PO	For post-anesthetic myositis
0.1-0.3 mg/kg	q8-12 hr	IV	Administer slowly or diluted as an infusion. Excitement and other side effects possible.
0.02-0.04 mg/kg/h	CRI	IV	
1-3 mg/kg	q12-q24hr	IV	Low doses for sepsis and cortisol replacement, high doses for immunemediated disorders
10-15 mg/kg	q6-q12hr	IV, PO Per rectum	Anorexia, depression, ataxia possible!
0.1 mg/kg	IV		respiratory depression
2-6 mg/kg/h	CRI		
4-12 oz/45 kg		via NGT	
2.5-5µg/kg	q12-q24	PO	Do not allow pregnant women to handle!
0.3-0.6 mg/kg	q4-q6h	IV, IM	Use with α$_2$-agonists to avoid excitement
0.01-0.03 mg/kg	Once	IV	Useful for maladjusted foals
0.005-0.01mg/kg	q1-q6h	SC	May cause colic
300µg/foal	q24-q48hrs	SC	Adequate response should be seen in 24hrs

Chapter 71 Drug Formulary – Equine Neonate

DRUG	TRADENAME	INDICATION
Nitazoxanide		Antiprotozoal
Norepinephrine		Vasopressor, refractory hypotension
Omeprazole	Gastrogard, Losec	Gastric ulceration
Oxyglobin		Anemia treatment
Oxytetracycline	Oxytet	Tetracycline antibiotic Contracted tendons
Oxytocin		Esophageal obstruction
Paramomycin	Humantin	Antiprotozoal
Penicillin-procaine G		β-lactam antibiotic
Pentastarch	Pentaspan	Synthetic colloid
Pentazocine	Talwin	Analgesia
Pentoxyfilline	Trental	Anti-inflammatory rheologic, anti-TNF
Pethidine	Demerol	Analgesic
Pentobarbital	Nembutal	Seizure control
Phenazopyridne	Pyridium	Urinary disinfectant
Phenylbutazone		NSAID, anti-inflammatory

Chapter 71 Drug Formulary – Equine Neonate

DOSE	FREQ	ROUTE	REMARKS
25-50 mg/kg		PO	May be effective in Rotavirus infection.
0.1-1.5 ug/kg /min	CRI	IV	Use in refractory hypotension in combination with an inotrope after iv fluids
1-4 mg/kg	q24	PO	May predispose to Salmonellosis
0.5 mg/kg	q24hr	IV	
1-10 ml/kg		IV	Can cause discoloration of urine and blood
6.6 mg/kg	q12h	IV	nephrotoxic, relaxes contracted tendons in larger doses!
3g per foal	q24h	IV	
0.1-0.2U/kg		IV	To resolve choke!
100 mg/kg	q24h	PO	Efficacy unproven for Cryptosporidium
22,000-44,000 U/kg	q12h	IM	IV administration causes seizure!
1-10 ml/kg	q48h	IV	Costly!
1-5 mg/kg	q6-q12	IV, IM	
7.5-10mg/kg	q8-q12h	IV, PO	Can cause sweating, tachycardia
0.3-0.6 mg/kg	q6-q12	IV, IM	Can cause apnea, ileus
2-10 mg/kg	q6h	IV	Apnea. Do not use with other barbiturate
4 mg/kg	q12h	IV	Urine discoloration, stains everything
2.2-4.4 mg/kg	q12-q48hr	IV, PO	GI ulceration! Kidney function

Chapter 71 Drug Formulary – Equine Neonate

DRUG	TRADE NAME	INDICATION
Phenobarbital		Anti-convulsant
Phenylephrine	Neo-Synephrine	Vasopressor
Phenytoin	Dilantin	Anti-convulsant
Polymyxin-B		Anti-endotoxic
Praziquantel		Tapeworm infection
Prednisolone-sodium succinate	Solu-delta cortef	Anti-inflammatory, shock.
Procainamide	Pronestyl	Supraventricular tachyarrhythmia
Propofol	Diprivan	IV anesthetic
Propranolol	Inderal	β-antagonist, ventricular arrhythmias
Psyllium		Bulk laxative
Quinidine		Atrial fibrillation
Ranitidine	Zantac	Anti-ulcer
Rifampin		Antibiotic
Romifidine	Sedivet	Analgesic, sedative
S-adenosyl-methionine		hepatic disease, cholestasis
Sodium bicarbonate		Anorganic acidosis, hyperkalemia
Sodium iodide		Actinobacillosis

Chapter 71 Drug Formulary – Equine Neonate

DOSE	FREQ.	ROUTE	REMARKS
2.5-10 mg/kg	q12h	IV	Respiratory depression
0.2-1 µg/kg/min	CRI	IV	
5-10mg/kg first 12h 20mg/kg		IV	Drowsiness, sedation
1000-6000 U/kg	q8-12h	IV	Nephro and neurotoxic
1.5 mg/kg		PO	
1-2.5 mg/kg	q6-q24hr	IV	Immunosuppression, adrenal suppression.
1 mg/kg/min	CRI	IV	May induce hypotension.
2-4 mg/kg		IV	after premedication, may cause apnea
0.03-0.05 mg/kg		IV	Hypotension
0.5-1g/100kg	q8hr	PO	For sand impaction or diarrhea
22 mg/kg	q2h	Via NGT	Neurologic, GI side effects, urticaria
6.6 mg/kg 1.5 mg/kg	q8h q8h	PO IV	
5 mg/kg	q12h	PO	May cause urine and feces discoloration.
0.04-0.12 mg/kg	as needed	IV, IM	
20 mg/kg	q24h	PO	Antioxidant
0.5-2 mEq/kg		IV, PO	Monitor K^+ levels! Do not give in respiratory acidosis!
100 mg/kg	q24h	IV	May have antifungal properties

Chapter 71 Drug Formulary – Equine Neonate

DRUG	TRADENAME	INDICATIONS
Selenium		Se deficiency
Sucralfate	Carafate	Gastric ulcers
Sulfadiazine-trimethoprim		Antibiotic
Sulfamethoxazole-trimethoprim	Cotrim	Antibiotic
Terbutaline	Brethine	Bronchdilator
Thiamine		Thiamine deficiency
Ticarcillin	Ticar	β-lactam antibiotic
Ticarcillin + clavulanic acid	Timentin	β-lactam antibiotic
Tramadol		Analgesic
Triple drip (guaifenesin-xylazine-ketamine)		Anesthetic
Vancomycin	Vancocin	Antibiotic
Vasopressin		Refractory hypotension
Vitamin C		Antioxidant
Vitamin E (natural form)		Antioxidant
Voriconazole	Vfend	Antifungal
Xylazine	Rompun	Sedation, Pre-anesthetic
Yohimbine		Prokinetic, antidote

Chapter 71 Drug Formulary – Equine Neonate

DOSE	FREQ.	ROUTE	REMARKS
2.5 mg/50kg	once	IM only	Can be overdosed!
20-40 mg/kg	q6h	PO	Do not give within 1-2 hours of other medications
30 mg/kg	q8-q12h	PO	
30 mg/kg	q12h	PO	
0.04-0.12 mg/kg	q8	PO	
1-10 mg/kg	q24h	PO, IV	
50-100 mg/kg	q6h	IV	
50-200 mg/kg	q6h	IV	
1 mg/kg	q6	IV, IM, Epidural	
2-6 ml/kg/h	CRI		1L 5% GGE 500 mg Xylazine, 1g Ketamine
6 mg/kg	q8	IV	for resistant Staph. aureus, C. diff. infection
0.2-0.6 U/kg 0.5-1.5 mU/kg/min	once CRI	IV IV	for CPR Hypotensive shock
100 mg/kg	q24h	IV	
20-50U/kg	q24h	PO	
3 mg/kg	q24h	PO	Costly
0.25-1.1 mg/kg	as needed	IV, IM	May cause collapse in unstable neonatal foals
0.1 mg/kg	q8-12h	IV	

DRUGS WITH NEUROLOGICAL EFFECT

DRUG	DOSE	ROUTE, FREQ	REMARKS
Diazepam	0.05-0.4 mg/kg	IV, Every 30 minutes	Not recommended for prolonged periods of time at higher doses
Midazolam	2-8 mg /hour/ 50kg foal	IV as a CRI after 5 mg bolus	Short half life
Phenobarbital	20 mg/kg initially 2-9 mg/kg	IV IV, IM q8-12h	Administer slowly (over 20 minutes) to effect! Monitor serum levels
Pentobarbital	2-10 mg/kg	IV, Q4-6h	Maybe repeated in 4-6 hours!
Phenytoin	5-10 mg/kg loading then 1-5 mg/kg	IV, PO q4-6h	May cause marked depression
Primidone	20-30 mg/kg	PO q12-24h	
Mannitol	0.25-1.0 g/kg	IV, q2-4h	For cerebral edema. Over 20-30 minutes
Hypertonic saline (3-7 %)	1-2 mL/kg	IV	For cerebral edema. Over 15-30 minutes! Monitor serum sodium levels (<150 mEq/l)
Magnesium-sulfate	50 mg/kg then 25 mg/kg/hour	IV	Monitor serum Mg levels

Chapter 71 Drug Formulary – Equine Neonate

DRUGS FOR USE IN CPCR

DRUG	DOSAGE	ROUTE	REMARKS
Epinephrine (Adrenaline)	0.01-0.02 mg/kg **0.5-1 ml/foal**	IV Intratracheal	**Can be repeated every 2 minutes**
Vasopressin	0.2-0.6 U/kg	IV	After 2-3 failed attempts with epinephrine
Sodium bicarbonate	1-2 mEq/kg	IV, PO	Give it after 5-10 min. of CPR
Atropine	0.01-0.04 mg/kg	IV, IM, SQ	Maybe used if no response to O_2 and epinephrine and vasopressin
Norepinephrine	0.1-1.5 µg/kg/min IV		After volume corrected and inotrope was given!
Dobutamine	2-10 µg/kg/min	IV	Infusion after correcting hypovolemia
Vasopressin	0.25-1.5 mUI/kg/min CRI	IV	Refractory hypotension
Doxapram	0.01-0.05 mg/kg/min	IV	Infusion, when mechanical ventilation is not feasible.
Dopamine	5-10 µg/kg/min	IV	Use only if other vasopressors are not available

CHAPTER 72
HEMATOLOGY AND CLINICAL CHEMISTRY normal values
United States (Mass Units)

	Premature Foals - Gestational Age		
Parameter	300-309 days Mean ± SE**	310-319 days Mean ± SE**	320-334 days Mean ± SE**
RBC (x10^6 /µl)	9.6 ± 0.5	10.1 ± 0.3	11.3 ± 0.2
Hb (g/dl)	13.1 ± 1.1	14.1 ± 0.5	13.2 ± 0.3
PCV (%)	41.0 ± 2.0	42.0 ± 1.0	43.0 ± 1.0
MCV (fl)	42.7 ± 1.4	42.2 ± 0.6	38.6 ± 0.7
MCH (pg)	14.0 ± 1.0	14.4 ± 0.4	11.8 ± 0.3
MCHC (%)	32.4 ± 1.7	33.8 ± 0.8	30.5 ± 0.7
Icterus Index (units)			
Tot. Plasma Pr. (g/dl)			
Fibrinogen (mg/dl)			
Tot. WBC (/µl)	5,000 ± 800	6,800 ± 1,800	4,900 ± 300
Neutrophils (/µl)	1,230 ± 260	1,540 ± 500	1,940 ± 460
Bands (/µl)			
Lymphocytes (/µl)	3,720 ± 650	5,090 ± 1,420	2,960 ± 270
Monocytes (/µl)			
Eosinophils (/µl)			
Basophils (/µl)			
Neut:Lymph ratio	0.33	0.30	0.66

Chapter 72 Hematology and Clinical Chemistry normal values U.S.

Term Foals - Postnatal Age	
1 day Mean ± SD	2-7 days Mean ± SD
10.5 ± 1.0	9.26 ± 0.8
14.4 ± 1.1	13.2 ± 1.2
40.0 ± 3.3	36.5 ± 3.1
40.2 ± 3.6	39.4 ± 2.3
13.6 ± 1.1	14.5 ± 1.1
36.0 ± 2.0	37.0 ± 1.1
40.0 ± 15	30.0 ± 15
6.1 ± 0.8 ***	6.4 ± 0.6
243 ± 74	310 ± 90
8,632 ± 2,570	9,075 ± 2,200
6,381 ± 2,225	6,528 ± 2,000
< 50	< 50
2,021 ± 660	2,203 ± 575
222 ± 160	305 ± 135
0	22
8	17
3.16	2.96

Chapter 72 Hematology and Clinical Chemistry normal values U.S.

Normal range = Mean ± 2 SE

* These values were compiled from available published and unpublished data.

** Values for 1st day of life.

*** Post nursing.

References:
1. Harvey JW, Asquith RL, McNulty PK, et al: Haematology of foals up to one year old. Equine Vet J 16(4):347-353, 1984.
2. Jeffcott LB, Rossdale PD, Leadon DP: Haematological changes in the neonatal period of normal and induced premature foals. J Reprod Fertil (Suppl) 32:537-544, 1982.
3. Medeiros LO, Ferri S, Barcelos SR, Miguel O: Haematologic standards for healthy newborn foals. Biol Neonate 17:351-360, 1971.
4. Sato T, Oda K, Kubo M: Hematological and biochemical values of Thoroughbred foals in the first 6 months of life. Cornell Vet 69:3-19, 1979.
5. Schalm OW, Carlson GP: The blood and blood-forming Organs. In Mansmann RA and McAllister ES (eds), Equine Medicine and Surgery, ed 3, Santa Barbara, CA, American Veterinary Publications, 1982, pp 377-414.
6. Rossdale and Partners: Normal values for Equine Neonates- http://www.rossdales.com/laboratories/reference-ranges.htm
Serum Biochemical Reference Values For
Normal Term Foals* (Postnursing)

Chapter 72 Hematology and Clinical Chemistry normal values U.S.

Parameter	Age 1 Day Mean ± SD	3-7 Days Mean SD
Sodium (mEq/L)	139.7 ± 6.0	39.5 ± 4.2
Potassium (mEq/L)	4.4 ± 0.9	4.5 ± 0.4
Chloride (mEq/L)	102.5 ± 3.0	101.3 ± 4.0
Bicarbonate (mEq/L)	22.9 ± 3.4	24.3 ± 2.1
Calcium (mg/dl)	11.7 ± 1.1	11.4 ± 0.8
Inorg. Phosphorus (mg/dl)	5.0 ± 0.85	6.4 ± 0.8
Magnesium (mg/dl)	2.2 ± 0.35	2.7 ± 0.15
Glucose (mg/dl)	136.0 ± 40	150.0 ± 30
BUN (mg/dl)	18.9 ± 4.3	13.6 ± 5.6
Creatinine (mg/dl)	2.3 ± 0.6	1.3 ± 0.3
Total Bilirubin (mg/dl)	2.9 ± 1.3	2.0 ± 0.5
Direct Bilirubin (mg/dl)	0.5 ± 0.2	0.5 ± 0.1
Indirect Bilirubin (mg/dl)	2.4 ± 1.1	1.6 ± 0.5
Alk. Phosphatase (iu/L)	1487 ± 452	871 ± 313
GGT (iu/L)	24 ± 7	42 ± 31
SDH (iu/L)	2.0 ± 0.9	2.0 ± 0.9
AST (SGOT) (iu/L)	154 ± 55	225 ± 60
LDH (iu/L)	487 ± 100	490 ± 100
Albumin (g/dl)	3.2 ± 0.4	3.1 ± 0.5
Globulin (g/dl)	3.3 ± 0.7	3.2 ± 0.5
A:G Ratio	1.0 ± 0.3	1.1 ± 0.4
Triglyceride (mg/dl)	82 ± 42	157 ± 74
Cholesterol (mg/dl)	246 ± 116	225 ± 60

* These values were compiled from available published and unpublished data.

Chapter 72 Hematology and Clinical Chemistry normal values U.S.

References:
1. Bauer JE, Harvey JW, Asquith RL et al: Clinical chemistry reference values for foals during the first year of life. Equine Vet J 16(4):361-363, 1984.
2. Gossett KA, French DD: Effect of age on liver enzyme activities in serum of healthy Quarter Horses. Am J Vet Res 45:354-356, 1984.
3. Rumbaugh GE, Adamson PJW: Automated serum chemical analysis in the foal. JAVMA 183:769-772, 1983.
4. Sato T, Oda K, Kubo M: Hematological and biochemical values of Thoroughbred foals in the first 6 months of life. Cornell Vet 69:3-19, 1979.
5. Schmitz DG, Joyce JR, Reagor JC: Serum biochemical values in Quarter Horse foals in the first 6 months of life. Equine Pract 4:24-30, 1982.
6. Varner DD, Vaala WE: Equine Perinatal Care. Part II. Routine management of the neonatal foal. Compend Cont Educ Pract Vet 8(2):581-594, 1986.
7. Bauer JE, Asquith RL, Kivipelto J: Serum biochemical indicators of liver function in neonatal foals. Am J Vet Res 50:2037-2041, 1989.
8. Rossdale and Partners- Neonatal Foals Normal Values. http://www.rossdales.com/laboratories/reference-ranges.htm

CHAPTER 73
HEMATOLOGY AND CLINICAL CHEMISTRY normal values
*European (Molar Units)

Neonatal Thoroughbred Foals (<36 hours old) (Rossdales)

**Clinical Pathology reference ranges – Means & ranges

Test	abbreviation	units	Mean	range
Total erythrocytes	RBC	$\times 10^{12}/l$	9.4	6.9-11.8
Packed cell volume	PCV	l/l	0.36	0.30-0.44
Haemoglobin	Hb	g/dl	13.2	10.2-15.4
Mean cell volume	MCV	fl	38.8	31.7-44.9
Mean cell haemoglobin concentration	McHc	g/dl	36.1	31.7-39.4
Mean cell haemoglobin	McH	pg	14.0	11.2-16.4
Total leucocytes	WBC	$\times 10^9/l$	8.8	6.2-12.4
Segmented neutrophils	Segs	$\times 10^9/l$	6.7	4.1-9.5
	Segs	%	75	58-85
Lymphocytes	Lymphs	$\times 10^9/l$	1.8	1.0-3.1
	Lymphs	%	21	14-37
Monocytes	Monos	$\times 10^9/l$	0.19	0.1-0.5
	Monos	%	2	0.5-5
Eosinophils	Eos	$\times 10^9/l$	0.1	0.1-0.2
	Eos	%	1	1-2
Platelets	Plts	$\times 10^9/l$	220	140-315
Plasma viscosity	PV	mPa	1.44	1.34-1.59
Total Protein	TSP	g/l	54	41-66
Albumin	Alb	g/l	31	25-35
Globulin	Glob	g/l	24	15-36
Alpha 1 globulin	x1 glob	g/l	0.9	0.5-1.5
Alpha 2 globulin	x2 glob	g/l	5.0	4.0-5.6
Beta 1 globulin	x1 glob	g/l	5.1	3.1-7.2
Beta 2 globulin	x2 glob	g/l	3.3	1.3-6.0
Gamma globulin	x glob	g/l	6.5	4.8-10.1

Chapter 73 Hematology and Clinical Chemistry normal values Europe

Test	abbreviation	units	Mean	range
Immunoglobulin G	IgG	g/l	11.7	6.9-18.6
Plasma fibrinogen	Fib	g/l	1.9	0.5-3.9
Serum amyloid A	SAA	mg/l	2.2	0-26
Aspartate amino transferase	AST	iu/l	157	111-206
Creatinine kinase	CK	iu/l	414	165-761
Lactate dehydrogenase	LD	iu/l	860	615-1110
LD isoenzyme 1	LD1	% total LD	5	2-7
LD isoenzyme 2	LD2	% total LD	20	17-24
LD isoenzyme 3	LD3	% total LD	42	36-46
LD isoenzyme 4	LD4	% total LD	28	21-34
LD isoenzyme 5	LD5	% total LD	5	2-10
Gamma glutamyl transferase	GGT	iu/l	21	10-32
Glutamate dehydrogenase	GLDH	iu/l	25	8-43
Serum alkaline phosphatase	SAP	iu/l	3341	2424-4544
Intestinal alkaline phosphatase	IAP	iu/l	824	528-1200
	IAP	% total SAP	23.7	<26
Urea	Urea	mmol/l	5.7	2.9-8.4
Creatinine	Creat	µmol/l	133	97-188
Bromsulphalein half time clearance	BSP	Seconds		
Glucose	Glu	mmol/l	3.1	2.1-4.1
Total bilirubin	TBili	µmol/l	55	16-94
Direct bilirubin	DBili	µmol/l	20	6-34
Bile acids	BAcids	µmol/l		0-8.0
Cholesterol	Chol	mmol/l		
Triglycerides	Trigs	mmol/l		
Lipase	Lip	mmol/l		
Amylase	Amyl	iu/l		
Calcium	Ca	mmol/l	2.9	2.7-3.2
Fractional urinary clearance	Ca	%		
Phosphate	PO4	mmol/l	2.0	1.6-2.5

Chapter 73 Hematology and Clinical Chemistry normal values Europe

Test	abbreviation	units	Mean	range
Fractional urinary clearance	PO4	%	0.3	0.02-0.53
Magnesium	Mg	mmol/l	0.8	0.6-1.1
Fractional urinary clearance	Mg	%		
Copper (serum)	Cu	µmol/l		
Copper (plasma)	Cu	µmol/l		
Zinc	Zn	µmol/l		
Sodium	Na	mmol/l	135	129-140
Fractional urinary clearance	Na	%		
Potassium	K	mmol/l	4.3	3.8-5.0
Fractional urinary clearance	K	%		
Chloride	Cl	mmol/l	97	90-103
Fractional urinary clearance	Cl	%		
Cortisol	Cort	nmol/l		
Fasting Insulin	Ins	µiu/ml		
Tri-iodothyronine	T3	nmol/l	8.4	<14
Thyroxine	T4	nmol/l	400	<800
Troponin	cTnI	ng/ml	0.46	0.18-0.79
Selenium	Se	µmol/l		

*Beaufort Cottage Laboraties
**Permission to reproduce courtesy of Beaufort Cottage Laboratories.

© Copyright 2011 Rossdales. All rights reserved.

All information is copyright of Rossdales and may be amended/updated at any time.

Please refer to our website for the latest information.
www.rossdales.com
www.rossdales.com/laboratories
www.rossdales.com/laboratories/reference-ranges.htm

Reference ranges on our iPhone/iPad app Rossdales Lab Guide, which is available (free) through the Apple AppStore:
www.rossdales.com/news/rossdales-laboratory-app-for-iphone-and-ipad-now-available.htm

CHAPTER 74
BLOOD GASES

Blood Gas Normals - Equine Neonates
(Lateral Recumbency)

	Arterial				
Age	O_2 mmHg (mEq/L)	CO_2 mmHg	pH	Base excess	HCO_3 (mEq/L)
Immediate post-foaling [2]	40-50	52-60	7.20-7.3	+2	24-26
2 hours [1]	68 ±10	49 ± 2	7.37 ± 01	+4	26 ± 2
4-12 hours [1]	75 ± 5	47 ± 2	7.39 ±.01	+6	28 ± 2
24 hours [1]	81 ± 6	48 ± 2	7.40 ±.01	+6	28 ± 2
1-3 days [1]	90 ± 6	48 ± 2	7.40 ±.01	+6	28 ± 2
4-14 days [1]	86 ± 5	45 ± 2	7.41 ±.01	+6	28 ± 1
Premature [2] - birth	39 ± 5	55 ± 4	7.27	-3	24 ± 1
(320-330 days gestation) - 1 hour	52± 4	48± 3	7.33	-1.3	25± 1

Values are expressed as mean ± SD

References:
1. Madigan, J.E.: Blood gas analysis in the equine neonate. Proceed Amer Assoc Eq Pract. 33rd Convention, pp 777-786, 1987.
2. Rose, R.J., Rossdale, P.D., Leadon, D.P.: Blood gas and acid-base status of spontaneously delivered, term induced and induced premature foals. J Reprod Fertil Suppl 521-528, 1982.

Chapter 74 Blood Gases

		Venous	
O_2 (mmHg)	CO_2 (mmHg)	pH (mEq/L)	HCO_3 (mEq/L)
---	---	---	---
42± 2	56± 2	7.33±.01	28± 2
42± 2	52± 2	7.38±.01	30± 2
42± 2	52± 2	7.38±.01	30± 3
43± 2	52± 2	7.38±.01	29± 2
38± 2	53± 2	7.38±.01	31± 2
---	---	---	---
---	---	---	---

CHAPTER 75
SERUM IMMUNOGLOBULINS VS AGE
IMMUNOGLOBULIN CONCENTRATIONS IN NORMAL THOROUGHBRED FOALS *

Serum IgG Concentration
(mg/100 ml)

Age	Mean	Range
Presuckle	15	0 - 38.5
24 hr postsuckle	1645	118 - 3180
2 week	974	213 - 1920
4 week	774	154 - 1680
6 week	817	270 - 1530
8 week	952	474 - 1530
10 week	1004	340 - 1480
12 week	1052	430 - 1630
Mare's Serum	2251	1544 - 2960
Mare's Colostrum	6408	162 - 13800

* Modified from Dr. Alex Ardans, Immunology Diagnostic Laboratory, VMTH, UC Davis. Ig concentrations measured by radial immunodiffusion (RID).

Chapter 75 Serum Immunoglobulins vs Age

	Serum IgG Concentration (mg/100 ml)	
Age	Mean	Range
Presuckle	18.8	10 - 48
24 hr postsuckle	52.1	14.5 - 115
2 week	41.4	14.5 - 96
4 week	40.7	21 - 65
6 week	58.1	27 - 124
8 week	79.8	38 - 144
10 week	93.9	30 - 155
12 week	105	52 - 215
Mare's Serum	222	89 - 290
Mare's Colostrum	221	27.6 – 454

CHAPTER 76
CARDIAC CATHETERIZATION PRESSURE MEASUREMENTS

TABLE 1a: Hemodynamics of normal foals

AGE h=hours d=days (n)	BODY WEIGHT (kg)	HEART RATE (bpm)	AORTIC PRESSURE (mmHg)	PULMONARY ARTERY PRESSURE (mmHg)	RIGHT ATRIAL PRESSURE (mmHg)	PULM ART WEDGE PRESSURE (mmHg)
2h(2)	45.4±2.4	83±10	95.7±11.9	40.3±4.7	3.1±0.6	7.5±2.5
4h(4)	45.4±2.4	84±2	85.0±2.9	41.0±2.8	4.4±1.2	9.0±1.9
6h(4)	45.4±2.4	84±2	91.3±2.4	36.3±2.7	5.5±1.2	9.0±1.8
8h(4)	45.4±2.4	81±3	90.6±1.6	32.4±2.4	5.5±1.6	7.7±1.2
10h(4)	45.4±2.4	80±1	87.5±1.4	30.3±2.6	4.1±1.1	7.2±1.4
12(7)	44.4±1.4	89±4	87.7±1.9	38.6±4.6	4.5±0.5	7.6±0.9
16h(4)	45.4±2.4	86±4	86.9±2.5	31.4±0.8	3.4±0.5	7.5±1.0
20h(4)	45.4±2.4	84±4	84.1±4.4	26.0±2.5	4.5±0.5	7.5±1.0
1d(4)	45.4±2.4	84±3	84.4±3.7	30.5±2.3	7.1±0.9	9.9±1.0
2d(9)	48.3±2.4	95±6	91.4±4.5	27.8±2.3	4.1±1.1	8.7±0.8
3d(9)	49.1±2.5	94±7	92.2±3.6	28.1±1.3	4.2±0.6	8.2±1.0
4d(9)	50.9±2.4	96±5	90.7±3.6	30.0±1.8	6.1±1.0	9.8±1.5
5d(7)	57.1±2.9	102±9	95.8±3.4	29.9±2.6	3.3±0.6	7.3±1.2
6d(7)	60.2±3.6	104±8	96.7±5.1	28.7±2.3	4.7±0.8	10.0±2.0
8d(7)	63.2±3.8	114±9	100.0±5.9	27.3±2.3	2.7±0.3	8.0±1.1
10d(5)	63.2±3.8	108±10	101.3±4.4	27.3±2.3	3.5±1.5	9.1±1.3
12d(4)	65.8±3.9	111±10	100.3±4.9	30.7±2.3	5.0±1.3	11.6±2.0
14d(4)	70.6±6.1	95±5	100.3±3.2	27.4±3.0	4.6±0.9	8.1±0.7

CHAPTER 77
CARDIOPULMONARY-CEREBRAL RESUSCITATION (CPCR) & Kit Suggestions

SEE INSIDE COVER FOR QUICK SUMMARY AND REVIEW

I. **FOALS AT RISK FOR ARREST**

   A. **SIGNIFICANT HYPOXEMIA**
      Dystocia
      C-Section
      Umbilical cord torsion

   B. **SHOCK**
      Septic
      Hypovolemic
      Obstructive
      Cardiogenic

   C. **Severe Metabolic Disorders**
      Marked acidosis
      Hyperkalemia > 6 mEq/L

TWO MAIN CAUSES OF ARREST IN FOALS
   1. Peripartum asphyxia - HYPOXEMIA
      Focus: oxygenate and ventilate
      Prognosis good if intervention is early
   2. Secondary to metabolic derangements /septic causes
      Focus: traditional ABC approach
      Prognosis poor (severely ill foal)

These are managed slightly differently, and carry different prognoses

SIGNS OF IMPRENDING ARREST
Bradycardia or asystole
   <40-60 bpm or irregular

Irregular to absent RR
   < 10 bpm, gasping

Mydriasis
   Sluggish or nonresponsive

Marked hypotension
> No pulse pressure
> Mean ≤ 40 mmHg

FORMS OF CARDIOVASCULAR ARREST
1. Asystole
2. Ventricullar fibrillation or pulseless ventricular tachycardia
3. Pulseless electrical activity (electromechanical dissociation)
4. Cardiovascular collapse (excessive vasodilation)

DURATION of resuscitation attempts
1. No survival reported in human patients after 30 minutes
2. **10 minutes is appropriate**

II. **HOW TO DO IT: 40-50 Kg foal example**
Step one: Preparation for (ideal is 3-5 people for the procedure)
#1 intubate and ventilate
#2 external chest compressions
#3 introduce iv catheter and start fluids
#4 attach ECG and prepare medications
#5 record

III. **CPR Steps**
A=Airway
B=Breathing
C=Circulation
D=Drugs and Fluids

A. ESTABLISH AIRWAY
1. Clean nasal and oral cavities, remove foreign objects (mucus, straw, blood, meconium)
2. Place 8-9 mm endotracheal tube
   a. Nasotracheal
   b. Orotracheal

B. BREATHING
1. Attach self-inflating AMBU bag with oxygen attached
2. Start with 20 breaths per minutes with oxygen

a. Vary 10-40 depending response or end tidal CO_2
   b. 2 breaths/ 10 chest compressions if using compression
   c. DO NOT USE: demand valve (barotrauma)
   d. DO NOT ELEVATE HEAD (decreased cerebral perfusion)

C. **CIRCULATION**
   1. **Fluids: 20 ml/kg boluses (less in immediate newborn)** (Plamalyte 148, Normosol R, Lactated Ringers, Colloids; see Chapter 22)
   2. **Begin chest compressions if** asystole or if the heart rate is less than 60 bpm within 30s of ventilation
      a. Lateral recumbency with back toward you
      b. Check for rib fractues first (fractured ribs to be on down side if present)
      c. 80 compressions per minute
      d. Allow time for diastole between compressions. EC: good luck
      e. Effectiveness should be evaluated (peripheral pulse, mucous membrane color, pupil size, End-tidal CO_2 (goal >15 mmHg,)
      f. If no evidence of blood flow, then change the compression technique (hand position, force, longer intervals between compressions
      g. Rotate people every 2 minutes

D. **DRUGS**
   Pharmaceuticals (consider if asystole or heart rate <60 BPM afer 30 seconds of ventilation and chest compressions).

   EPINEPHRINE
   1. First line of drug for CPR
   2. Potent alpha and beta adrenoreceptor agonist
   3. Generates the greatest coronary and cerebral blood flow
   4. Associated with the best resuscitation rates

5. **Traditional low dose is 0.01 mg/kg (1:1000; 0.5-1 ml/50 kg)**
6. **Intravenous, intraosseal, intratracheal**
7. Intracardiac is **not** recommended (myocardial laceration, ventricular tachycardia, coronary vessel thrombosis)
8. **Dose can be repeated every 3-5 minutes**

VASOPRESSIN (ADH)
1. Synthetic arginine vasopressin indicated after 2-3 - attempts of failed epinephrine
2. Long half life, use only once
3. **Dose: 0.2-0.6 U/kg (10-30 U/foal; 0.5-1.5 ml IV)**

OTHER DRUGS - LIMITED INDICATIONS
1. Bradyarrhythmias, bronchoconstriction
   a. Atropine (0.01-0.02 mg/kg)
   b. Glycopyrrolate (0.001-0.002 mg/kg)
2. **Electrolytes – EC: controversial**
   a. Calcium (1-10 mg/kg) may improve cardiac contractility
   b. Sodium bicarbonate (1-2 mEq/kg) if severe acidosis present
   c. Magnesium sulfate (14-28 mg/kg) may be useful in cases of ventricular or junctional tachyarrhythmias
3. **Glucose** (3-5mg/kg/min) if severe hypoglycemia (<50mg/dl; 2.8 mmol/l) present - avoid hyperglycemia
4. **Corticosteroids** in septic, anaphylactic shock or in suspected adrenal insufficiency
   a. prednisolone Na-succinate 1-2.5 mg/kg,
   b. dexamethasone Na-phosphate 0.05-0.2 mg/kg) **EC:** controversial
5. **Class III antiarrhythmic drugs** severe ventricular tachyarrhythmias unresponsive to Lidocaine and Magnesium sulfate
   a. Amiodarone 5mg/kg
   b. Bretylium 5 mg/kg,

IF CPCR fails thus far:

Epinephrine: 1 mg (1 cc of 1:1000) doses, 0.01-0.02 mg/kg

Vasopressin if epinephrine fails after 2-3 doses: 1 cc (20 units)

If not due to dystocia/c–section/ prolonged delivery
Can try atropine 0.02 mg/kg
Stagger with epi

If prolonged (> 5 min) use sodium bicarbonate (0.5 mEq/kg, slow)

E. INSTRUMENTS
1. ENDOTRACHEAL TUBE
   a. 7 -12 mm (internal diameter) Bivona®, 45-50 cm length.
      For naso-tracheal intubation
   b. variable for minis (3-5 mm)
2. AMBU BAG
3. 1 LITER RESERVOIR BAG
4. FACE MASK
5. BAIN CIRCUIT
6. IV SETS (infusion)
7. BLOOD GLUCOSE CHEMISTRY STICKS
8. IV CATHETERS
9. O_2 REGULATOR - Pressure gauge and flow rate gauge on O_2 tank (make sure it's full)
10. LONG BLADED LARYNGOSCOPE
11. MISCELLANEOUS
    a. Superglue, 2-0 (00) nonabsorbable suture material with needle
    b. Tape - 3" Elasticon® and white adhesive 1/2 inch
    c. Shaver, Betadine soap and solution
12. SMALL SURGERY SET
13. STOMACH TUBE - Harris flush or enema tubes (intra-esophageal) 24 French 60 inch

14. DRUGS AND FLUIDS
    a. Epinephrine - 1:1000
    b. Polyionic fluids (Plasmalyte 148, Normosol R, Lactated Ringers) and colloids (Hetastarch, Oxyglobin, Dextran, Pentastarch)
    c. Vasopressin (20U/ml)
    d. 5% $NaHCO_3$
    e. Atropine injectable (0.5 mg/ml)
    f. Glycopyrrolate (0.2 mg/ml)
    g. Lidocaine (20mg/ml)
    h. Calcium borogluconate 23%
    i. Magnesium sulfate (500mg/ml)
    j. 1% Dextrose
    k. Amiodarone (50mg/ml)
    l. O_2 NASAL CATHETER
        a). 14 French 40 cm. Oxygen Catheter (0-airlife-Amer. Hosp. Supply)
15. DEFIBRILLATOR

References:
1. Magdesian KG.: CPCR. Personal communication. 2012.
2. Fielding CL, Magdesian KG: .Cardiopulmonary cerebral resuscitation in Neonatal foals. <u>Clinical techniques in Equine Practice</u>. Vol.2. No.1. pp 9-19. 2003.
3. Palmer JE Neonatal foal resuscitation.<u>Vet Clin North Am Equine Pract</u>. 2007 May;23(1):159-82
4. Corley KT, Furr MO: Cardiopulmonary resuscitation on the newborn foal. <u>Comp. Vet. Ed</u>. 22:957-966, 2000

CHAPTER 78
LIMB DEFORMITIES – INTRODUCTION
by Hans Castelijns

Hans Castelijns is a veterinarian and farrier who is exceptional in his knowledge and experience with foals. See end of chapter for consulting information. Please consult his web site for further information about foal hoof and limb management.
http://www.mascalcia.net/articoli/a2000_28a.htm

I. GENERAL

A. "Correct" leg conformation is important to obtain a good price at the sales, sustain a successful training regimen in the young adult, to attain a high score at shows, and perhaps most important, to prevent lameness during a long career of the sport or racehorse.

B. Leg conformation, and associated defects, is heavily influenced before birth by genetics of the parents.

C. The mare's influence is of course both genetic, although it usually takes several offspring to notice, and environmental, therefore management of the mare is an important factor.

Obese mares (during pregnancy), tend to have a higher incidence of foals with angular deviations at birth. This higher incidence, specifically at the level of the carpal and tarsal joints, with a lot of "windswept" foals (one hock varus the opposite valgus), could be due to reduced uterine space caused by excessive abdominal fat.

II. EVALUATION OF LIMB CONFORMATION

A. Evaluation of the foal for it's conformation at, or soon after, birth is useful in all foals and essential in high risk cases: twins, prematures, dystocias, and previous history of limb problems from foals of similar breeding.

B. Evaluation should take into account:
  1. That a foal is not an adult:
     a. A base wide, outwardly rotated stance of the front legs is perfectly normal in lighter breeds, as it increases stability of these long legged,

narrow breasted babies[1], and tends to "correct" itself with time.

    b. This stance should not be confused with a valgus fetlock when seen from the front. In fact the best view for catching angular, and especially rotational deviations, of the front limbs is the skyline view, looking down from the shoulder to the toe, evaluating how the radius aligns with the cannon bone and the cannon bone with the pastern and the hoof.

2. The age of the foal.
   a. Growth plate closure times can be defined functionally, radiologically and histologically (Table I). For correction purposes, the first are essential.
   b. Distal growth plates (proximal of PII, proximal of PI, distal of MC/MTIII) close functionally within the first 3 months, followed by the distal GP of the tibia and finally the distal GP of the radius[2]
   c. Food intake changes naturally with age; developmental orthopaedic disease (D.O.D.) is due mostly to excess, not only of protein but also of energy (carbohydrates). Limiting energy intake takes a different approach in the new born as opposed to a 3 month old, which is grazing on lush spring pastures and/or might have access to crib feeding.

3. Body condition score and weight.
   a. An upright pastern is normal in the lightweight newborn; the fetlock should naturally extend further (drop) with increase in body weight.
   b. The breed. For example: Quarter horses and Andalusians are already "stocky" at birth and have higher incidence of varus deviations than, for instance, thoroughbred foals. A slight inward rotation of the lower hind leg is as lot more serious in a Standardbred trotter than in other breeds as it will probably lead to a cross gaited movement and interference at lower to medium speeds in future training.

C. Evaluation should be performed viewing the foal/limb:
1. **From the side** to spot abnormalities in the **sagittal plane** (flexural deformities).
2. **From the front** or the **back** to spot angular deviations in the **frontal plane**.
3. **From above** to look for axial rotations in the **horizontal plane**.
4. Bear in mind that the same foal, indeed the same limb, often presents a combination of flexural, angular and rotational deformities.

Table I. - Growth plate activity and closure times in months.[2]

Growth plate:	End of fast growth (months)	Radiological closure (months)
Distal tibia	8	17-24
Distal radius	8-10	20-42
Distal MC/MTIII	3-4	6-15
Proximal PI	2-3	12-15
Proximal PII	2-3	8-12

CHAPTER 79
LIMB DEFORMITIES -FLEXURAL DEFORMITIES (Sagittal plane)

A. **Definitions.**
1. As seen from the side, each joint may extend normally, less than normal (hypo-extension), or more than normal (hyper-extension).
2. While there is a large and fanciful vocabulary to describe flexural (and angular) deformities such as "club foot", "knuckling", "over at the knee", the terms hyper and hypo-extension are preferred for clarity.
3. When evaluating from the side, bear in mind that new born foals naturally have less extension at the DIP and fetlock joints than adults, as they weigh a lot less.
4. When detecting a flexor deformity, it is useful to decide whether the defect is:
    a. Moderate; not an immediate threat to the well being of the foal, with a good chance of spontaneous self-correction or easy to correct by conservative means.
    b. Severe; probably not self-correcting, causing discomfort or tendency to worsen; needs immediate attention.
    c. To determine severity in the case of hypoextension, manipulate the lower limb to test the joint's ability for extension, palpate the tension created thereby in the flexor tendons and the common digital extension tendon.

B. **Management and treatment of flexural deformities.**
These include: exercise or exercise restriction, bedding, bandaging, oxytetracyclines, specific hoof care techniques like trimming or gluing on extensions to the hoof and surgery.
1. Exercise
    a. <u>Exercise should be restricted (stall rest) in the case of hypo-extensions (contractions)</u>, as rest relaxes the flexor muscles and diminishes the vicious cycle of contraction - pain - further contraction.
    b. Exercise tones up the muscles in the case of flexor flaccidity.[3]
2. Bedding
    a. Foals are born with a conically inverse hoof, i.e. the distal border of the hoof is narrower than the

coronary band and furthermore the bottom of the hoof is covered with the equipodium or "feathers" which wears off with normal exercise on normal ground.
- b. Deep bedding nullifies a lot of the functions of corrective trimming and of glue-on extensions
- c. A good practice is to move the bedding to the sides of the stall during the day time, keeping only a thin, packed layer in the middle, where the foal can "feel the ground".

3. Bandaging
   a. Robert Jones type bandaging is appropriate in severe cases of hypo-extension of joints, as bandaging relaxes flexor musculature.
   b. Bandaging is more effective if done up to the elbow, but more difficult to keep nicely in place and therefore has to be checked regularly.
   c. Do not splint, or use rigid tubing, unless you are really experienced and willing to monitor the foal continuously. Foals are very lively and thin skinned, serious pressure sores are too often the result of splinting and/or casting.
   d. **Bandaging relaxes the flexor muscle-tendon units so it should not be applied in cases of hyper-extensions (flexor flaccidity).**

4. Oxytetracyclines (OTC)
   a. May be used in the treatment of contractions in foals (hypo-extensions).
   b. Often quite effective in the newborn or days old foals, less so in older foals; Not entirely risk free (nephrotoxicity).
   c. Dosage is 3 grams / 50 kg foal, preferably in 500ml of saline fluid.[4]
   d. Should be born in mind that OTC treatment is systemic and therefore might not only resolve a specific hypo-extended joint or joints but may also cause hyper-extension of the previously normal joints.

5. Farriery treatments include trimming, gluing on dorsal, palmar or plantar extensions and the use of heel or toe wedges.

Chapter 79 Limb Deformities – Flexural Deformities (Saggital Plane)

    a. Foal cuff type shoes on the market include Mustad Baby Glu (cyanolitic glue), Dallmer (Dallric in the U.S.A.) foal shoes (epoxy glue), and Ibex foal shoes (cyanolitic glue).
    b. All these foal shoes can also be applied with polyurethane adherents (superfast, adhere from Vettec) or Polymethylmetacrylates (PMMA's like Equilox, Bond N' Flex, Top Gum etc.)
    c. All glues except cyanolitic ones release heat, care should be taken to protect the hairline with duct tape.
    d. The hoof's surface needs to be mechanically cleaned (sand paper) and dried (hairdryer) if wet.
    e. All cuff type shoes should be removed within 7-8 days after application on the newborn or days old foal, as they will not allow for hoof expansion, because foal hooves grow twice as fast as adult hooves and are narrower at the bottom then at the coronary band in the newborn.

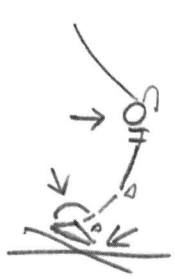

Flexor laxity

    f. A useful tip is to write the application, or the recommended removal, date on the shoe (Table II).
    g. Polyurethanes and PMMA's can also be used by themselves to create dorsal, lateral and medial extensions, but not for plantar/palmar extensions (you don't want to glue on the bulbs or the frog!)
7. Surgery is discussed for each specific condition.

Table II .Foal shoe removal times relative to the foal's age on application

Age (days)	Remove within (days)
1	7
7	10
20	14
45	20

I. TREATMENT OF SPECIFIC FLEXURAL DEFORMITIES

A. Hyper-extended DIP joints (flexor flaccidity)
1. This condition is often underestimated ("it will self correct"). The toe of the hoof will eventually grow long enough to touch the ground, leaving the distal phalanx in a negative plane, and subluxated relative to the second phalanx. The following consequences have been described as a result of this condition:
   a. Inflammation of the fetlock suspensory apparatus.
   b. Displacement of the distal metatarsal epiphysis.
   c. Flattening of the articular surface of the proximal sesamoids.
   d. Flattening of the proximal articular surface of PI.
   e. Marginal elevation and entheseophyte formation on the dorsal aspect of the fetlock joint.
   f. Remodelling of the extensor process of PIII.
   g. Under slung and contracted heels.
   h. Reluctance to move with further developmental consequences.[3]
2. Moderate /severe can be distinguished by observing the foal when moving:
   a. Does the toe touch the ground when taking a stride?
   b. Are the bulbs excoriated?
   c. Are there signs of curb?
3. Plantar (palmar) extensions.
   a. Plantar extensions will relieve pressure on the dorsal, pinched aspects of partially cartilaginous tarsal bones.
   b. Exercise tones up the flexor musculature.
   c. Do not bandage, even in the case of rubbed, excoriated bulbs.
   d. Glue on plantar (palmar) extensions, which will immediately lift the bulbs **off** the ground and force the toe **on** the ground.
   e. Bulb lesions can then be treated with local antiseptic.
   f. Before applying the shoe, shorten the toe and trim the under-run heels lightly.

EC My favourite plantar extension is a large fitting Dallmer D2 shoe, with a frog support plate screwed in, so as to relieve the under-run heels.

Chapter 79 Limb Deformities – Flexural Deformities (Saggital Plane)

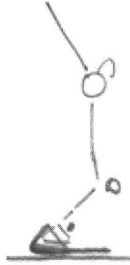

B. Hypo-extension of the DIP joints (club feet).
1. To judge severity, look whether the heels.
2. touch the ground when the foal moves.
3. Extend the joint manually whilst palpating the deep digital flexor tendon as part of evaluation.
4. Stall rest.
5. Reduce bedding during the day time.
6. Bandaging should be considered.
7. A dorsal extension can be made out of resin (Superfast-Vettec)
8. In those cases where the heels do not touch the ground and manual extension is painful, glue on a cuff shoe (e.g. Dallmer B), attaching an aluminium plate with screws to this shoe.
    a. The dorsal extension should be at least the length of the hoof (total length of plate equals 2x hoof length), with the toe of the plate slightly curled up, so as to limit stumbling and hooking into the bedding.
    b. At the heels the plate should be bent downwards providing an initial heel raise, equal to the amount of space seen under the heels of the foal at rest, before shoeing.
    c. Every 2 days the plate should be taken off (unscrewed) and the heel-raise diminished, until after ±6 days it can be eliminated.
    d. Initially, raising the heels breaks the vicious cycle of pain reflex - further contraction.

e. After 7-10 days the shoe is removed, the hoof trimmed and, when necessary, a slight dorsal extension (without heel raise) reapplied.

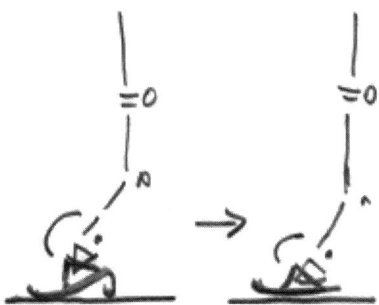

C. Hypo-extension of the fetlock(s)

1. Severe cases are defined by the fetlock moving dorsally from the vertical (knuckling).
2. Bandaging is useful.
3. If several joints are affected, oxytetracycline can be considered in the newborn. (3 gr. in 500 ml saline)
4. Raising the heels with a glue-on shoe with a screwed on wedge releases the DDFT tension, thereby leaving only the suspensory ligament and the superficial digital flexor tendon to bear the foal's weight on the fetlock which will therefore tend to come down.
5. Stall rest is important to prevent, or diminish, pain on fetlock extension.

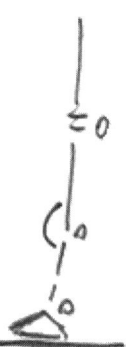

D. Hypo-extension of the carpus

1. Moderate cases (dorsal radius-MCIII angle of 180°-187°) can be turned out for free exercise, a slight lowering of the heels, sparing the toe, seems to be of some help [1]
2. With larger hypo-extension of the carpus (dorsal angle between radius and MCIII > 187°), a lot of tension is

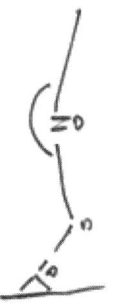

created in the common digital extensor tendon (CDET), which can easily rupture with too much exercise.
3. A ruptured CDET is easily recognised by a large, soft swelling over the dorso-lateral aspect of the carpus and the characteristic "throwing" movement of the hoof during ambulation of the foal.
    a. These foals should have stall rest, compact bedding, and bandaging up to the elbow, prognosis for ruptured extensor tendons is quite good.
4. More severe cases (>200° dorsal angle), which do not improve over 1-3 weeks with bandaging and rest and which show trouble standing, are candidates for tenotomy of the ulnar flexor tendon(s), as a salvage procedure.[4]

E. **Hyper-extension of the carpus.**
   EC: This is not a good conformation for racehorses as it may predispose to slab fractures of the carpal bones.
   1. In severe cases (dorsal angle < 170°), check for incomplete ossification of carpal bones (dorso-palmar X-Rays). If this is the case:
      a. Exercise can be too hard on the immature bones.
      b. Bandaging, although usually recommended, will weaken the flexor muscles even more.
      c. Palmar extensions might be of use in combination with stall rest on firm bedding.
   2. In moderate cases and with complete ossification of carpal bones:
      a. Shorten the toe.
      b. Turn out for exercise.

F. **Hypo-extension of the tarsus (sickle hocks)**
   1. The hock flexs dorsally and extends plantarly, i.e. although it is technically a hypo-extension it is more of a "flaccidity" deformity, often accompanied by hyper-extension of the DIP joint and curb.

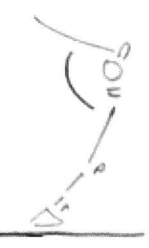

2. In premature foals and severe cases (strong signs of curb, difficulty in extending the joint), check for collapsed or incompletely ossified tarsal bones (latero-medial X-rays).
3. In the case of incomplete ossification:
   a. Give stall rest on firm bedding.
   b. Apply a large bearing surface behind the foot using a plantar extension shoe, this helps in extending the hock and relieving the dorsal aspect of the tarsal bones
4. Foals with well calcified tarsal bones:
   a. Benefit from exercise.
   b. In the case of curb and/or a tendency to raise the toes of the ground, apply plantar extensions.

References:
1. Curtis,S.: From Foal to Racehorse. Newmarket Farriery Consultancy. Newmarket,1999.
2. Betsch,J.M.: Reconnaissance, évaluation et gestion des déviations angulaires du poulain. Pratique Vétérinaire Equine, volume 37, 45-59,2005.
3. Hertsch,B.: The Hoof and How to Protect It Without Nails. Helmuth Dallmer publisher, Salzhausen-Putensen, 84-87,1996.
4. Boussauw, B.: Le anomalie dell'arto angolari e di flessorie: diagnosi e trattamento veterinari. Infor Mascalcia n°125, pag. 21-27, 2007
5. Castelijns, H.: Tecniche moderne di mascalcia per la prevenzione e la terapie delle zoppie nel cavallo. Tesi di Laurea, Facoltà di Medicina Veterinaria di Perugia. Pag.12, 1998.
6. van Heel, M.C.V.; Kroekenstoel, A.M.; van Dierendonck, M.C.; van Weeren, P.R.; Back,W.: Uneven feet in a foal may develop as a consequence of lateral grazing behaviour induced by conformational traits. Equine Veterinary Journal, volume 38, 7,646-651 2006.

CHAPTER 80
ANGULAR AND ROTATIONAL DEVIATIONS – GENERAL

I. GENERAL

A. Angular deviations (in the frontal plane) are defined as:
   1. **Valgus** whereby the segment of the limb, immediately distal to the affected joint/growth plate, is deviated laterally.
   2. **Varus** whereby the limb segment below the deviation is deviated medially.
   3. Bear in mind that the same limb may present valgus and varus deviations at different points e.g. carpus valgus with fetlock varus.

B. Varus and valgus deviations can be observed by:
   1. Viewing the limb from the front or the hind (often useful for evaluating fore limbs too).
   2. Viewing the limbs from above, positioning oneself close to the shoulder or the hip of the foal.
   3. On the fore limbs, and to judge cannon bone – pastern alignment, by picking up the fore limb at the distal end of the cannon bone, whilst letting the digit hang down freely.
   4. A long ruler or a farrier's rasp can be useful as a visual guide, when in doubt.
   5. Dorso-palmar/plantar x-rays permit accurate measurements, the assessment of ossification of carpal bones and the exact area where deviation takes place; the use of long cassettes is recommended. (Assessment of ossification of tarsal bones is best done with latero medial x-rays of the hock.)
   E.C.: Beware of assessing a fetlock as valgus, on an outwardly rotated fore limb. For there to be a valgus fetlock, the pastern Varus deviations tend to get worse with growth, when left untreated, valgus deviations tend to self correct with widening of the upper body.

C. Treatment of angular deviations depends on active growth plates and includes:

1. **Trimming**:
   a. Correct hoof flares on the side of the hoof to which the lower limb deviates to.
   b. Lower the hoof on the side the distal limb deviates to, only if this side is too high.
   c. Trim the frog, which is comparatively larger in a foal than in an adult horse, asymmetrically – more on the side the limb deviates to.
   d. Thin the hoof wall on the side of the deviation.
   e. Ideally it is better to trim a little often, than a lot at long intervals.
   f. With short hooves and/or larger deviations, there is a limit to what you can achieve with trimming.
2. **Lateral or medial extensions** to the hooves.
   a. With polymers like polyurethanes (e.g. superfast, adhere) or polymethylmetacrylates (PMMA) (Equilox, Bond n'Flex, TopGum etc.)
      i. Polyurethanes like Superfast are quick setting and wear resistant.
      ii. PMMAs have excellent adhesion, but should be reinforced with glass-carbon or Kevlar fibers, to increase their resistance to wear.
   b. With foal shoes; respect foal shoe removal times, relative to the foal's age (see guidelines in section.
3. **Surgery.**
   a. Periosteal stripping under general anesthesia on the "hollow" side, at the growth plate where the deviation takes place, that is, on the side which has an angle of less than 180°.
   b. Transcutaneous growth plate stimulation with an 18G, 40mm needle. This can be done with local anesthesia, surgical prep of the overlaying skin and approximately 10mm deep stabs into the growth plate, on the side where growth needs to be stimulated (concave side),moving the needle in a fan shaped pattern through the single cutaneous perforation into the underlying

periostum.[1] Advantages of this technique relative to periosteal stripping are that it can be done at the farm, and it doesn't cause as much periosteal reaction or scarring.
- c. Transphyseal bridging with screws[2], screws and wire, screws and plates under general anesthesia.
- d. Periosteal stripping, or transcutaneous stimulation of the growth plate, aims at increasing growth on the ipsilateral side, does not over-correct, is repeatable after a 6 week interval, and depends on an active growth phase of the treated physis.
- e. Transphyseal bridging is a growth retardation procedure on the side with a larger angle than 180°, the implants have to be removed (2nd surgery) as they may over-correct and they still work at slower (later) phases of physeal growth.[3]

4. **Combination of surgery and hoof extensions**.
- a. Periosteal stripping or transcutaneous growth plate stimulation work for 4 to 6 weeks and are synergetic with hoof extensions on the opposite side of the limb, e.g. lateral stripping of the distal physis of the radius and medial hoof extension for the correction of severe carpus valgus.

D. **A rotational deviation** (in the horizontal plane) is defined as an axial rotation of a limb segment relative to the segment proximal to it.
1. It can be inward or outward relative to e.g. inward rotation of the digit relative to the cannon bone.
2. Rotations can best be observed from above, looking downward along the limb.
3. Rotations of the digit, relative to the cannon bone, can be judged by picking up the limb loosely at the distal end of the cannon bone, and letting the digit hang.
   - a. Observe the direction of the frog, relative to a line perpendicular to the ground.
   - b. Rotate the hoof capsule gently, it will rotate more, and with greater ease, in the direction of the rotation of the digit.

E. Treatment of rotational deviations.
1. Only rotations of the digit relative to the cannon bone can be corrected by trimming or hoof extensions.
2. Trimming or hoof extensions should extend the toe-quarter area of the hoof, opposite to the direction of the lower limbs rotation e.g. a lateral toe extension, to correct an inward rotation of the digit relative to the cannon bone.
3. Outward rotations of the entire fore limbs from the elbow down, present at birth and in the first weeks – months of life, tend to self-correct with growth and widening of the thorax, and should therefore not be treated with hoof modifications in the first 6 months.
4. Inward rotations tend to get worse with growth, and should be treated more aggressively than outward rotations, which have a tendency to self-correct.

II. TREATMENT OF SPECIFIC ANGULAR AND ROTATIONAL DEFORMITIES.

Lower limb growth plates, around the fetlock, close functionally a lot earlier than the distal plates of the tibia and radius; priority should therefore be given to get the lower limbs well aligned at the fetlock within the first 3-4 months of the foal's life. (See table I chapter II).

A. Fetlock varus.

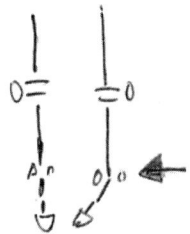

1. Frequent condition in all breeds, including trotters, warmbloods, Andalusians and heavy breeds but also of the hinds of thoroughbreds.

2. Can be masked, upon superficial evaluation, by valgus carpus or hock, or by outside rotation of the entire limb.
3. Needs conscientious treatment within the first three months, because of lower growth plates closure times. Tends to worsen with growth.
4. Can be present at birth (check for latero medial laxity at the fetlock).
5. Often acquired during growth in heavy, wide breasted foals or as a consequence of weight bearing on the opposite limb to an injured limb.
6. Trim medially, save hoof laterally.
7. Extend with a polymer extension to the lateral side.
   a. Ideally to the extent to where the outside of a hoof, belonging to a normal digit, would reach.
   b. Extend the whole side wall, including the heels.
   c. Beware of pinching or burning the coronary band at the heels with the fast setting and heat producing polymers.
   d. Do not let it grow forward too much, as it will then become a lateral toe extension, favouring outward rotation of the digit. Trim regularly.
8. Extend with a lateral extension foal shoe.
   a. With large degree of varus (>3-4°), present at birth, or acquired from overload on one limb, apply lateral extension cuff type foal shoes, as these can usually extend further than extensions out of pure polymer, they also "pull on" the whole hoof, not only the side wall.
   b. Wide lateral extensions with foal shoes, which can have as much ground surface as the hoof itself, are also called for when the fetlock varus belongs to a limb which has an added varus at the carpus or hock.

   e.g. "Windswept" foals which are born with one hock varus and the opposite valgus, often have a varus fetlock on their varus hocked limb, both joints react well to a wide lateral extension, applied in the first days after birth.

- c. When using cuff type shoes, set the cuff a bit wide on the side of the extension, as the hoof wall there tends to be a little straighter.
- d. Respect foal shoe removal times (table II, chapter III).
- e. Do not raise and then extend the lateral wall, only extend it.
9. Surgery
   - a. Stripping or transcutaneaous stimulation of the medial aspect of the distal growth plate of the cannon bone and/or the proximal G.P. of the first phalanx.
   - a. Take dorso palmar x-rays to decide, and as a baseline to judge improvement.
   - b. In the author's experience, periostal stripping of these growth plates results in more periostal reaction and visible swelling than stripping of the higher growth plates.
   - c. To be done in the first three months of life.
   - b. Transphyseal bridging of the lateral aspect of the distal G.P. of the cannon bone, can be attempted for severe deviations (> 4-5°), and when time is running out (10-14 weeks of age)

B. Fetlock valgus.

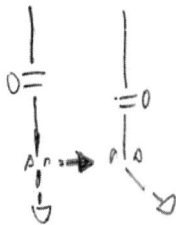

1. True fetlock valgus is a rare condition.
2. Check by hanging the limb.
3. Tendency to self correct permits less aggressive treatment.
4. Check for latero medial laxity at the fetlock in the newborn.
5. Trim laterally, save medially.
6. Small medial extensions with polymers may be of help.

Chapter 80 Angular and Rotational Deviations - General

       a. Do not have extension on the medial wall in the toe area, as this easily causes inward rotation of the digit.
7. Surgery is rarely called for
       a. Lateral stripping or physeal stimulation of distal GP of MC/MT III and/or of proximal GP of PI.
       b. Medial transphyseal bridging of distal GP of MC/MT III.
8. Do not over correct!

C. Inward rotation of the digit, relative to the cannon bone.

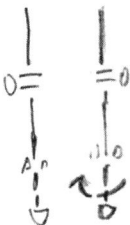

1. Frequent condition, often acquired during (fast) growth.
2. Contributing factors may be:
       a. Stocky heavy breeds or individuals.
       b. Hilly paddocks.
       c. DIP hypo extension (club foot): most club feet are also turned (rotated) inward.
       d. Mistaken "correction" of outwardly rotated, base wide stance of entire limb.
3. Trim <u>medial toe</u>, sometimes reduce <u>lateral heel</u> flare, save or leave extra hoof at the lateral toe area.
4. When not enough hoof is available, extend <u>lateral toe</u> with polymers.
5. Keep monitoring the condition as it tends to grow worse with growth and increase in width/weight.

D. Outward rotation of the digit, relative to the cannon bone.

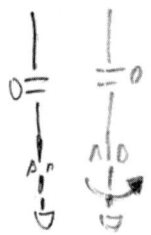

1. Rare condition on the fore limbs, more frequent on hind limbs.
2. Check your diagnosis by hanging the limb, looking for the way the frog points and manipulating the hoof outwards and inwards.
3. Tendency to self correct, treat less aggressively.
4. Trim lateral toe, reduce flare on medial heel if present, save medial toe.
5. Extend medial toe slightly with a polymer if the hoof is worn too much in this area.
6. Monitor, do not over correct.

E. Carpus valgus.

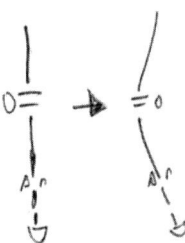

1. One of the most frequent conditions, usually present at birth.
2. Tendency to self-correct (Wolf's law [4]) is dependent on:
   a. Degree of angular deviation; up to 10° deviation causes faster growth on the concave side of the distal growth plate of the radius, larger degrees of valgus benefit from treatment, as excessive one sided pressure on the growth plate may actually retard growth there.
   b. Age: the younger the more self-correction is possible; however distal growth plate of the

radius is one of the latest physa to close functionally.
3. Other considerations:
   a. Extra cellular articular cartilage matrix, undifferentiated at birth, differentiates in pressure and tension resistant areas in the joints at a fast rate in the first 6 months of life, slower thereafter. It is therefore useful to get correct alignment as soon as possible.[5]
   b. A slight degree (2-3°) of valgus at the carpus might be physiological, as it allows for perpendicular weight bearing of the lower limb, in the stance phase at speed.
4. Check for lateromedial laxity at the carpus at birth.
   a. If present, and there are other reasons to suspect dysmaturity, x-ray for complete ossification of carpal bones.
   b. If incompletely ossified, bandage and give stall rest.
   c. Medial extensions for 1 week with a cuff type shoe, helps prevent lateral crushing of the carpal bones.
5. If at birth valgus at the carpus is larger than 10-12° with no laxity (x-ray, use visual guides like rulers):
   a. Extend medially with a cuff type shoe for a week.
   b. Foals can be turned out normally with these shoes.
   c. A polymer extension afterwards, if still needed.
6. If valgus is between 5° and 10° at birth (with no laxity), extend medially with polymers or cuff type shoes.
   a. Polymer extensions have the advantage that they do not have to be removed as quickly in the very young foal, as cuff type shoes.
   b. Prevent the medial extension from growing too far forward as it will create inward rotation of the digit; trim extension at the medial toe and re-apply at the medial heel.

c. Round off borders well to prevent striking injuries, although in the author's practice these are almost unheard of.
7. Evaluate cannon bone – digit alignment.
   a. Do <u>not</u> apply medial extensions for correction of valgus carpus if the fetlock is varus!
   b. Do <u>not</u> leave the medial side higher than the lateral side when extending medially; the extension will amplify the latero-medial height imbalance, twisting the digital joints and causing varus fetlock and inward rotation of the digit.
8. After 5-6 weeks of age medial extensions by themselves increase the likelihood of deviating and/or rotating the digit inwards.
9. At this age, and if there is the slightest hint of a medial deviation of the digit, it is advisable to combine medial extension with:
   a. A lowering of the medial hoof wall.
   b. Periostal stripping or transcutaneous physeal stimulation on the lateral side of the distal growth plate of the radius, as these will work in synergy, and reduce the risk of creating a varus fetlock.
10. Both medial extensions and lateral GP growth stimulation (distal radius) are repeatable in the case of severe (>15°) carpus valgus defects.[6]
11. Severe (>15°) carpus valgus in 0-3 month olds, and large (10-15°) carpus valgus in foals 3-6 months old, may benefit from medial transphyseal bridging.

    E.C. An early approach, combining repeated medial extensions with lateral distal radius G.P. stimulation, can obtain satisfying results in up to 20° valgus at the carpus.

F. Carpus Varus

Chapter 80 Angular and Rotational Deviations - General

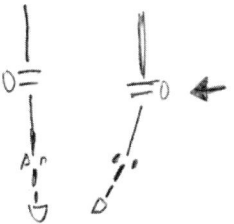

1. Rare condition.
2. May be present at birth, or acquired on the opposite limb to an injured one.
3. Keep in mind that 2-3° valgus is normal for the carpus; by this token, a straight radius – MC III alignment, could be considered as "varus".
4. Needs aggressive, early treatment, as the foal's development tends to worsen the condition.
5. Start with a lateral extension at birth:
   a. Cuff type shoe initial week
   b. Followed by a polymer extension.
6. If needed, medial stimulation of the distal GP of the radius.
7. There is less concern that lateral extension of the hoof will cause fetlock valgus, instead of straightening the carpus varus, as with the opposite correction (medial extension for carpus valgus creating fetlock varus).

G. **"Offset" carpus**

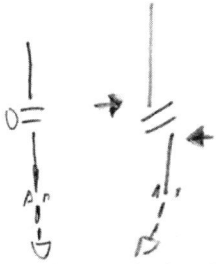

1. This condition is correctly described as a valgus radio carpal joint, in combination with a varus carpal – metacarpal joint.
2. The combined angular deviations are characterized by:

445

a. An "oblique" carpus, as seen from the front, whereby the two rows of carpal bones are not parallel to the ground.
b. Distal radius ending on the medial aspect of the proximal carpal bones.
c. Proximal MC III originating below the lateral aspect of the distal carpal bones. (Radius and MC III are not in line)
d. A ruler applied to the medial side of the carpus will project downwards to the outside of the hoof, while this is neither the case in a true carpus valgus, or in a normal carpus; in the first case the line will fall to the inside of the hoof; with a normal carpus it will fall approximately to the middle of the hoof.

3. The condition was considered by the author to be congenital (and indeed is frequently present in the affected foal's dam), a recent report, however seems to imply that it can also be acquired.[7]
4. Objective, baseline, deviations can be established with dorso palmar x-rays of the carpus.
5. Offset carpii may cause the following problems in the (young) adult performer:
    a. Medial splints, as the MC II (medial splint bone) is overloaded by the medially displaced distal radius, leading to entheseophyte formation at the proximal third of the interoseous ligament.
    b. Over 5 times larger incidence of carpal lesions in racing Thoroughbreds than with normal, or slightly valgus carpal conformation.
    c. Hang phase of the stride, is characterized by an initial lateral deviation of the hoof – lower limb from the sagittal plane, followed by a medial deviation before setting the hoof down. This "S" shape of the suspension arc of the limb, is readily seen in movement from the front, and heavily penalized in dressage competitions.
6. Correction of radio carpal valgus, in combination with carpo-metacarpal varus, can be attempted by:
    a. Lateral growth stimulation (stripping or transcutaneous stimulation) of the distal physis

of the radius, in combination with a <u>lateral</u> hoof extension.
   b. Lateral growth stimulation of the distal physis of the radius, in combination with medial stimulation of the distal physis of the MC III.[8]
   c. A combination of a. and b.
7. In any case it is prudent to keep the lower limb from increasing it's medial deviation (carpal-metacarpal varus) by:
   a. Trimming; saving the lateral hoof while rounding off the medial side.
   b. Lateral extensions with polymers.
   EC.: Do not confound carpus valgus with "offset knees", as the approach to the hoof is diametrically opposed; medial extension in the case of carpus valgus; lateral extension in the case of "offset" carpus.

H. Outward rotation of the entire front limb.

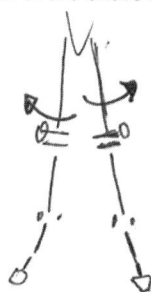

1. Natural in lightly built breeds at birth ("A" frame stance).
2. Does not need correction in the first 6 months of life, as it tends to self correct with widening of the breast.
3. May erroneously lead to valgus fetlock diagnosis.
4. At a walk foals may set down their foot on the outside wall.
5. Hoof shape generally remains symmetrical.

Chapter 80 Angular and Rotational Deviations - General

6. (Gently) pushing a balled fist, between the elbow and the ribcage of the foal, will rotate the entire limb inwards to a more "normal" stance.
7. This exercise, together with adduction exercises of the forwardly stretched limb, are useful physiotherapy for this condition, perhaps better not started before 12 months (and therefore outside the scope of this chapter).

I. Windswept: Valgus + opposite varus hocks

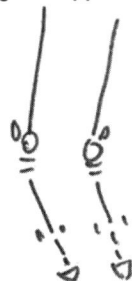

1. Varus hocks are much more frequent than varus carpii, usually as part of a condition known as "windswept", whereby both hocks are deviated in the same direction, one valgus one varus.
2. The condition is attributed to intrauterine positioning; the author has variously tried to find correlations with gestation length, dam's age, hind feet first presentation at birth etc., without significant results.
3. Windswept foals, not only have angular deviations of both hocks, their whole pelvis is usually tilted downwards on the side of the bowed (varus hocked) leg.
4. Newborns often have problems standing and ambulating on the varus hind, the hoof can quickly become severely distorted.
5. Valgus and varus hocks are treated similar to the carpii.
6. Distal tibial growth plates close slightly earlier than distal growth plates of the radia (functionally at ± 8 months).
7. Correction in the newborn consists of:

Chapter 80 Angular and Rotational Deviations - General

    a. A large lateral extension on the hoof of the varus-hocked limb, with a glue-on cuff type foal shoe.
        i. Don't glue the lateral side of the cuff on too tightly, as the lateral wall is often atrophied.
        ii. There is often also a degree of D.I.P. hyper-extension present (flexor flaccidity); if this is the case, extend the shoe both laterally and plantarly.
    b. A usually smaller, medial extension on the hoof of the valgus hocked limb; the size of the medial extension depends on:
        i. The amount of valgus deviation of the hock, keeping in mind that in most light breeds, a 2-3° valgus of the hock, is more "normal" than straight (in the frontal plane) hocks.
        ii. That there is no varus fetlock on the same limb: hind limb fetlocks need even more precocious correction when varus than front limbs. In the case of varus fetlocks, align MT III and digit before correcting the valgus hock.

8. Lateral extensions on the varus limbs of windswept newborns with cuff type foal shoes:
    a. Dramatically improve their stance and ambulation.
    b. Can be followed, after a week and shoe removal, with a trim and a lateral hoof extension with a polymer.
    c. Can be used again in the 3-4th week of life if necessary.

9. Be aggressive in treating any varus deviation (hock, fetlock) on a hind limb of a trotter, as this will lead to cross gaited interferences, when in training.

10. As is the case with the carpii, valgus hocks tend to self correct, varus tends to correct less spontaneously and needs more attention.

11. Valgus angular deviations of the hock respond to the usual surgical techniques:

a. Lateral periostal stripping, or transcutaneous physeal stimulation, at the site of the distal growth plate of the tibia.
b. Medial transphyseal bridging, which can also be done with a single lag screw.
12. Varus hocks can benefit from surgery at the distal growth plate of the tibia by:
    a. Medial stripping or physeal stimulation.
    b. Lateral transphyseal bridging.
13. Surgery for the valgus hock is recommended if:
    a. There is no progress with hoof extensions in the first 4 weeks.
    b. Hock after 4 weeks is still more than 10-12° valgus.
    c. The fetlock of the same limb is varus (lateral tibia growth plate stripping + lateral hoof extension in this case!)
14. Surgery for the varus hock is recommended if:
    a. There is no progress with hoof extensions in the first 4 weeks.
    b. Hock after 4 weeks is still more than 6-8° varus.
15. Surgery is synergetic with hoof extensions which should be applied regardless.

Hans Castelijns D.V.M - Farrier equine podiatry consultant and referrals Loc. Valecchie n°11/A, 52040 Cortona (Ar)- Italy Tel + Fax ++39 0575 614335 - Mobile ++39 333 7716663

References:
1. Colles, C.M.: Physeal Stimulation for the Correction of Angular Limb Deformities. Proceedings BEVA Congress 2006 page 319.
2. Von Saldern, F.C., Thorpe, P., Zieg, H., Hyde, V. and O'Keeffe, A.: Transphyseal Bridging using Single Screw Placement for the Correction of Angular Limb Deformities in Foals and Yearlings. Proceedings BEVA Congress 2006, page 319.
3. Auer, J.A.: Angular limb deformities, Flexural limb deformities. Chapters 89-90, pp 1130-1165, Equine Surgery 3rd edition, Saunders Elsevier, St. Louis MO, 2006
4. Wolff, J.: The law of bone remodelling. Berlin, Spring-Verlag. 1986

5. Brama, P.: Functional adaption of articular cartilage: the formation of regional biochemical characteristics during the first year of life in the horse. Dynamics of equine articular cartilage. Utrecht 1999 Chapter V pp 75-88.
6. Betsch, J.M.: Reconnaissance, evaluation et gestion des deviations angulaires du poulain. Pratique Vétérinaire Equine n° special 2005, Vol 37, pag. 45-59
7. Santschi, E.M., Leibsle, S.R., Morehead, J.P., Prichard, M.A., Clayton, M.K., Kenlen, N.S.: Carpal and Fetlock Conformation of the Juvenile Thoroughbred from Birth to Yearling Auction Age. Equine Vet. J. (2006) 38 (7) 604-609.
8. Auer, J.A.: (2007) Personal communication.

Manufacturers:
Dallmer-Foal shoes: www.dallmer.de email: hufshuh@dallmer.de
Vettec adhere – superfast – polyurethane polymers :
www.vettec.com
Mustad hoof care Baby Glu foal shoes www.mustadhoofcare.com
email: mail@mustardhoofcare.com
Equilox Polymethylmetacrylate polymers: www.equilox.com email: equilox123@aol.com
TopGum Polymethylmetacrylate polymers www.top-gum.com
email: jpripb@wanadoo.fr
Ibex Foal shoes: email: ibexequine@aol.com
Hans Castelijns can be contacted by e-mail at the following address for consult on management and treatment of foals with flexural, angular and or rotational deviations.

Consult is fee based, contact Christiana Stawski for details at christiana@alice.it

INDEX

Abscess
    rhodococcus equi, 146, 295
    umbilical, 204,205
Abdominal distension, 46
    associated with necrotizing enterocolitis 169
    associated with the uroperitoneum, 192
    associated with the meconium, 126
    atresia coli, 218
Abdominal pain, (See Colic)
    enteritis and obstruction and, 167, 253
    gastric ulcers and, 177
    meconium retention and, 131
    strangulating hernia and, 207
Abdominal paracentesis
    method, 255
Abdominal radiographs, 313
Abdominal ultrasonography, 296-302
    ruptured bladder and, 298
    method, 296
Absorption
    carbohydrate, 146
Absorption of colostral immunoglobulin, 28
Acepromazine, 261, 263
Acetylcysteine enema, 26
    method, 127
Acid-base status,
    case example of, 107
    evaluation of, 99-100
    sepsis and, 126
    venous 56, 59
Acidosis,
    diarrhea and, 171
    goat's milk and, 120
    paraenteral nutrition and, 11
    respiratory distress and, 246
    prematurity and, 51
    respiratory (see hypercapnea)

Actinobacillus equuli, 135
ACTH,
    adrenal insufficiency and, 51, 53, 381
Acute abdominal pain, (See Pain)
Adenovirus, 138
Adhesions
    intestinal, 253
Adrenocortical insufficiency, 51, 53
Aerosolized medications, 360-361
Afterbirth (see Placenta)
    containment for Salmonella control, 152-153
Aganglionosis, 218
Agalactia, 118
    Domperidone, 118
Airway,
    hydration, 359
    suctioning of, 368
    therapy, 358
Albuterol, 363
All in one parenteral nutrition, 111
Allantoic fluid
    ultrasound, 275-276
Ambu bag, 70,71
    CPR and 417
Amikacin, (see aminoglycosides)
Amino acid solutions,
    for TPN, 112
Aminoglycosides
    dose, 381, 375
    septic arthritis and, 200-202
    toxicity and, 188
    use and precautions, 152, 376-377
Aminophylline, 381
Amniotic fluid
    L/S Ratio, 244
Amoxicillin,
    dose, 381

Ampicillin
    dose, 375, 381
    in sepsis, 376
Anaphylaxis,
    epinephrine and, 389
    plasma and, 40
Anemia
    in neonatal isoerthyrolysis, 182
    indications for transfusion, 183
    Fell Pony Syndrome and, 164
Anesthesia, 263
    for dystocia, 20-22
Angular limb deformities, 422-452
    hypothyroid and, 239
Aniridia, 217
Anomalies (see Congenital Anomalies)
Anterior uveitis, 136
Antibiotics (see antimicrobials)
Anti-endotoxin plasma, 38
    salmonella control and, 153
Anti-RBC alloantibodies
    colostrum and, 182
    neonatal isoerthyrolysis and, 185
        mules and, 182
    plasma donor and, 40
Anti-Rhodococcus equi hyperimmune plasma
    administration, 148
    source, 137
Anticonvulsants
    therapy, 158-159
    use in sepsis, 143
Anti-erythrocyte alloantibodies (see Anti-RBC alloantibodies)
Antimicrobial therapy
    aminoglycosides (see aminoglycosides)
    CNS infection and, 158
    doses for, 381
    guidelines, 374
    in diarrhea, 173

    post birth use and, 370
    probability and susceptibility in sepsis, 137
    schedule and daily plan, 91
    therapeutic monitoring, 377
    transport of foal and, 63
    trough levels, 377
Antiserum (see Plasma)
Antitoxin
    tetanus, 6,25,142
Aortic arch, persistence of, 211
Apnea, 58 (See Resuscitation)
    seizures and, 155
Arabian foals
    abiotrophy and, 220
    epilepsy, 156, 157
    immunodeficiency and, 162
Arrhythmias, (See Electrocardiography and see Resuscitation)
Arterial blood gas
    daily monitoring and, 26, 61
    factors affection, 58
    methods of obtaining, 345
    minimum data base and, 89, 90
    normal values, 411
    oxygen use and, 60, 93
    post foaling use, 26
    resuscitation and, 71
Arterial samples (see Arterial Blood Gas)
Arthritis, septic
    arthrotomy, 201, 202
    diagnosis, 199
    diarrhea and, 197
    omphalophlebitis and, 285-286
    treatment, 187-189
Asphyxia, 1
    differential, 57
    oxygen needs and, 55
    respiratory distress and, 244

resuscitation and, 81
seizures and, 155
Aspiration pneumonia, 4
    meconium, 5
Asymptomatic ulcers (see Gastroduodenal Ulcers)
Atelectasis
    hypercapnia and, 59, 261
    hypothyroid and, 240
    hypoxemia and, 52, 55, 57
    prematurity and, 52
    radiography and, 243, 313
    respiratory distress and, 243
Atresia
    ani, 46, 218
    coli, 46
    recti, 218
    tricuspid, 211
Atrial fibrillation, 329
Atrial septal defect, 211
Atropine,
    bradycardia use in, 265
    cardiac arrest use in, Front Cover, 75
    dose, Front Cover, 383
Auscultation,
    lung, 55
Autosomal trisomy, 225
Bacteremia
    diarrhea and, 166, 171
    in septicemia, 135
    pneumonia and, 138
    omphalophlebitis and, 205
    open gut and, 1
Bacterial
    infections, 135
Bain circuit, 71, 420
Banamine®, (See Flunixin Meglumine)
Barium
    enemas, 316

    gastrointestinal contrast study and, 257
Bedding
    diarrhea and, 174
    nursing care and, 96
    transport of the foal and, 63
Behavior
    change of sepsis, 124
    normal, 47
Belgian foals
    anridia and, 217
    bleeding disorder and, 235
    junctional mechanobullous disease and, 221
Beta2 sympathomimetics, 362
Bethanecol
    dose and uses, 383
Bicarbonate, 110, 110
    calculating amount to give, 105
    emergency dose, Front Cover, 386
    respiratory distress and, 246
    resuscitation and , 76, 419
    (also see Acid-base status)
Biosecurity, 356-357
Birth
    normal events of, 17
Bismuth subsalicylate
    dose and use 389
Bladder
    radiography, 181
    urinary rupture, 192-196, 199
Blindness
    neonatal maladjustment syndrome and, 131
    post seizure and, 124
Blood administration, 347
Blood chemistry
    normal values, 408
Blood clotting (see hemostatic disorders)
Blood cultures
    diarrhea and, 171

    method, 335
    minimum data base and, 88
    resuscitation protocol and, 72
    salmonella and, 151
    sepsis and, 136
Blood donor, 40, 184
Blood gas, (see Arterial blood gas)
Blood/plasma donors, 40
    R. equi, 148
Blood pressure, 45
Blood sampling techniques, 344, 345
Blood type
    cross match, 347
    NI and, 184
Body temperature
    regulation, 66-67
    transient tachypnea syndrome and, 139, 247
Body weight, 2, 8
Bottle feeding, 91
Botulism, 140
Bradycardia, 74, 76, 80
Bronchodilator drugs
    nebulization and, 359, 362
Bruxism, 177
Bucket (see feeding)
BUN,
    elevation in diarrhea cases, 171
    elevation in renal disease, 189
    monitoring in parenteral nutrition, 92, 114
Butorphanol
    dose, 383
    in colic cases, 258
    in mares, 21
    in meconium retention cases, 129
Calcium
    mammary secretions and, 10
Caloric requirements (see Parenteral Nutrition)
Candidiasis, 143

Carbohydrate intolerance, 166
Cardiac arrest, 74-76
Cardiac catheterization, 211
    normal values, 415
Cardiovascular status
    evaluation of, 74
Carpal bones
    incomplete ossification, 51, 96
Cataracts, 95, 216
Catheter, IV (see Intravenous Catheters)
    daily care, 95
    parenteral nutrition and, 92
    selection and placement, 341
Catheterization,
    bladder 89
    cardiac, 211, 415
Cefotaxime,
    meningitis treatment and 142
Ceftiofur, 385
Ceftizoxime, 385
Ceftriaxone, 385
Cephalothin, 385
Central nervous system
    drugs use for problems in, 403-404
Cesarean section,
    anesthesia for, 3, 22
Cephalosporins (see specific drugs)
Cerebellar abiotrophy, 220
Cerebral edema
    therapy, 133-134, 403
Cerebrospinal fluid collection, 337
    in meningitis, 141, 142
    normal values of, 339
Charcoal, activated
    dose, 385
    in diarrhea, 173
Chemical restraint, 354
Chemistries (see Blood Chemistries)

Chest
    therapy, percussion and vibration and,
Chest radiographs (see thoracic radiography)
Chloramphenicol
    dose, 385-386
    in meningitis, 158
    in sepsis, 137
Cimetidine
    ulcers and, 178
Cite® Foal IgG, 33
Cleft palate, 218
    differential diagnosis, 125
    exam for, 48
    signs of, 54, 218
Clenbuterol, 22, 387
Clinical pathology (also see Blood Chemistries)
Clinical signs
    of ill foals, 124
Clostridium difficile, 168, 356
Clostridium perfringens, 167
Clotting tests (see Hemostasis)
CNS (see Central Nervous System)
Colic,
    in clostridium perfringens type C, 167
    in necrotizing enterocolitis, 169
    in Salmonellosis, 151
    maternal, 3
    meconium retention and, 126
    ulcers and, 177
Colon torsion, 255
Colostrometer®
    IgG and, 28
Colostrum, 28
    amounts to feed, 29, 91, 118
    daily plan and, 91
    impending parturition and, 13
    specific gravity, 28
    supplementation, 29

Coma
 sepsis and, 136
 hyperbilirubin and 185
Combined immunodeficiency, 162
Complete blood count
 uses, 2, 8, 26
 in minimum data base and, 88
 normal values, 405
Conformation
 assessment of, 422-450
Congenital anomalies, 216-228
 seizures and, 156
Conjunctivitis, 44, 209
Constipation, 124
Continuous positive airway pressure, 59
Contracted foal syndrome, 220
Contracted tendons, 47
Convulsions (see Seizures)
Corneal abrasion
 prevention, 96
Corneal dermoid, 216
Corneal ulcers
 prevention, 345
 treatment, 208
Coronavirus, 170
Corticosteroids
 And fetal lung maturation, 15
 in shock, 85
 induction of parturition and, 15
Cortisol, plasma
 immaturity and, 57
Coughing, 45
Coupage,
 physical therapy and 139, 245
 resuscitation and, 70
CPCR- CardioPulmonary Cerebral Resuscitation, see front cover, 416
Cranial nerves, 47

Cranial trauma
    signs of, 155
Creatinine,
    aminoglycoside use and, 372
    increase without renal disease, 103, 133,189
    normal values, 208
    peritoneal fluid and bladder rupture,193
    renal disease and, 190
    urachal rupture and, 194
Creatinine kinase
    in CSF, 339
    in maladjustment syndrome, 133
    in white muscle disease, 229
Critical care patient
    daily plan, 91
    monitoring, 91
Cryptorchidism, 225
Crytosporidium
    diarrhea and, 162, 167
    treatment, 397-398
CSF (see Cerebrospinal Fluid)
Cyanosis, 55
Cystitis
    urachal infection and, m 192, 194, 205-206
Cytobin®
    for hypothyroidism, 240
Daily nursing care, 95
Dandy-Walker syndrome, 156
Death,
oo dam, 5
sudden 168
Decubitus sores, 111, 134
Dehydration,
    and diarrhea, 170
    azotemia, 188
    estimation and correction of, 98-110
Depression
    and septic arthritis, 198

hypothyroidism and, 239
ill foals and, 88, 124
poor nutrition and, 111
ruptured bladder and, 192
septicemia and, 136, 142
Tyzzers hepatitis and, 143

Detomidine,
sedation and, 261, 262
for ultrasound exams and 269

Dexamethasone,
Immune mediated disorders, 236
induction of parturition and, 15
lung maturation and, 15

Dextrose
initial evaluation and, 89
resuscitation and, 421
transport of foal and, 63

Diaphragmatic hernia, 219
differential and, 127
radiography, 314

Diarrhea
causes of, 166-168
fluid therapy and, 99
hyponatremia and, 103
gastric ulcers and, 176
in septicemia, 144
parenteral nutrition use indications and, 111
salmonella and, 151
septic arthritis and, 197

Diazepam,
anticonvulsant therapy, 158
dose, 387-388
restraint and 262, 354

Digestive tract inoculums, 26

Dilantin (Phenytoin)
dose, 399-400

Disinfectant
methods, 356-357

Disseminated intravascular coagulopathy, 38, 236
DMSO,
    adhesion prevention and, 256
    brain edema treatment, 133
Dobutamine,
    Anesthesia use and, 265
    dose, 387
    in shock, 83
    in renal failure, 189
Dopamine
    dose, 387
    use not suggested in foals, 84
Doppler tail
    blood pressure, 45, 82
Dopram™ drip (see Doxapram)
Doxapram
    for hypercapnia, 60
    in resuscitation, 389
Drug therapy,
    formulary and general principles of use, 374
Ductus arteriosus
    and reversion to fetal circulation, 212, 244
    chemical closure, 53
Dummy foal (see Neonatal Maladjustment Syndrome)
Duodenal-pyloric stenosis (also see gastroduodenal ulcers)
    clinical signs, 176, 256
Duodenal stricture, 176
Dysmature (see prematurity)
Dysphagia,
    botulism and, 140
    hyperbilirubinemia and, 185
    temporary pharyngeal paresis and, 48, 218
    tetanus and, 141
    white muscle disease and, 229
Dystocia, 20
    anesthesia for, 21
    high risk foals and, 4

Dysuria,
    ruptured bladder and, 192
E.Coli
    diarrhea and, 167
    sepsis and, 135, 197, 336
ECG, (see Electrocardiography)
Echocardiography
    practical approach to, 308, 309, 322
Ectropion, 216
Edema (see Pulmonary Edema)
Electrocardiography, 328-333
    arrhythmias, 329
    patent ductus arteriosus and, 212
Electroencephalgram, 157
Electrolyte imbalances, 98-110
    ruptured bladder and, 193
Emergency drug doses, see Front Cover
Endocrine problems, 239-241
    assessment of fetal well being, 8
    hypoadrenocorticism, 240
Endotracheal tube (see Nasotracheal Tube)
Endoscopy (see Gastroduodenal Ulcers)
Enema
    acetylcysteine, 26, 129
    fleet, 130
    precautions, 130
Enteral nutrition, 117-123
    (see Feedings also)
Enteritis
    colic and, 168, 253
    differential diagnosis, 253
    radiography, 315
    ultrasound and, 297-301
Enterocolitis, 151, 168, 169, 317
Entropion, 208, 216
Epidural block
    dystocia and, 21

Epinephrine,
    dose in resuscitation, (see front cover), 75, 85, 389
    use in cardiac arrest, 75
Episcleral hemorrhages, 44, 124, 136, 208
Equine herpes 1,
    congenital 138
Esophageal stricture and stenosis, 219
Estrone sulfate, 8
Examination of foal (see Physical Examination)
Eye, 208-210
    congenital anomalies of, 216-217
        (see entropion)
    corneal ulcers and, 208
    daily care of, 96
    examination of, 47
Facial asymmetry
    autosomal trisomy and, 255
Factor VIII deficiency, 235
Failure of passive transfer
    definition and treatment, 4, 29, 34, 35
Fecal occult blood, 177
Feeding 117-121
    amounts of milk and, 91, 117, 122
    firm stools and, 120
    frequency, 99, 117
    ill foals and, 120
    milk types, 109-111
    orphan, 118
    preventing septicemia and, 371
    via tube, 99, 332
Fetal circulation, reversion to, 244
Fetal measurements and ultrasound, 268-278
Fetal electrocardiography (see Electrocardiography)
Fetal monitoring, 8
    heart rate, 270
    ultrasonography and, 268-278
Fever
    gastric ulcers and, 177

    ill foals and, 124
    sepsis score, 144
    septic arthritis and, 198
    septicemia and, 136, 151
    transient tachypnea and 45, 139
Flexor contractures, 220, 425-435
Flexor tendon laxity, 425
Fluconozole, 143
Fluid,
    intake, 99
    therapy, monitoring of, 99
Fluid, intravenous 98-110
    Composition chart of 109
    hyperkalemia, 103
    hypernatremia and, 103
    hypokalemia, 103
    hyponatremia, 103
    in parenteral nutrition,
    maintenance, 100
    resuscitation and, 104-106
    types, 99-101
    therapy guidelines, 98-110
Flunixin meglumine, 174, 180
    Colic pain use, 248
    dose, 389
    pain control meconium, 129
Foal Rejection, 122
Foal handling methods, 359
Foal heat, 166
Foaling area contamination, 370
    hygiene, 1
Fractional excretion
    renal, electrolytes, 189
Fractured ribs, 244, 251-252
    and diaphragmatic hernia 249
Gastric distension
    radiography and, 315
Gastric emptying

time of, 316
Gastric reflux,
    ulcers and, 177
Gastric ulcers (see Gastroduodenal Ulcers)
Gastroduodenal Ulcers, 176-181
    clinical syndromes of, 176
    endoscopic findings, 178
    radiography, 178
    perforation and, 176
    surgery for, 257
    treatment of, 178-180
Gastrojejunostomy, 257
Genetic disorders, 216-228
Gentamicin (see Aminoglycosides)
Gestation
    length, 10, 17
    prematurity and, 50
Glucose
    CSF values, 339
    energy from, 261
    foal transport and, 63
    hypoglycemia with diarrhea, 232
    levels during resuscitation, 76
    seizures and, 158
    solutions for parenteral nutrition 114
Gluaraldehyde coagulation test for IgG, 33
Glutathione peroxidase activity, 229
Goat's milk, 120
    acidosis and, 120
Goiter, 239
Hemophilia, 35
Handling foals (see foal handling methods)
Hand washing
    in infection control, 356
Heart
    fetal, 270
    foal distress and, 18
    murmur, 211

Hematology
- normal sounds, 44
- rate, newborn normal, 18, 19
- resuscitation and, 74
- (see Echocardiography and Electrocardiography)

Hematology
- normal values, 405-406

Hematuria, 189

Hemolytic anemia, 92
- neonatal isoerthyrolysis and, 182-183
- white muscle disease and, 230

Hemostatic disorders, 235-236

Hepatitis
- serum, 42
- Tyzzer's disease and, 143

Hernia
- diaphragmatic, 219, 257
- differential diagnosis, 248
- scrotal, 248
- umbilical, 206

Herpes, Equine I (see Equine Herpes I)

High meconium retentions (see Meconium Retention)

High risk foals, 2, 11

Hereditary junctional mechanobullous disease, 221

Humidification therapy, 359

Hydration
- assessment of, 102, 171

Hydrocephalus, 221

Hygiene, (see Biosecurity)

Hypercapnia,
- causes of, 59
- doxapram for, 60

Hyperglycemia
- Insulin and 391
- parenteral nutrition and, 115

Hyperimmune plasma (see Plasma)

Hyperkalemia
- cases of, 101

insulin treatment of, 391
treatment in renal failure, 103, 190
with bladder rupture, 193
with white muscle disease, 230
Hyperkalemic periodic paralysis
    differential with tetanus,
Hyperlipidemia
    hypoglycemia and, 232
    with parenteral nutrition, 116
Hyperphosphatemia
    phosphate enema and, 130
Hyperthermia,
    drugs and 384
    malignant hyperthermia 224
    seizures and, 158
Hyperventilation
    transient tachypnea and, 139
Hyphema, 67
Hypoadrenocorticism
    premature and dysmature, 240
    therapy for, 240-241
Hypocalcemia, 106
    differential from tetanus, 141
    seizures and, 155
Hypochloremia
    in ruptured bladder, 193
    renal disease and, 190
Hypoglycemia, 232-234
    and transport of foal, 63
    change of condition and, 92
    diarrhea and,
    differential with botulism, 140
    foals at risk, 232
    glycogen branching enzyme and 222
    in neonatal maladjustment syndrome, 132
    in septicemia, 136
    seizure-like activity and, 156
    symptoms, 156

Tyzzer's disease and 143
Hypokalemia,
    metabolic acidosis and, 103
    parenteral nutrition and, 114
Hyponatremia,
    causes of, 103
    enema use and, 130
    renal dysplasia and, 190
    ruptured bladder and, 193
Hypopion, 125
Hypothermia, 60
    and hypoglycemia, 232
    correction of, 67
    prematurity and, 51
    septicemia and, 136
    transport and, 64
Hypothyroidism,
    angular limb deformities and, 239
    forms of, 239
    respiratory insufficiency and, 240
    treatment of, 240
Hypoventilation,
    doxapram and, 60
    hypercapna and, 59, 245
    hypoxemia and, 57, 261
    oxygen use and, 245
    prematurity and, 51
    respiratory distress and, 243
Hypovolemia,
    clinical markers of, 102
    echocardiography detection and, 324
    tachycardia and 77
Hypovolemic shock, 81, 85, 291
Hypoxemia
    causes of, 57-58, 81, 416
    septicemia and, 135
    respiratory distress and 243
    therapy, 58

Icterus,
- in neonatal isoerthyrolysis, 124
- in Tyzzer's 143
- kernicterus, 185

IgG,
- colostral, 28
- milligrams dose for plasma transfusion, 29
- plasma us, 41,
- prematurity and, 52
- sepsis and, 58

IgM
- presuckle sample for CID, 162

Ileocolonic aganglionosis, 218

Ileus
- necrotizing enterocolitis 169
- need for parenteral nutrition, 111

Immaturity (see Prematurity)

Immunodeficiencies, 162-165
- Fell pony, syndrome, 164

Immune mediated thrombocytopenic bullous pemphgoid, 236

Impactions, 254

Inguinal (scrotal) hernias, 225

Induced parturition, (see Parturition also)
- premature foals and, 52

Infections (see also septicemia)
- antimicrobial use and, 26, 137
- bacterial, 26
- botulism, 140
- delayed gut closure and, 370
- herpes I, (see equine herpes)
- IgG level and, 32
- Immunodeficiencies and, 162
- Listeria, 143
- meningitis, 142
- plasma therapy and, 37, 38
- rhodococcus, 146-149
- salmonella, 135

seizures and, 144, 155
  sepsis score and, 144
  septicemia, 135
  septic arthritis, 201
  tetanus, 141
  umbilical, 290
  viral, 130
Intestinal protectants, 173
Intestinal strangulation, 257
  radiography, 313
  ultrasound 296
Intra-articular antibiotics, 200
Intracranial pressure, 157, 337
Intravascular catheters
  arterial, 342
  daily care of, 92
  management, 343
  placement, 341
  preparation, 342
  venous, 341
Intravenous fluids (see Fluids)
Intubation (see Nasotracheal and Nasogastric)
Intussusception,
  Ultrasound, 297
In utero infection, 26, 135
Iodine
  thyroid problems and, 239
Iridocyclitis, 209
Isoproterenol, 362
Ivermectin, 39, 166
Joint infection, (see Arthritis, septic)
Joint-ill (see Arthritis, septic)
Jugular pulses 44
Junctional mechanobullous disease 22
Kaolin
  in diarrhea, 173, 391
Kernicterus, 185
Ketamine, 264, 393

Kidney (see Renal)
Kyphosis 47
Labor,
    induction, 13-15
    stages of, 1, 17-18
Lactose tolerance test, 171
Lameness, 224, 422
    septic arthritis and, 198
Lasix, 189, 389
Lecithin/sphingomyelin
    in respiratory distress, 244
Leukopenia
    clostridium perfringens and, 167
    enteritis, 254
    salmonella and, 151
    septicemia, 135
Lipids,
    emulsions in parenteral nutrition, 112
Liver (see also Hepatitis)
    abscesses, 205
    drug metabolism and, 374
    fatty 112
Low meconium retention, 127
Low risk foals, 1
Lung (see also Thoracic and Respiratory
    function test with oxygen, 93
    fetal ultrasound 275
    maturity and corticosteroids, 15
    respiratory distress and, 243-245
    surfactant and, 244
    ultrasound 291, 292, 295
Luxated lens, 217
Lymphopenia,
    EHV-1 and, 139
    immunodeficiencies and, 162
Lysosomal storage disease, 156, 232,
Maladjustment syndrome (see neonatal maladjustment syndrome)

Mammary secretions
    and impending parturition, 10-12
    electrolyte composition, 10-12
Management,
    approaches to newborn, 1, 370
    to prevent neonatal infection, 370
Mannitol, 147
    cerebral edema and, 134, 157
    dose, 134, 393
    seizure treatment and, 157
Mares (see Maternal)
Mares milk substitutes (see milk)
Mare vaccination, 5
Mare's match, 119
Maternal conditions
    risk factors and, 2

Maturity
    assessment of, 14, 50
Mechanical ventilation (see also Positive Pressure Ventilation)
    need for, 59, 60, 93
Meconium
    routine enema and, 25, 127
Meconium aspiration, 138
Meconium retention
    clinical signs, 16, 129
    prevention, 130
    radiography and,
    treatment, 129
    weed whacker wire and, 129
Meglumine,. Flunixin (see Flunixin Meglumine)
Meningitis
    cerebrospinal fluid and, 337
    diagnosis, 142
    treatment, 142
Meningoencephalitis
    seizures and, 156

Metabolic Acidosis 104, 245 (see Acidosis)
Metamucil, 174
Metaproterenol, 362
Metronidazole, 168, 395
Microphthalmia, 216
Midbrain syndrome, 155
Milk,
- amounts to feed, 117, 122
- cows milk, 30
- mare's production of, 117
- milk replacers, 119

Milk of magnesia
- for high meconium retention, 129

Mineral oil, 129, 173, 395
Minimum data base, 88
Mucous membranes
- cyanosis and, 88
- evaluation of, 124, 236

Murmurs,
- normal newborn, 44
- patent ductus arteriosus, 308
- tetralogy of fallot, 309
- tricuspid atresia, 211, 214, 323
- ventricular septal defect, 214, 309
    - ultrasound of, 310

Mutoclopramide
- dose, 395
- for delayed gastric emptying, 179

Myocardial depression, 324
Myoclonus, congenital, 221
Myoglobin in urine
- white muscle disease and 229

Nasal intubation
- in resuscitation, 417
- method, 318-319

NSAID, 85 (see specific agents)
Nasogastric tube
- feeding foals, 17

method and types of tubes, 332
Nasolacrimal duct obstruction, 216
Nasotracheal intubation, 318
Navel (see Umbilicus)
Navel ill (see Omphalophlebitis)
Nebulization
    bronchodilators, 362
    medications, 361
Necrotizing enterocolitis, 168-169
    Clostridium perfringens typce C, 167
    radiography of, 316
    ultrasound
Neonatal isoerthyrolysis (NI)
    blood transfusion and, 184, 346
    clinical signs, 182
    hypoglycemia and, 185, 232
    in mules, 182
    prevention 186
    serial tube agglutination test of colostrum, 183
Neonatal maladjustment syndrome
    clinical signs and treatment, 131-133
    other conditions and, 131
    seizures and, 133
Neonatal salmonellosis (see Salmonellosis)
Nephron hypoplasia 190
Neurologic
    cranial trauma and, 155
    examination, 47-48
    (see also, brain edema, botulism, meningitis, neonatal maladjustment syndrome, seizures, white muscle disease)
Neutropenia, 51, 136, 165, 168, 237
Neutrophil/lymphocyte ratio 3, 51
Neutrolphilia,, 136
Newborn foals,
    Immediate post birth evaluation of, 18
Non-steroidal anti-inflammatory drugs,
    (see also specific agents)

    use in colic 256
    diarrhea therapy and, 174
    ulcers and, 176, 180
Norepinephrine, 265
Normal foals,
    post birth parameters, 18
Nosocomial infection, 356
Nursing care,
    daily, 95-96
Nutrifoal™ milk replacer, 332
Nutrition support
    convalescing foals and, 120, 121
    diarrhea and, 92
    enteral, 117
    feedings of milk, 113
    parenteral nutrition 92, 111
Nutritional myodegeneration (see White Muscle Disease)
Obstetrical equipment, 21
Oliguria
    acute renal failure in, 102, 189
Omeprazole, 179, 397
Omphalophlebitis,
    ultrasound and, 290
Ophthalmology (see Eye)
Opisthotonos
    maladjustment syndrome and, 131
    tetanus and, 141
Oral feedings (see Feedings)
Orphan foal,
    feeding method, 118
Osteomyelitis, 205
    radiography of, 200
    signs of, 185
    septic arthritis and, 197
    ultrasound of, 303-306
    umbilical infections and, 197
O2 therapy, (see Oxygen)
Oxygen
    administration guidelines, 52, 61

    CardioPulmonary Cerebral Resuscitation and 416
    conditions requiring, 4, 57, 88
    insufflation, 93
    methods, 58-60
    respiratory distress and, 77, 246
    resuscitation and, 416
    shock, 81
Oxygen administration equipment, 95
Oxytocin
    induction of parturition and, 13
    choke, 397
Pain control,
    lameness and, 202
    flexural deformities, 425
    meconium retention and, 126
Parasites
    diarrhea and, 106-107
Parenteral nutrition 111-116
    administration, 112-113
    all in one bag, 112, 114
    catheter types, 92, 113
    for diarrhea, 174
    indications for, 11
    problems with, 104, 115
    simple set up, 114
Parrot mouth (pragmatism), 219
Partial thromboplastin time (PPT), (see Hemostasis)
Parturition
    detection of, 10-12
    induction of, 13-15
    normal, 17-19
Passive immunity
    assessment of, 32-36
Passive transfer,
    colostrum evaluation and, 28
    definitions of, 34
    tests for, 32-34
Patent ductus arteriosus, (see also Ductus Arteriosus)
Patent foramen ovale, 211, 312
Patent urachus

examination for, 46
  ill foals and, 206
  infection and non infected, 206
  ultrasound for, 281-282, 286
Penicillin
  dosages, 380-381
  in sepsis, 26, 137, 142, 200
Penis,
  persistent membrane over glans penis, 219
  persistent preputial ring and, 46, 249
  urethral mucous plug and, 46
Pentobarbital
  in seizures, 397
Percussion (see Respiratory Therapy)
Perforating ulcers, 176
Peritonitis
  omphalophlebitis and, 205
  perforating ulcers and, 176
  ruptured bladder and, 194
Persistent fetal circulation, 57
Petechial hemorrhage
  examination for, 44, 124
  with sepsis, 126
Pharyngeal paralysis syndrome, 45, 48, 125
Phenobarbital dose, 159, 354, 399
Phenylbutazone
  colic and, 258
  gastric ulcers and, 180
  relative safety, 174
Phenylephrine, 362
Phenytoin
  dose, 399-400
Physical exam
  daily monitoring and, 91
  foal, 43-49
  mare, 8
Physical restraint, 354
  Madigan squeeze induced somnolence, 353
Placenta
  post foaling examination, 25

    premature separation of, 4, 14, 15
    ultrasonography and, 268
    weight of, 2
Plasma,
    administration of, 41
    adverse reactions with, 42
    anti-endotoxin, 38
    anti-Rhodococcus equi, 148
    commercial sources of, 38, 39
    hepatitis and, 42
    indications for use, 35, 37
    platelet rich plasma, 39
    storage of, 40
Plasmapheresis, 40, 148
Platelets, 93, 235
Pneumatosis intestinalis, 317
Pneumonia
    cleft palate and, 45, 52, 139, 218
    lung sounds and, 49
    meconium aspiration, 4, 5
    oxygen needs and, 55
    radiography and, 313-314
    respiratory distress and, 139, 244
    viral, 138
Pneumothorax, 251, 364
Poor growth
    hypothyroid and, 239
Positive pressure ventilation, 364
    methods, 366
    principles, 364
Post foaling evaluation, 25
Postural drainage, 71, 358
Potassium (see Fluids)
Predict A Foal, 10
Pregnant mare,
    risk factors in, 2, 3
Prekallikrein deficiency, 235
Prematurity 50-54
    adrenocortical insufficiency and, 51, 76
    clinical signs, 50

    equine herpes I and, 139
    gestation length and, 50
    outcomes, 52
    parenteral nutrition and, 111
    poor colostrum absorption and, 41
    respiratory distress and, 139, 244
    risk of infection and, 135
    treatment, 53
Premature placental separation, 4, 13, 14, 244
    maladjustment and, 131
Premature ventricular contractions, 4, 13, 14, 244
Preputial ring or membrane, 249
Prerenal
    failure versus renal failure, 188
Primary apnea, 69
Primidone, 160, 403
Procainanide
    for atrial fibrillation, 77
Progesterone, 8
Prostaglandin
    induction of labor and, 14, 119
Prothrombin time, 217
Pulmonic stenosis, 199
Pyloric stenosis, 253, 256, 315
    radiography of, 315
Radiography,
    Abdominal 314
    Thoracic 313
Ranitidine, 167
    dose, 399
    gastric ulcers and, 178
Renal disorders 188-191
    biopsy for, 190
    congenital disorders, 190
    creatinine levels, 189
    fractional excretion of electrolytes,189
    management, 190
    post renal, 188
    prerenal disorders, 188
    ureter defect, 192

urinalysis and, 189
Renal
    dysplasia, 190
    hypoplasia, 190
Respiratory (see also Blood gas and hypoxemia)
    character
        abnormal, 43
        normal, 43
    rate
        abnormal, 43
        normal, 43
Respiratory distress syndrome 243-247
    diagnosis, 243
    differential diagnosis, 247
    insufficiency and hypothyroidism, 240
    management, 245
    oxygen use and, 93, 245
    prematurity and, 244
    radiography and,139, 313
    sepsis in, 138, 139
    surfactant and, 243
Respiratory failure, 246
Respiratory stimulant, 385
Respiratory therapeutics 358
    chest percussion and, 358
    nebulization, 361, 362
    postural drainage and, 358
    systemic and airway hydration, 359
Restraint, 63, 351
    squeeze induced somnolence and 352
Resuscitation, 416, front cover
Rhodococcus equi 146-149
    diarrhea and,
    immunoprophylaxis and,
Rotavirus, 6, 169, 398
Ruptured bladder, 192 (see Bladder, rupture)
Rupture of common digital extensor tendon,220, 425, 430
Rye neck, 47
Salivation
    Fell pony syndrome 164

gastric ulcers and, 177
Salmonella, 151-154
    asymptomatic shedders, 151
    control measures, 152
    neonatal, 152
Salmonella bacterin, 153
Sand
    diarrhea and, 166
Scleral injection, 208
    in early salmonellosis, 44, 151
Scoliosis, 47
Scrotal hernia, 225, 248, 253
Second degree AV block, 329
Sedation and anesthesia 261-267
    Acepromazine 263
    Diazepam 262
    Xylazine 262
Seizures
    anticonvulsants and, 158-159
    apnea and, 155
    blindness and 124
    bromide 159
    causes of, 155, 157
    corneal ulcers and, 208
    diagnosis, differential, 155-156
    evaluation of, 156
    foal transport and, 64
    prognosis, 160
    septicemia and, 144
    treatment, 157
    Tyzzers 143
Selective IgM deficiency (see Immunodeficiencies)
Selenium, 26, 229, 230, 401
Sepsis score, 144
Septic arthritis 197-203 (see Arthritis, septic)
Septicemia 135
    antimicrobial use, 137, 370
    blood cultures, 136, 335
    causative agents, 135, 136
    clinical path, 136 (see also Sepsis score)

    diarrhea and, 136
    IgG levels and, 136
    maladjustment syndrome and, 131
    minimum data base, 88-89
    omphalophlebitis and, 205
    parenteral nutrition and, 111
    plasma therapy for, 37
    pneumonia and, 138
    prevention, 370
    respiratory distress and, 244
    septic arthritis and, 197
    sequel to, 138
Serum immunoglobulin (see IgG)
Serum hepatitis (see hepatitis)
Shock (see also Anaphylaxis and Resuscitation)
    assessment of, 81
    emergency drug dosages, front cover, 76
    resuscitation, 74
Sick foals
    signs of, 88
Single radial immuno-diffusion, 28, 32, 33
Small for gestational age, 5, 50, 61, 232
Small intestine,
    ultrasound of 296-301
Sodium bicarbonate (see Acid-base)
Softcheck, 11
Solu-delta cortef, 399
Squeeze induced Somnolence, 353
Stall
    disadvantages and advantages in critical care, 354
    management of limb deformities and, 425
Spinal fluid
    normal and abnormal, 339
    techniques of obtaining, 337
Sternal position, 57, 64, 72, 93, 95, 335,
Steroids (see Corticosteroids)
Stranguria, 124
    cystitis and, 192, 205
    ruptured bladder and, 192
Strongyloides westeri, 166, 172

Strongylus edentatus,, 172
Strongylus vulgaris, 172
Strychnine
 differential for tetanus, 141
Suctioning
 traceal, 368
Sucralfate
 dose in gastric ulcers, 179, 401
Surfactant
 corticosteroids to pregnant mare and, 15
 deficiency, 57, 244
 prematurity, 51, 244
 replacement, 53
 respiratory distress and, 56, 243
Synovial fluid
 culture of, 199
 normal vs infected, 198, 307
Synthroid®, 240
Swan-Gantz thermodilution catheters, 245
Swollen joints, 124, 136, 197
T3, T4 (see Thyroid)
Tachycardia, 77, 78, 329, 330
Talwin®, 262, 397
Tarsal bones, 51, 428, 431, 433
Teeth grinding
 ulcers and, 177
Temperature
 neutral thermal environmental 66
 normal, 43
Terbutaline,
 dose, 401
 nebulization, 362
 respiratory therapy, 362
Tetanus 141
 antitoxin, 25
 differential diagnosis, 141, 230
 immunization, 26
Tetracycline
 contracted tendons 397, 425, 426, 430
 dose, 397

in sepsis, 137
  nephrotoxicity and, 188
Tetralogy of fallot, 309
Thermal loss (see Temperature)
Thiabendazole, 166
Thoracic (see Radiography)
Thrombocytopenia,
  In DIC , 236
  Immune mediated, 39. 236
Thyroid
  hypothyroid, 239
  limb problems 239-240
  normal values, 242
  respiratory insufficiency and, 240
  thyroid stimulation hormone, 239
Ticarcillin, 137, 401
Timentin, 401
Titrets
  test of milk electrolytes, 11
Tocolysis, 21
Trace minerals
  milk replacer and, 117
  TPN and, 114, 115
Trachea
  aspirate in sepsis work up,
  suctioning of,
  wash, technique,
Transient hypogammaglobulinemia, 164
Transient tachypnea syndrome, 45, 139, 247
Transport of ill foal, 63
Transtracheal aspiration (see also Trachea)
  technique, 320-321
Trauma
  cranial (see Neurologic)
Tricuspid atresia, 211, 214, 322, 323
Triglycerides
  serum, 408
  TPN, 92, 116
Trimetroprim sulfa
  CNS infections and, 142

dose, 401
in sepsis, 170
Truncus arteriosus, 211
Tube (see Nasogastric and Nasotracheal)
Twins
    septicemia and, 136, 244, 268
Ulcers (see corneal and Gastroduodenal)
Ultrasonography 268-312 (see also Echocardiography)
    Abdominal, 296-302
    Cardiac, 308-312
    Fetal,, 268-281
        transabdominal, 268
        uteroplacental unit, 278
    Echocardiography, 308-312
    Thoracic, 290-296
    Musculoskeletal, 303-307
    Umbilical, 281-290
Umbilical 204-208
    abnormalities of, 125
    abcsessation of, 204
    acute diffuse edematous, 205
    daily care of, 96
    examination of, 46
    hernia and, 206-207
    patent urachus and, 193, 206
    post birth care, 18, 25, 96
    ultrasound of, 281-290,
Umbilicus, (see Umbilical)
Unreadiness for birth (see Prematurity)
Urachus (see also Patent Urachus)
    patent, 206
    rent in, 194
    ultrasound of 287
Urinalysis
    normal, 189
    specific gravity, 189
    urachal infection and, 205
    volumes of urine, 81, 91
Uroperitoneum 192, (see also Bladder, rupture)
Ureter defect, 194

Urethral mucous plug, 46
Urine output, 81, 91
Urinary catheters, 97,194, 195
Urination, 46
Uteroplacental unit, ultrasound of, 278
Uterine inertia, 20
Uveitis 47
    in septicemia, 136
Vaccination,
    for Rhodococcus equi, 148, 149
    mare, 5
Vaginal discharge of mare, 3, 268
Valgus, 27, 422, 423, 433-450
Valium® (Diasepam)
    dose, 387
    during transport, 64
    restraint, 354
Varus, (See Limb Deformities- 422-433
Vascular anomalies (see Cardiac anomalies)
Venous blood gas (see Blood gas)
Ventilation (see also hypercapnea)
    continuous positive airway pressure, 306
    mechanical ventilation, 59, 364
Ventricular
    arrhythmias, 75, 76, 419
    septal defect (VSD) 212
Vertebral fractures
    radiography and, 314
Viruses 169
    Adenovirus, 138, 162
    Corona virus, 170
    equine herpes I, 6, 165
    equine herpes virus 4, 6
    rotavirus, 169, 177
        vaccine, 6
        diarrhea and 167
    west nile virus, 6
Virogen rotatest, 169
Vitamins
    E-selenium, 26, 85, 229

Levels, 230
post birth use and, 26
Volvulus
differential diagnosis 253
large intestine, 46
radiography of, 255, 315
small intestine, 296, 315
Von Willebrand disease, 235
"Wander-barker" (see Neonatal Maladjustment)
Water intoxication
enemas and, 130
Weakness
botulism and, 140
cardiac abnormalities and, 211
meningitis, 142
white muscle and, 229
Weed Whacker line for meconium, 129
Weight
body, 2, 91
White foal, 218
lethal (see Ileocolonic aganglionosis)
White muscle disease
clinical signs, 229
differential from tetanus, 230
treatment, 230
Wry Mouth, 47, 220
Xylazine (see chapter 51 Sedation and Anesthesia)
anesthesia with ketamine, 22
butorphanol, 21, 157
colic, use in, 259
dose, 394, 401
seizure control limitations and, 64, 159
in dystocia, 21
in seizure control, 64, 159
restraint and, 306
diazepam and, 262
Zinc sulfate turbidity, 33